Women's Health

Your Guide to
a Healthier and
Happier Life

DISCLAIMER

This book is intended for general educational purposes only. It is not to be used as a personal health guide. A health-care professional should provide you with specific information about your health, since each person's life involves so many variables. This book is not to be used for diagnosis, prescription or treatment of disease or any health disorder whatsoever.

First printed February 1998

10   9   8   7   6   5   4   3   2   1

Manufactured in the United States of America

Publisher's Cataloging-in-Publication
(Provided by Quality Books, Inc.)

Newman, David E., 1963-
        Women's health: your guide to a healthier and happier
life / David E. Newman, Holly Stevens.--1st ed.
        p. cm.
        Includes index.
        Preassigned LCCN: 97-77581
        ISBN: 0-9661346-5-6

1. Gynecology--Popular works. 2. Women--Health and hygiene. I. Stevens, Holly A., 1965- II. Title.

RG121.N49   1998   618
                                     QBI98-55

Women's Health

Your Guide to a Healthier and Happier Life

David Newman, MD
Holly Stevens, MD

DEDICATION

I dedicate this book to my wife, Sylvia Newman, Ph.D.,
for her patience and assistance,
and to my children, Kevin, Nicole and Andrew,
for being my most special gifts in the world.
I love them all and hope my daughter
benefits from the information within this book
when the time comes.

–D.N.

For my family.

–H.S.

CONTRIBUTORS

DAVID NEWMAN, M.D.
PMS, Difficult Periods & Pelvic Pain;
Pelvic Infections & STDs; Menopause; Pre-Pregnancy Consult;
Third Trimester; Labor and Delivery;
Pregnancy After 35; Infertility

HOLLY STEVENS, M.D.
Cancer Screening and Prevention; First Trimester

RICHARD BOESEL, M.D.
Contraception; Breast Health; Incontinence;
Second Trimester of Pregnancy

JACKIE COTTON, M.D.
Caring for Your Baby

BECKY AND MARK DeLEGGE, M.D.
Nutrition & Weight Loss

WARREN OVERBEY, M.D.
First Trimester

WESLEY ROBINSON, M.D.
Pain Management in Labor

BARBARA TARKIN, Ph.D.
Adolescence; Adult Stresses

PRE-PUBLICATION ENDORSEMENTS

"An Eye-Opening Look at Women's Health Through All Changes and Challenges of Life. The refreshing Mix of First-Rate Medical Information and Clear, Concise Conversational Style Can't Be Beat."

Dr. Charles Hammond
Professor and Chairman, Dept. of OB/GYN
Duke University

" I find the Section on Incontinence to be Superbly Written and Presented in a Fashion that can Easily Be Understood by the Lay-Reader. It Opens Diagnostic and Therapeutic Options in a Logical, Non-Threatening Manner and Allays Concerns About This Most Embarrassing Quality of Life Issue."

Dr. Keith Stone
Professor and Chairman, Dept. of OB/GYN
University of Florida

Dunn and Associates are using the statements to promote the value of the book with the back cover. Dunn and Associates is an award winning graphic arts firm that specializes in book cover designs and are contracted to complete the book cover by December 15th.

"You are Covering a Vast Amount of Material with Concise, Graceful prose".

Michael Ames
Temple University Press
1601 North Broad Street
Philadelphia, PA 19122-6099
215/204-8787

'I find it an Interesting, Well-Written and Comprehensive Guide'

Belinda Budge
Senior Editor, Harper Collins Publishers
77-85 Fulham Palace Road

PREFACE

We hope you and every woman in your family, from pre-teens through the elderly, will use this book as your first reference to guide you through the challenges you face in your life-long development. Life is filled with transitions. While we cannot make each transition stress-free, our goal in developing this book is to provide you with good information to help you manage the changes and stresses.

Keep this book handy in your home library, and refer to it frequently to help you through the most common problems you face at each stage of life. Of great importance is the material on adolescence. We very directly encourage abstinence, but if a young woman is going to be sexually active, she must know the physical and emotional risks. The very first chapter includes a list of ways to avoid date rape. If we are able to help one young woman get through adolescence without experiencing this trauma because of information she read in this book, the entire project will have been worthwhile. As obstetricians and gynecologists in private practice, we see the anguish of too many young women who experienced rape as adolescents, and we know how it harms their adult relationships.

Our desire to help you understand pregnancy, menopause and a full array of other matters is evident from the front cover to the last page of this book.

Many women shared very personal experiences with us so you will realize that you are not alone as you face many difficult situations. Please use this book to become better educated. The more you learn, the more confident you will be as you face decisions about your health and well-being. This book helps you live a "healthier and happier life" by empowering you to be proactive and responsible for your health.

We wish you the best in life: the ability to love and laugh, feel compassion for yourself and others, and to enjoy something about each and every day.

ACKNOWLEDGMENTS

We want to thank the doctors who contributed chapters to this book. Their expertise and experience make this book so useful to many women. These contributors include Richard Boesel, M.D., Warren Overbey, M.D., Barbara Tarkin, Ph.D., Wesley Robinson, M.D., Jackie Cotton, M.D., and Becky and Mark DeLegge, M.D. We also thank Keith Stone, M.D., and Charles Hammond, M.D., for their endorsements.

We acknowledge Jeannie Marendt DeSena for her editorial contributions, Jamie Raynor for her book design and layout, Sylvia Newman for her editorial reviews and for the numerous interviews she conducted, Kathi Dunn of Dunn & Associates for the cover design, Susan Kendrick for the back-cover material she developed, and Laure Anselin for her organizational assistance.

Special acknowledgment goes to all of our patients, our professors and the pioneers in our field who came before us.

We are grateful to Dan Poynter, who shared many insights into the publishing process through his personal counseling and his book, *The Self-Publishing Manual*.

David Newman, M.D.
Holly Stevens, M.D.

CONTENTS

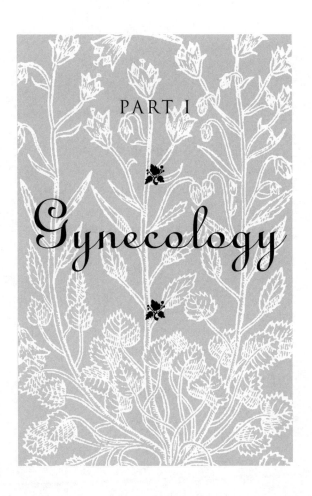

PART I

Gynecology

Life is Change.

Change is Stress.

With Education You Can

Understand and Anticipate

the

Changes of Life,

Reducing

Your Stress.

CHAPTER ONE

ADOLESCENCE

Growing, Changing, Choosing Wisely

During puberty and your teenage years, changes occur not only in your body, but also in your emotions, your relationships with other people, your thinking skills, and your understanding of yourself and the world around you. Although change can be frightening and confusing, it is a natural and necessary part of life. There are many ways you can help yourself accept the new developments and learn to deal with them in ways that are healthy and productive. When you are prepared for changes and can anticipate what these will mean, you are less frightened or overwhelmed by these new experiences and feelings.

One important tool for reducing the stress associated with adolescence is education – reading and learning about these changes before and during the time they are occurring. You can get information and education from many different places, including books, computer information services, your doctor, and your parents or other adults you know and trust, such as teachers, coaches and religious leaders. Your friends can also help you during adolescence by being emotionally supportive. They may be experiencing very similar things in their lives. It is important to remember, however, that no matter how much you like and trust your friends, there are some questions to which they do not know the answers. It is best to rely on several different sources of information, especially when you are dealing with complicated or difficult issues.

The purpose of this chapter is to explore what occurs during your teenage years, beginning with the changes in your body and the way they make you feel. This chapter addresses issues related to your health, such as nutrition, sleep, alcohol and drugs, and mental health. This chapter also explores sexuality and what this means for you as a teenager. Next this chapter examines the changes that occur in your relationships with your parents and your peers, both male and female. The final section covers issues of sexual assault, including stranger rape, date or acquaintance rape, sexual molestation and incest. Some of these issues may be uncomfortable to read about, and I suggest you talk about these issues and your feelings with your parents or other adults you trust.

> " I hate having acne. It's so ugly and hard to get rid of. Once it goes away, the next day it's there again. It's so frustrating. Then there's the topic of weight. Everyone wants to be a certain weight, but you never can get yourself to that weight. I hate it when people or the doctor asks me how much I weigh. I'm always afraid I'll weigh too much and they'll tell me I'm overweight."

How Physical Changes Affect Your Body Image

Puberty is the time in your development when your body begins to change from a young girl to a woman. Puberty signals the beginning of adolescence – the stage in your life that leads to adulthood – and is a time of many changes. For most girls, some of these changes are exciting and desired, but other changes are uncomfortable and may be a source of embarrassment and confusion. The major physical changes associated with puberty include the appearance of pubic and underarm hair, the development of breasts, and the onset of your menstrual cycle. Other changes include changes in your complexion (such as acne), gains in height and weight, and changes in the overall shape and appearance of your body.

These physical changes take place at different times and in different ways for each teenager. For some, the developmental changes in their bodies occur earlier than for others. For most girls, puberty begins between the ages of 9 and 14. There is nothing you can do to speed up or slow down your rate of development, for this is a biologically determined process. It is natural and normal to want to compare your development with that of your friends and classmates. However, please remember that every girl develops at her own pace, and being ahead of – or behind – your peers in physical development has nothing to do with what kind of person you are or what kind of woman you will become. Girls who develop much earlier and much later than their peers may feel awkward and embarrassed about being in a different phase of development than the majority of their friends. It is important to remember that eventually everyone's body goes through all of the physical changes associated with puberty.

Throughout your life as a female, you are bombarded with images and fantasies of what the "perfect" woman is supposed to look like. These images are displayed in magazines, in movies and television and are reflected in our culture's fascination with women who are beautiful and thin. It is tempting to believe that being beautiful and thin are the keys to being happy. The reality is that all of our bodies and faces are different and beautiful in their own ways, and whether you are tall or short, thin or not depends to a large extent on your genes. Your physical appearance says nothing about your other attributes, such as your intelligence, your special talents, your sense of humor, your moral standards or your personality. Some teenage girls feel so strongly that they have to "measure up" to a standard of beauty that they engage in very dangerous behaviors such as starving themselves to reach a certain weight. It is important to recognize your limitations as well as your assets, and to concentrate on becoming a well-rounded and competent person, rather than on becoming a certain size or measurement. You have a problem if you are so preoccupied with your weight that you starve yourself or purge (vomit or use laxatives after eating), or if you are even considering these things. It is unhealthy to focus your thoughts only

" I got my first period when I was 11. I thought it was really cool at first. It made me feel older. Only one other of my friends had gotten her period, so I was one of the first."

on your weight, food or calorie and fat intake. If you do these things, you must let someone help you. Self-starvation and purging are considered eating disorders and are very serious conditions. (Chapter 3, "Nutrition and Weight Loss," discusses them in depth.) With proper intervention and early detection, you can avoid serious and permanent consequences of eating disorders. Talk about these feelings and behaviors with your parents, your doctor or another adult you trust in order to prevent yourself from developing a disorder that can lead to serious medical and psychological complications.

If you do not feel comfortable talking with an adult you know, use your local telephone book or telephone information and find the number for community mental health services, adolescent health services or special clinics that deal with eating disorders.

No one is perfect, not even movie stars and models, and it is important for you to recognize and appreciate the many wonderful things about you as a person. Perhaps you have a special talent in music, art or athletics; or maybe you are a kind and giving person; or perhaps you excel in academics or in working with the elderly or with young children. Whatever your physical appearance, you are much more than your reflection in a mirror. Teenage boys may appear to be interested only in a girl's appearance, but when asked, boys acknowledge they are more interested in girls who are nice and who have high expectations and standards for themselves. (And boys are worrying about their own appearance and development!) It is important to feel good about your appearance, but it is more important to feel good about your personality traits, your standards of behavior and your other accomplishments. After all, your physical appearance can and will change with time, but time cannot take away all of the other qualities that make you the special person you are.

How You Can Build a Healthy Body

You carry many of the habits you establish during your adolescence into adulthood. Therefore, the good and healthy habits you form now not only help you look and feel your best as a teen, but they also insure you will look and feel your best in the future.

EAT GOOD FOODS

One of the best things you can do for your body and your health is to try and eat foods that are good for you. Everyone likes "junk food," and in moderate amounts there is no reason you can't eat foods that have less nutritional value. However, your body is growing and developing in leaps and bounds right now, and it needs foods that provide nutrients, vitamins and minerals. Try to eat foods from the basic food groups every day, such as fruits and vegetables, protein (chicken, beef, fish), carbohydrates (pasta, bread, rice) and dairy products (milk, yogurt), and try to drink plenty of water. Eating nutritious foods gives your body the energy you need and helps keep you healthy.

GET ENOUGH SLEEP

Another good thing you can do for yourself is to get proper amounts of sleep every night. During sleep, your body refuels and rejuvenates itself. Most teenagers need at least eight hours of sleep each night, and some teens need even more than that. Enough sleep allows you to function well in school and have the energy to do all the things you like to do. When you get the right amount of sleep, you also help keep your body and your mind healthy. Let your doctor or parents know if you regularly have sleep problems, including **insomnia** (regular and consistent problems falling or staying asleep) and excessive fatigue or sleepiness. Sometimes sleep disturbances indicate other problems, and it is important to find out what is causing the disturbance.

KEEP POISONS OUT OF YOUR BODY

You also need to be aware of the health hazards of using alcohol, drugs and nicotine. Not only are these products illegal for teenagers to use, but they can also be extremely dangerous to developing minds and bodies. Treat your body with the respect it deserves, and stay away from toxic chemicals. You may feel a lot of pressure from others to use or experiment with alcohol, drugs or cigarettes. Some teens give in to this pressure, or they decide to use these substances to make themselves feel "cooler," more sociable, or less depressed or anxious (more on this later). But when you use these chemicals at an early age, you do damage to your body and your mind, and you run the risk of

Adolescence: Growing, Changing, Choosing Wisely

developing an addiction. Think about the choices in front of you and make decisions that benefit you not only now, but also in the future. People who like themselves do not engage in dangerous behaviors, because they see themselves as valuable and want to keep themselves healthy and free from poisons. Alcohol, drugs and nicotine are poisonous to your body and should be avoided.

LOOK OUT FOR YOUR MENTAL STATE

Another aspect of your health is your mental health, meaning your emotional and psychological well being. Due to the hormonal changes in your body, you (and your friends and family) may notice an increase in moodiness or changes in your mood. You may feel very happy and upbeat at times, and then quickly find yourself sad or angry. Almost all teens report feeling irritable and unhappy at times, and many report their moods seem to shift rapidly. Some changes in mood are expected in adolescence, and most of these changes can be linked to events or circumstances in your life. For example, you may be feeling positive and happy and then find out your parents will not allow you to do something you were counting on being allowed to do. It is normal to then experience anger, frustration or disappointment. Do not be alarmed if you notice changes in your mood that are connected with events in your life. However, if you find your moods are very unstable or seem to have no connection with events in your life – or if you find you are always experiencing the same intense emotion (such as sadness, anger, irritability) regardless of what is happening in your life – something other than normal teenage mood shifts may be occurring. You should share your concerns with your parents, guidance counselor or other adult, or contact a local mental-health center or hotline number.

It is normal for every person to occasionally feel "down in the dumps," sad or even depressed. Such feelings can last from several minutes to several hours, but they usually go away. More intense emotional responses can occur after a tremendous loss (such as the death of a loved one, a family divorce, etc.) or a traumatic event (such as being a victim of a crime, being in a car accident, etc.). Again, this is a normal response to a life circumstance. However, if you are experiencing intense feelings of anger, irritability, worry or depression that are affecting the activities of your daily life, this may be the signal you need some assistance in dealing with an emotional problem. Some of the signs and symptoms to look for are:

🦌 *A decrease in your energy or motivation*
🦌 *Major changes in your eating or sleeping patterns*
🦌 *Withdrawal from your friends and family*
🦌 *A decrease in your ability to concentrate or do school work*
🦌 *Intense feelings of sadness, anger, irritability or worry that do not go away*
🦌 *Thoughts of suicide*
🦌 *Self-destructive or self-injurious behavior (cutting on yourself, abusing drugs or alcohol, self-starvation, etc.)*
🦌 *Extremely risky or dangerous behavior*

If you experience these difficulties, you must get help. You can do this by talking with your parents, the parents of a friend you like and trust, a teacher or school counselor, your doctor, or your pastor, priest, rabbi or other religious leader. You also can contact your local mental-health center or call a hotline number. Emotional or psychological problems are very treatable, but they can lead to more serious consequences if you do not get the help you need. Just as you would see your doctor for a physical problem, it is important to see a mental-health professional if you are having emotional problems.

Sexuality: What You Should Know
EXPLORING YOUR FEELINGS
Interest in the Opposite Sex

In addition to the physical changes of adolescence, other changes are occurring inside you. Chemical and hormonal changes taking place contribute to the start of your menstrual cycle, and these hormonal changes may also produce feelings of physical attraction to others. Just as we are bombarded with images of women as beautiful and thin in the media and in our culture, we are also exposed to images of sexuality and sexual activity. It is normal during adolescence to become interested in peers in a sexual way and to have dreams or fantasies that have some sexual content. Very often during adolescence, girls develop crushes on peers or even adults in their lives whom they look up to and admire. Some girls are described as "boy crazy" because it seems all they can think about is boys, to the exclusion of their family, friends, schoolwork and other interests. While an interest in boys is normal and healthy, you should recognize it is just one part of adolescence. You should not allow an interest in boys to become the only interest or goal in your life.

Same-Sex Attractions

During this time of sexual awakening, some teenagers feel strong attractions to peers of the same sex. In addition, some teenagers feel sexual attractions to both boys and girls. **Homosexuality** is defined as having sexual attraction to and engaging in sexual behavior with members of your same gender, while **heterosexuality** is defined as attraction to and sexual behavior with members of the opposite gender. **Lesbians** are women who engage in sexual relationships with other women. Men who engage in sexual relationships with other men are called **homosexuals** or **gays**. **Bisexuality** is defined as having sexual attractions to and engaging in sexual behavior with members of both genders (male and female).

Lesbians, male homosexuals and bisexuals make up a minority of the population, but people who define their sexual orientation as something other than heterosexual are not considered by the medical or mental-health community to be sick, crazy or mentally ill. It is important to remember that during adolescence, many different and new feelings and sensations are emerging. Many heterosexual adults report that during their adolescence they experienced intense and loving feelings (often with a sexual attraction) toward a person of their own gender. In addition, a substantial number report engaging in sexual behavior with someone of their own gender. Adolescence is a time of identity development and exploration, and having feelings of attraction toward others of the same sex is not considered abnormal. Nor, however, do such feelings and behaviors during this developmental period mean that an adolescent is going to develop into a homosexual or bisexual adult. Human sexuality and the development of a sexual orientation are complicated processes that often are not completed until a person is well into adulthood. The development of a sexual identity is based on the interaction between many factors, including genetic contributions, environmental factors and individual personality and experiences.

If you are experiencing feelings of attraction toward a same-sex peer, or feel you are different from your same-sex peers in terms of your sexual preferences, you may have conflicting feelings. Many people and institutions in our culture view homosexual relationships as wrong or abnormal, and you may be very frightened and confused. Many adult homosexuals or bisexuals say their adolescence was a particularly difficult period in their lives, as they struggled to sort out their sexual identity in a culture that defines "normal" as being attracted to members of the opposite gender. You may find it difficult to talk about your feelings to your friends, your parents or other adults you know. Furthermore, you may feel isolated, different and afraid. Most communities have support groups and organizations for teenagers who are unsure about their sexual orientation. You can look in your local telephone book, computer information services or local teen health services for organizations that serve the gay and lesbian population in your area.

> " I feel like I'm in a pinball machine. There are so many changes that I'm going through, both emotionally and physically. I'm not at any one emotional level. Sometimes I can handle what's going on, sometimes not."

Regardless of your sexual orientation, the goal of adolescence is to develop into a healthy, happy adult and be able to engage in healthy and safe relationships with others. While this may be more difficult for homosexual adolescents than for heterosexual adolescents, it is important to remember that sexuality and sexual identity define only part of who you are as a person, and loving and accepting yourself are the cornerstones to a healthy adulthood.

BEGINNING TO DATE

Depending on the rules and standards in your family, you may begin dating during adolescence. The purpose of dating is to learn how to interact with peers and, through a process of trial and error, to learn what qualities in others are most important to you and make for the healthiest and happiest relationships. When you begin dating, you also begin to learn about making sexual decisions. It is normal to be physically and sexually attracted to other people and to want to act on those feelings. However, it is also normal to be confused and frightened by sexual feelings, because these are new feelings for most teenagers. While many teens are taught sex education in school, these classes usually focus on the physical and biological components of reproduction and on the related health issues, such as sexually transmitted diseases. Equally important but not often discussed are the feelings, attitudes and beliefs that accompany the biological and medical aspects of sexual activity. If you are like other teens, you may find yourself in a situation of understanding what sexual activity is, but not understanding your own sexual feelings and behaviors. That is why it is important to recognize and understand the way you feel about sex.

" My parents didn't really set an age when I could start dating. They just said that once I was mature enough, it would be all right to date."

DECIDING ABOUT SEXUAL ACTIVITY

There is an incredible amount of pressure on teens to participate in sexual activity. This pressure comes from our culture and the media, and it also comes from peers who may imply the way to become popular with others is to engage in sexual behavior. Sexual urges can be quite strong during adolescence, and so can the influences of the media and peers. At times, it can feel very difficult to resist such pressure, and many adolescents do choose to become sexually active during their teenage years. You may think everyone except you is having sex, or you may be afraid the person you are dating will break up with you if you do not have sex. Deciding whether or not to become sexually active as a teenager is a big decision – and one that should not be made for the sake of popularity or for the sake of keeping a boyfriend interested in a relationship. As you make this very personal decision, you need to consider your and your family's moral and religious beliefs, as well as your age, maturity level and other factors. While it seems that sexual activity is not something many teenagers would care to discuss with their parents, it is important to understand how your parents feel about this issue and to get their perspective. Believe it or not, they were once teenagers, too! Even though times have changed from when your parents were teenagers, they, too, had to deal with their developing sexuality and relationships with others.

" I've thought about becoming sexually active, but now I think I made the right decision to wait until I'm married and truly in love, because I don't want to have a child until I'm 100-percent ready for one. I know women who have had children at a young age who had to quit school and get a job to support their children as well as themselves. I just don't want to live like that."

Adolescence is a good time for you to learn how differently men and women approach relationships. For many women, the ideal way to show love to another person is by doing acts of kindness and thoughtfulness; likewise, women often feel that a man who does kind and thoughtful things is expressing his love. Many young men, on the other hand, want to show a woman they care for her by having sex. This very common conflict that carries into adult relations. Now is the time to help young men understand how to express love without having intercourse. A relationship based on love and communication will last much longer and be much happier than one based on sex alone.

There are alternatives to sexual activity, particularly **abstinence** (refraining from sexual activity) and **masturbation** (self-stimulation). Both of these are healthy and normal alternatives to becoming sexually active, but you do not hear as much about them from your friends or the media.

Abstinence involves a decision to postpone having sex until you are married. By remaining a virgin, you avoid pregnancy and sexually transmitted diseases, and more importantly, you assure the relationship you develop with a partner is one based on friendship and love, not simply a hormonal urge.

Masturbation provides a sexual outlet without risk of pregnancy or disease. You may be able to reach an orgasm with your imagination alone, or through stimulation with your hand or a vibrator. You will notice the area of your vulva with greatest sensitivity is the very top where the two labia join. The junction of the labia covers a small lump of tissue called the clitoris. With orgasm, the vaginal muscles contract rhythmically, and a small amount of fluid is released.

Everyone wants to feel loved and cared for, and there are many ways of expressing this. While sexual feelings are very powerful, if you have sex with someone, it changes your relationship with that person. For couples in a long-term, committed and stable relationship, sex can increase the intimacy and attachment they feel. For other couples, having sex can interfere with the communication and feelings the couple has for one another. Having sex may also change the way your feel about yourself. Many young women report they felt disappointed after their first sexual experience. Sometimes, after deciding to have sex, a couple splits up and the girl often feels used or exploited, and she may even acquire a bad reputation among peers. The most intimate act of your life can become an item for gossip, and this can be a very unpleasant experience. Being sexual is a big responsibility, and many teenagers are not emotionally prepared for the consequences of having sex. If you do choose to become sexually active, you alone are responsible for protecting yourself from an unplanned or unwanted pregnancy by using birth control, and you also must protect yourself from contracting a sexually transmitted disease. Before becoming sexually active, you should seek medical advice about birth control and sexually transmitted diseases from your doctor or health-care provider or from local clinics and agencies that provide this information. Most of the information you may learn from peers will be wrong, and relying on incorrect information about pregnancy and sexually transmitted diseases can have life-altering and life-threatening consequences.

The topic of sexually transmitted diseases is covered in its own chapter, and I encourage you to read it as soon as you finish this chapter. One point is important to mention here: The younger you are, the more easily you can contract a sexually transmitted disease from sexual contact with an infected person. As you age, the lining of the vagina develops a protective barrier that lowers the chance you will catch an infection through intercourse. If a man with gonorrhea or chlamydia – and he may not know he has it – has intercourse with a 14-year-old and a 30-year-old, the 14-year-old is three times more likely to become infected than the 30-year-old. Infections at this young age can result in chronic pelvic pain, infertility or, in severe cases, an abscess that requires a hysterectomy to cure. Hysterectomy involves removal of the uterus and means you can never become pregnant.

Sometimes, after deciding to have sex, a couple splits up and the girl often feels used or exploited, and she may even acquire a bad reputation among peers. The most intimate act of your life can become an item for gossip, and this can be a very unpleasant experience.

Your First Gynecological Exam

You should see a family doctor or gynecologist for gynecological care when you begin to think about sexuality, start puberty or become sexually active. At the latest, you should have your first gynecological exam by age 18. Women need regular exams for cancer screening, contraceptive counseling and other health-maintenance reasons.

At the first visit, you can just meet the doctor; let him or her know this is your first visit. After the initial discussion, you have the option of proceeding with an exam, or scheduling it for sometime later. During the initial discussion, I review normal anatomy and development. I also establish with both you and your parents that I consider you an adult, and that you have the right to tell me things I will not repeat without your permission. Also, at the first visit I request permission from your parents to start you on birth control without informing them if you and I feel it is in your best interest. I encourage you to speak to your parents about any plans to be sexually active, but my first job is to make sure you have someone to come to for good medical care and protection. I feel that if you become sexually active and do not use protection, you are very immature. If you are sexually active and have obtained protection, you are showing maturity and using judgment. Obviously the ideal situation is to choose abstinence, but we all know that abstinence is not the choice of all young women.

At a gynecological exam, you first speak with your doctor while dressed. Then the doctor leaves the room while you undress and put on a gown. In some offices the gown is made of cloth, while in others it is made of paper. When the doctor returns, he or she examines your head, lungs and heart while you are sitting. You then lie back with your legs flat on a pullout portion of the exam table for a breast exam and abdominal exam. In a breast exam, your doctor presses your breast tissue with his or her fingers, feeling for a mass the size of a marble. The abdominal exam allows the doctor to check your uterus, liver and spleen for enlargement. Then the end of the table is pushed in, and stirrups, in which you place your feet, are pulled out. You need to move your bottom to where it feels like it is just off the end of the table. Your doctor then places a hand against your thigh, gently opens your labia and inserts a plastic or metal speculum into your vagina. This instrument holds the vaginal walls apart so the doctor can see your cervix, the portion of the uterus that protrudes into the top of the vagina. During this part of the exam, try to concentrate on letting your bottom muscles relax, avoiding the natural desire to tighten up. If you are relaxed, the speculum can be inserted with minimal pressure. You should not feel any pain with a pelvic exam; if you feel discomfort, please let your doctor know. If your doctor always causes you pain while performing a pelvic exam, you should consider finding another doctor.

With the speculum in place, the doctor does a test called a Pap smear by passing a tiny wooden spatula over your cervix, then inserting a small swab into the cervical canal. The spatula and swab are placed on a glass slide and sent to a lab. Results are ready in about two weeks. A Pap-smear result can range from normal to atypia (atypical findings that may lead to a repeat of the Pap smear), to (mild, moderate or severe) dysplasia to cancer. Dysplasia is a precancerous condition that is treated so that you do not develop cancer; it is discussed further in Chapter 8, "Cancer Screening & Prevention."

After the Pap smear, the speculum is removed. Your doctor then places a gloved, lubricated finger into your vagina in order to evaluate your uterus and ovaries. Once this is done, your exam is over and the doctor leaves the room. You are given a wipe to remove any excess lubricant, and you can get dressed. When you are dressed, your doctor returns to discuss your exam and make plans for your care. You now have begun a relationship with a doctor who can care for you through the challenges of your adult years, from childbearing on into menopause and beyond.

How Your Relationships Change
LESS PATIENCE WITH FAMILY

During adolescence, it is normal to want to start spending more and more time with your friends, and less and less time with your family. While you may enjoy this change, your parents and siblings may not understand why or how they have suddenly become so much less important in your life. They may not know why you are suddenly dressing differently, using expressions they have never heard before or preferring to be with or talk to friends instead of them. Even though you may have felt close to your parents in the past, you may suddenly feel they do not understand you and can no longer relate to the issues and problems you are dealing with. You may feel they are embarrassing to be around, and you may resent their interest in your life and your friends. Many teens feel their parents are being "nosy" when they ask questions about what is going on in their lives. The less you tell your parents about your life, though, the more worried they become and the harder they try to get information about your life from other sources. It is especially important during your teenage years to try and keep the lines of communication open with your parents. They will not necessarily approve of all of your decisions, but the more open and honest you can be with them, the more they are able to understand and try and offer some guidance and some support. If you tell them nothing, they have nothing to offer in return, and then you may find yourself struggling alone to make decisions and understand what is happening in your life. Every parent and teen have to work to find a way for the teenager to maintain some privacy and the parent to feel informed and involved in the teenager's life.

As confusing and frightening as adolescence is for you, it is just as confusing for your parents. They are watching their child turn into an adult, and whether you are their oldest child or their youngest, this transformation is never easy. They are used to being in control of your life, taking care of you and making decisions for you – after all, that has been their job since you were born. All parents are concerned about the decision-making skills and values of their teenagers, and they want you to be safe and happy and to make good decisions. The more they see you making good decisions for yourself about school, friends, values and behavior, the more responsibility they are able to turn over to you, and the better they (and you) feel. If it seems as though every time you and your parents get into a discussion you or they become angry or upset or do not seem to be listening, perhaps a neutral person can help. This person may be a relative (aunt, uncle, older cousin, and grandparent), a person who knows you and your family (a minister, priest or rabbi), or a trained counselor. Sometimes this person can help teenagers and their parents re-establish their communication and begin talking again about the issues that are important and the decisions that need to be made.

Your relationships with your siblings also change during your

> *The more your parents see you making good decisions for yourself about school, friends, values and behavior, the more responsibility they will be able to turn over to you, and the better they (and you) will feel.*

teenage years. In the past you may have spent time with your younger siblings, but now you may not want to have a younger brother or sister tagging along with you and your friends, or being in the room while you are on the telephone. Try and remember that your adolescence is difficult for your brothers and sisters and whatever that you are going through is not their fault. Especially with younger brothers and sisters, you may need to make an extra effort to spend some time with them so they do not feel left out. They are watching you and taking cues from you about how to be a teenager when their turn comes. They may not understand what you are doing or what you are feeling, but they still want to be a part of your life. You may find it easier to talk with older brothers and sisters who have already gone through some or all of their adolescence, and they may be a source of support and information for you.

MORE INTEREST IN FRIENDS

One of the biggest changes in adolescence is how much more important your friends and your peer group become in your life. You may find yourself more concerned with what your friends think about you and your choices than you used to be. It is normal to want to be like your friends. Your desire to be like them may mean you decide to change the way you dress, the words you use and the kinds of things you are interested in. It is also normal to want to carve out a unique identity for yourself, and this may mean you feel different from your friends. One of your goals during adolescence is to find a happy medium between being like your friends and being your own person. It is also important to remember that friendships during this part of your life can feel very intense, and some of the friends you make during your teenage years will be the friends you keep for the rest of your life. Other relationships will feel very important for a short period of time, but will change or fizzle out over time.

One important thing to remember is that you need to get to know people well before you share your thoughts, your feelings or your body with them. Many teenagers have trouble keeping a confidence; they may gossip or tell others things about you that are not true. They may also try and convince you to engage in behaviors you know are wrong or not good for you. It takes a strong person to resist the pressure from peers to engage in dangerous, illegal or inappropriate behavior. You will have occasions where you must do what you believe is right, even though your friends may not agree with you. It is important to find friends you feel comfortable with and who have proven they have your best interests at heart. Likewise, it is important to be a trusted and good friend to others. No matter how important your friends are to you, however, you may sometimes find yourself disagreeing with decisions they make or behaviors they engage in. Sometimes this may mean the relationship is over, while other times it is still possible and desirable to maintain the friendship.

A FEW WORDS ABOUT SPECIAL RELATIONSHIPS

You read earlier in this chapter about dating and relationships with peers. Sometimes during adolescence, people have steady relationships with just one person. It is normal to want to be in such a special relationship and be part of a couple. It is also normal to want to spend time with this special person, either on the telephone or in person. However, it is important to maintain your relationships with other peers while you are dating someone and to not become dependent on a boyfriend to fill all of your time and to be with you for all of your activities. While it may feel flattering if a boyfriend wants you to spend all of your time with only him or to end your relationships with others, doing so is not healthy. In healthy relationships, each member of a couple has other friends and interests he or she pursues without the other partner. These interests may include sports or recreational activities, volunteer work, extra-curricular activities at school, religious activities or other things you enjoy doing. If you have a boyfriend, you should work to keep a balance in your life; allot time to your family, your friends, and your interests and activities, as well as your boyfriend.

It is normal and natural for two people to occasionally disagree or to have arguments. Most people can work through their differences by talking about the problem and finding a way to resolve it by compromising or negotiating. When couples argue about things, one or both people can become angry; their feelings may be hurt, or they may hurt their partner's feelings. Hitting or physically hurting one another is never OK for couples. If you and a boyfriend have been physically aggressive with one another, this is a very strong signal that something is very wrong in the relationship. Most often, the girl is the one who is being physically hurt or forced into sexual activity by a boyfriend. If this is happening to you, you may feel ashamed or embarrassed, or you may feel you deserve to be hurt. There is never a good reason to hurt someone. If your partner is hurting you, you must get help. Being hurt in a relationship is called abuse, and in healthy and loving relationships, people do not get physically hurt. You can get help from trusted adults in your life, or you can find numbers in your local telephone book for battered women's shelters, police or sheriff's departments, hotlines and mental-health centers. If someone you know is in an abusive relationship, you have a responsibility to your friend to help make sure she is safe from harm. In this situation, you may have to violate a confidence, but you should alert her parents, a school guidance counselor or someone you trust to help her with this situation.

What You Should Know About Sexual Assault

Sexual assault involves rape or other sexual activity that is non-consensual, meaning one person does not give consent or want to participate in the sexual activity. Force or violence may or may not be involved, the perpetrator may or may not be someone you know, and the sexual activity may or may not involve sexual intercourse. Sexual assault occurs when a person (usually female) is forced to have sexual activity with someone (usually male). Women can be sexually assaulted by strangers or by men they know. These men may be friends, dates or other men the woman has had prior contact with.

RAPE

Common Scenarios

The most common situation where a woman is forced into sexual activity is **"date rape"** or **acquaintance rape**, when the victim knows the person who rapes her. These types of rapes occur frequently on college campuses or in other social situations where men and women have a lot of contact with each other. Date or acquaintance rape can occur to teenagers in high school or even to girls who are not yet in high school.

One factor that contributes to date or acquaintance rape is the use of alcohol and other drugs, which impair judgment and may lead you to pass out or be less careful about what you are doing and who you are with. It is important to always know the people you are with and where you are going, and to be prepared for an emergency by carrying extra money in case you need to find transportation home or to call someone to pick you up. You can go out with groups of people or on double dates until you get to know someone well enough to trust him, or you can go to parties with a friend you trust not to leave you stranded or alone. You must be able to strike a balance between having fun and trusting your friends and acquaintances, and being careful about your own safety. Even when alcohol and drugs are not involved, and even when a woman is careful about her own safety, rape can still occur, but it is important to minimize the chances you will become a victim of sexual assault.

12 WAYS TO AVOID DATE RAPE

Sometimes sexual assault is unavoidable, and a woman is never to blame if she is assaulted; however, if you use common sense, you can keep yourself out of situations where date rape is more likely to occur.

- 🐌 *Do not lose control of yourself, whether with drugs or alcohol.*
- 🐌 *Avoid sending sexually suggestive messages (by dressing in revealing clothing, by talking about sex, and by being overly physical with your dates).*
- 🐌 *Recognize and avoid situations that are likely to lead to sex on a date (parking on a dark road, going into someone's bedroom at a party).*

& *Avoid being alone with one or more men, particularly if they are drinking.*

& *Always be prepared to get yourself home from a date – have change for a phone call and someone to call.*

& *Consider carrying something for personal defense, such as a whistle, pepper spray or a personal attack alarm.*

& *Decide before you go on a date how far you're willing to go sexually, and do not send misleading messages.*

& *Be confident in your right to say no, and do not back down.*

& *Recognize that when a man keeps insisting, he's about to pressure you for sex – be clear that he has gone too far, and get out of the situation.*

& *Be careful about even kissing someone you don't know well, because he may then think it is OK to demand more.*

& *Think twice about dating someone who is three or more years older than you are.*

& *Clearly and confidently understand that if a man buys you a very expensive dinner, he has bought a very nice meal; he has not bought the right to any sexual activity with you.*

Rape can occur to anyone at any time and in any place, but it is important to be mindful of some basic safety issues. For example, walking alone at night in dark or deserted areas, opening the door of your home without checking to see who is there, accepting a ride with someone you do not know, or becoming intoxicated or high are all examples of not being careful about your own safety. However, whether or not a woman is acting cautiously, *she never deserves to be attacked or sexually assaulted.*

The Trauma

During a rape, a woman may or may not be threatened with a weapon, or she may or may not be beaten up or physically hurt. Whether or not a weapon is used or physical harm is inflicted, it is still a sexual assault. The nature and extent of physical injuries or the type of force or weapon used do not make the assault any less traumatic for the victim.

After being sexual assaulted, many women experience a traumatic reaction, meaning they may feel numb or unable to feel or make decisions. They may be unable to function, their eating and sleeping patterns may be disrupted, and they may have many conflicting and intense emotions and feelings. Immediately following a sexual assault, it is very important to seek help. No one is able to deal with the effects of such a trauma by herself, and no one should have to go through this kind of trauma alone. If you are the victim of sexual assault, you should tell your parents or another trusted adult. You should notify the police and be examined by a doctor whether or not you think you have sustained any physical injuries. The sooner you do this following the assault, the faster law-enforcement agencies can do their job in terms of finding and charging the person who did this to you, and the sooner you can begin the process of healing, both emotionally and physically. If you do experience a rape, you should not bathe or douche before you go to the emergency room for an exam, as samples of vaginal fluid may help police convict the perpetrator of this very serious and damaging crime. You can also contact a local rape-crisis center for assistance.

Many women are reluctant to notify law-enforcement officials following a sexual assault. They believe they will be blamed for the assault or it will be assumed they "asked for it" to happen. Many women avoid the police because they are embarrassed and ashamed. The decision about whether or not to involve law-enforcement is a personal one and is based on many factors. You should not make this decision alone, particularly immediately following the trauma when your thinking and decision-making skills are poor. Most police departments have specially trained female officers who deal with cases of sexual assault, and you will not be blamed or held responsible for being the victim of a terrible crime.

The Importance of Counseling

If you have been the victim of sexual trauma, you need the support of your family and friends. You may also need the assistance of a trained counselor or mental-health professional to help you deal with the psychological and emotional effects of an assault. If you do not seek professional help after such a trauma, problems may arise later in your life, particularly in the areas of intimate relationships, trust, self-esteem and sexuality. If you have been sexually assaulted in the past and have never told anyone, you may benefit from counseling with a professional, even if the assault occurred years ago. I see many women in their 30s who are having major problems relating emotionally with their partners. With questioning, I find many of them had a very disturbing sexual experience as a young adult. They ball up the event, comprehending it with the understanding of an adolescent, and bury it deep in their soul. Over the years, after they have families of their own, this ball is like a bad seed that suddenly grows to consume them. They become angry and depressed, and are confused about why their relationships are suddenly going bad. If you experience such a trauma, please get professional guidance to help you deal with it before you try to bury it deep in your soul. While discussing a rape may seem too painful in the short term, in the long term, I promise you it provides tremendous relief.

If you have been sexually assaulted in the past and have never told anyone, you may benefit from counseling with a professional, even if the assault occurred years ago.

MOLESTATION

There is another type of sexual assault, called sexual molestation, sexual abuse or incest. **Incest** is defined as sexual activity that takes place between an adult and a child or teenager in the same family. **Sexual abuse** or **molestation** involves sexual activity between children and adults, usually an adult the child knows, such as a friend of the family, a relative or a person in the community. The reason these types of sexual activity are considered sexual assault is that the adult is in a position of power and he (or she) uses this power to engage a child in sexual activity. This type of sexual abuse involves all forms of sexual activity such as fondling (touching), oral sex and intercourse. Sexual abuse is against the law; if it occurs, the responsibility and the blame always rest with the adult. All adults know this type of activity is wrong. The job of adults is to protect children from harm, and children can be very severely harmed physically and emotionally if they are sexually abused.

When an adult is sexually molesting a child, he will sometimes threaten the child with harm if the child tells anyone, or he may treat the child in special ways that the child likes, even though the child may not like the abuse. Most children feel powerless to stop the abuse. They are afraid to tell anyone, because they are afraid something bad will happen, or they are afraid they will get the adult in trouble. If you are being sexually abused, or if you know someone who is being abused, you must tell someone what is happening so the abuse can be stopped. You may be able to tell one or both of your parents, another relative, your doctor, a teacher or guidance counselor, or another trusted adult. Or you can call your local police department or social service agency.

Immediately after telling someone what has happened or what is happening, you will have a lot of different emotions, and there may be some disruptions in your family. (If someone in your family is abusing you , you or that person may have to leave your home for some period of time.) It is very important to get counseling at this time, because sexual abuse can have a very severe impact on how you feel about yourself, your body, your attitude toward sex, and your ability to establish and maintain healthy and loving relationships with others in the future. In addition, others in your family may need professional counseling to assist them with this trauma. The sexual abuse of children is a serious problem, but it can be stopped. You can get help if you let someone know this is happening to you.

Keeping These Changes in Perspective

Many changes and stresses happen to you during adolescence. It is very important to remember as you grow and develop into a woman that you are not alone and that many sources of information, help and support are available if you need them. The key to having a successful adolescence is to make sure you understand what is happening to you and why, and to take steps to keep yourself healthy and safe. No one expects you to do this alone, but each adolescent must make the choices and decisions facing her for herself. Some of the choices you make as a teenager can have consequences that will stay with you for the rest of your life, so it is important to weigh your choices carefully and make decisions that are right for you.

While you are exercising this new right to make your own decisions, allow yourself to make some mistakes. No one is perfect, and the younger you learn this, the better you will handle the many mistakes you are bound to make from now on. Your goal should be to learn from your mistakes as well as your accomplishments.

Additional Resources
Books

- **Reviving Ophelia: Saving the Selves of Adolescent Girls,** *Mary Pipher, Ph.D.,* Ballantine Books, 1994.

- **The Shelter of Each Other: Rebuilding Our Families,** *Mary Bray Pipher, Ph.D.,* Ballantine Books, 1997.

- **Schoolgirls: Young Women, Self-Esteem, and the Confidence Gap,** *Peggy Orenstein,* Anchor, 1995.

- **Meeting at the Crossroads: Women's Psychology and Girls' Development,** *Carol Gilligan and Lyn Mikel Brown,* Ballantine Books, 1993.

- **Teens Talk About Sex: Adolescent Sexuality in the '90s,** *Roper Starch,* Worldwide, 1994.

- **The Secret Trauma: Incest in the Lives of Girls and Women,** *Russell D,* Basic Books, 1986.

- **Sex and America's Teenagers,** The Alan Guttmacher Institute, 1994.

- **For Children Who Were Broken (Women),** *Elia Wise,* Berkley Publishing Group, 1991.

- **Food Fight: A Guide to Eating Disorders for Pre-Teens and Their Parents,** *Janet Bode,* Simon & Schuster, 1997. *Reading Level: Ages 9-12.*

Organizations

- **National Drug Abuse Hotline** (800) 662-4357
- **CDC AIDS Info** (800) 342-2437
- **National Runaway Hotline** (800) 621-4000
- **National Hotline for Missing & Exploited Children** (800) 843-5678

- **Youth Crisis Hotline** (800) 448-4663

- **American Academy of Child & Adolescent Psychiatry**
  3615 Wisconsin Avenue NW
  Washington, DC 20016-3007
  (202) 966-7300
  Fax (202) 966-2891

- **Streetcats Foundation**
  267 Lester Avenue, Suite 104
  Oakland, CA 94606

Internet Sites

- **http://www.villing.com/JFK_Health_World.htm**
  Health World's mission is to help children build healthy lives. The hands-on interactive exhibits, discovery zones, classrooms and more bring to life an environment that is exciting and supplements the health education efforts of schools, families, youth organizations, health care and social associations.

- **http://www.psych.med.umich.edu/web/aacap/**
  This is the site of the American Academy of Adolescent Psychiatry. This site helps educate parents and families about psychiatric disorders affecting children and adolescents. The Academy publishes "Facts for Families" – more than 52 informational sheets that provide concise and up-to-date information on such issues as the depressed child, teen suicide, helping children after a disaster, discipline, learning disabilities, and child sexual abuse. Thousands of these publications are distributed weekly, and the "Facts for Families" has been cited and recommended by such publications as Better Homes & Gardens, Ladies' Home Journal and USA Today.

- **http://www.adaa.org**
  This site of the Anxiety Disorders Association Of America (ADAA) – which promotes the prevention and cure of anxiety disorders and seeks to improve the lives of all people who suffer from them – provides educational material and additional links.

- **http://www.siecus.org/pubs/fact/fact0006.html**
  The web site of SIECUS, the Sexuality Information and Educational Council of the United States, features a parents' area and links, and offers more than two dozen publications to the public. This address takes you to SIECUS' "Sexual Orientation and Identity" fact sheet.

CHAPTER TWO

ADULT STRESSES

Weathering Life's Storms With Grace

You can expect changes and stresses to be part of your life as an adult woman. This chapter explores the many developmental changes that often occur throughout adulthood, including: living alone; establishing a relationship with someone; marrying; rearing children; caring for aging parents and dealing with the death of parents; facing the end of marriage, either because of divorce or the death of a spouse; and aging, which brings with it changes in your health and physical capabilities. Some of these changes can be expected and anticipated, while others occur suddenly and without warning. In any case, one thing you can count on throughout the course of your life is change. The natural course of life involves changes in yourself, your relationships, your physical capabilities, your behaviors and your emotions. Anticipating and welcoming change allows you to remain flexible and, to some degree, in control of the direction your life takes. Fighting against change or refusing to acknowledge change can lead to disappointment, anger and feelings of being overwhelmed and out of control. When you understand these life-cycle changes and their effect on you, you will deal with stress in a healthier way and adapt better to whatever new situations you face.

Living Alone

Many women live alone for at least some period of their adult lives, and others live alone throughout the course of their adulthood. In past generations, women lived with their parents (or other caretakers) until they found life partners, but this is no longer the case.

While some women choose to live alone, others find themselves living alone prior to marriage or after the end of a marriage. Single living can be an enlightening and wonderful journey, or it can be lonely and frightening. If you are single, it is up to you to create a life that is fulfilling and secure.

PROVIDING FOR YOUR PHYSICAL SAFETY

All women who live alone, whether single by choice or through circumstances, are solely responsible for their own security. Protecting yourself may seem like a daunting task, but living alone simply means that you must be mindful of where you live, work and play to ensure your physical safety. When you choose a residence, think about things that affect your security. For example, is the lighting adequate where you park your car and around your home? How easily could an intruder get into your home, and what deterrent measures are available? Does the apartment complex or community have a security guard? Should you consider installing an alarm system? Make sure you know the basics of self-defense, and follow common-sense safety guidelines, such as not inviting strangers into your home. Certain pets can offer additional security. When you live alone, it is a good idea not to broadcast that fact. Your answering-machine message does not need to disclose who lives with you, and you can use your first initial rather than your first name in your telephone-book listing. While it is not necessary to become overly paranoid, it is always important to take precautions to protect yourself.

LOOKING OUT FOR YOUR
ECONOMIC WELL-BEING

Another aspect of security is financial security. All women have the responsibility for their financial security, whether they live alone or with a partner. Educate yourself on financial issues and options with books, online services or consultations with professionals in the field of money management or finances. Many home-computer programs have household-budgeting features as well as other options for managing your money. It is important to have both short-term savings (for household emergencies) as well as long-term savings for retirement. If you enter into living arrangements or business arrangements with others, be sure that you are protecting yourself financially. Often it is worthwhile to obtain legal or financial advice up front to protect yourself from being harmed financially later on. Many women find it difficult to be assertive about protecting their interests because they do not want to offend or anger others, but your top priority should be the protection of your interests and assets.

FORGING CONNECTIONS WITH OTHER PEOPLE

Some women find living alone stressful because they often feel lonely and are confronted with household or automotive responsibilities that they do not feel capable of managing. Whether you are single by choice or because of the loss of a spouse through death or divorce, you need a social network of friends and family whom you feel comfortable with and can ask for assistance. This not only helps combat feelings of loneliness, but also provides you with support and help, all of which serve to reduce your stress. Our society has seen a tremendous increase in mobility and a decrease in extended-family and community relationships, which makes it more difficult – but not impossible – to meet people and establish a social network wherever you are living. If you have relocated or live in an area where you have no existing support network, there are numerous ways you can meet people and reduce boredom and loneliness. These include volunteer work (contact your local United Way office for a complete rundown of volunteer opportunities), pursuing hobbies, taking continuing education classes at a local community college or university, and participating in civic groups, clubs or religious organizations. Think about the kinds of activities and interests that you have; by involving yourself in things you like, you meet others with similar interests. In addition, if you live alone, consider adopting a pet. Pets make wonderful companions, and research has shown that people who have pets report less depression and stress. Whether you are living alone temporarily or permanently, by taking responsibility you can enjoy a fulfilling and secure life.

Marriage
CHOOSING THE LIFE PARTNER FOR YOU

For most people, marriage signifies an emotional, legal and spiritual commitment to another person. Prior to marriage, it is important for you and your partner to work on establishing your relationship. Spend time together; learn about each other's likes and dislikes, feelings, behaviors and values. During this "courtship" phase, it is easy to overlook or not notice flaws or negative characteristics in someone you care about. The phrase "love is blind" is most certainly true during this beginning phase of a relationship. In addition, you may not feel free to express differences of opinion, or to say or do things that you think would upset your partner. During this initial stage of your relationship, it is normal to feel very physically attracted to your partner; you may feel emotionally and physically excited by the thought or presence of your partner. These feelings can be very intense, and very pleasurable.

At some point, a relationship moves into a second phase. You become more comfortable expressing dissenting opinions or disagreeing, and the level of excitement in the relationship may change. During this second phase, you continue to learn more about each other and about yourself in terms of decision-making, values, priorities and behaviors. You feel that you know your partner very well and are ready to make a commitment. Usually this commitment is expressed through an engagement, which may be formal or informal and signifies for friends and family your intent to marry.

It is sometimes difficult to know if the person you have chosen to marry is the "right one." Each of us is compatible with many other people. You must identify your own priorities, needs and expectations, and seek a relationship that will fulfill them. However, no one person can satisfy all of your needs or make you completely happy, and you should not depend on another person for your total fulfillment or happiness. Many marriages end because one or both partners are disappointed that marrying someone did not make everything in their lives better. Having unreasonable expectations of your partner prior to getting married may later cause difficulty in the relationship.

Many religious denominations ask their followers to engage in pre-marital counseling. This marriage preparation may involve talking with a clergy member and taking written inventories regarding expectations and behaviors that you and your partner hold for yourselves and each other. A trained mental-health professional also can lead you through this process. The purpose of this counseling is to identify potential problem areas in a relationship, to make sure you and your partner know each other well, and to teach you some strategies for dealing with potentially problematic issues. Issues that tend to cause problems typically involve sexual attitudes and practices, financial issues, relationships with families of origin, child-rearing and expectations regarding domestic responsibilities. If you and your partner are from different religious, cultural or ethnic backgrounds, there may be additional complicating factors that you should be aware of prior to marriage.

TYPICAL TROUBLE SPOTS FOR COUPLES

- ♠ *Sexual attitudes and practices*
- ♠ *Financial issues*
- ♠ *Relationships with families of origin*
- ♠ *Child-rearing*
- ♠ *Division of domestic responsibilities*
- ♠ *Differences in religious, cultural or ethnic backgrounds*

BUILDING A LIFE TOGETHER

Wedding plans are often made during the engagement period, and many couples choose to marry in a public ceremony in the presence of friends and family who witness their lifelong commitment to one another. Although it is normal to be nervous prior to your wedding, this time is one of great joy and expectation. Following the marriage ceremony, couples traditionally go on a honeymoon trip before settling into married life. Newlyweds often find that the excitement and intensity they enjoyed prior to marriage give way to a more predictable and stable routine. This change may be frightening if you assume that you made a mistake in marrying your partner because you no longer feel tremendous excitement and passion. Actually, it is normal and expected for you and your spouse to establish routines, and for the intensity and excitement of courtship to evolve into a sense of security and stability as your marriage progresses.

Building and sustaining a healthy and happy marriage takes a tremendous amount of work, energy and commitment. It does not just happen on its own, nor does it happen just because two people love one another. Marriages can be particularly hard to sustain in our culture, where they are threatened by other demands and circumstances of our times – such as financial pressures and physical distance from extended family. While no one marries with the expectation of failure, the divorce rate in the United States hovers at about 50 percent; in other words, half of all marriages end in divorce. This statistic may be frightening and overwhelming, but it may also push you into working harder on your marriage. Like everyone else, you want to be happy in your marriage – to feel respected, loved and taken care of, and in return, to help your partner feel the same way. For a marriage to be successful, it has to be the most important and central commitment of your life, superseding all other commitments and demands. Solid and healthy marriages demand that couples genuinely respect and like their partners, and believe that they are dependable, honest and compassionate.

One of the first tasks of a healthy marriage is learning to attach to each other and look to each other first to meet your needs. You both must separate emotionally from your families of origin – the parents and siblings you grew up with – and attach to your new family – each other, and the children you may someday have. As you do this, you must find new ways to maintain emotional ties with your extended families within the context of your marriage. In addition, you both have to begin thinking in terms of "we" and "us," and not solely in terms of "I." Commitment to a marriage means forging a bond that comes through intimacy and shared experiences. This process needs to continue throughout the life of a marriage, not just at the beginning, because you continue to grow and change as you mature. When you have children, it becomes even more important for you and your spouse to work to maintain your sense of yourselves as a couple. It is easy to focus much of your marital time and energy on child-rearing, losing sight of your needs to spend time together as a couple and to maintain intimacy. Couples in healthy marriages rely on each other for emotional support and nurturing. This mutual dependence is particularly important in our society, where people frequently live apart from their extended families or may feel isolated

" We want to have a few years together first so that when we have kids we can look back and say, 'You know, we used to have so much fun!' We really want to build strong foundations on us before we involve anyone else."

in their communities or in their workplaces. Focusing exclusively on the needs of children in a family means that the needs of the adults may not be met, which can lead to anger, disappointment and frustration in a marriage.

Inevitably, you have to confront crises during the life of your marriage partnership. These may be financial crises, deaths of loved ones, illnesses, natural disasters or other stressful events that affect your marriage and family. You and your partner must find a way to deal with these crises in healthy and adaptable ways; otherwise, your marriage may be destroyed. Crises can provide opportunities for you to develop strengths and resources you never knew you had; a crisis may serve to bond you together and enhance your attachment. You must find ways of coping with monumental stresses, as well as with the smaller, day-to-day stress that everyone faces. Disappointment, hurt feelings and disagreements are also a part of marriage, and you and your spouse have to find a way to argue and express disagreement without damaging the foundation of trust you have built and without using violent or abusive tactics. Maintaining a sense of humor and playfulness in a marriage can help you survive both the large and small problems that you will inevitably face.

HOW TO FIGHT FAIR

🪶 *Avoid using cruel statements or ones that will "hit below the belt."*

🪶 *Do not bring up a laundry list of past complaints or experiences, but rather stick with the issue at hand.*

🪶 *If one or both partners seem to be losing emotional control, take a "time out" and agree to meet in a designated time to continue the discussion.*

🪶 *Follow basic problem - solving steps of identifying the problem, generating solutions, evaluating solutions and choosing one for implementation.*

🪶 *Do not make disparaging remarks about your partner's appearance, family of origin or sexual capabilities.*

One important strategy for coping with marital and family issues and crises is communication. This may sound simplistic, but it can be very difficult to keep the lines of communication open with your partner, particularly during a crisis and couples must work at communicating with one another. Open lines of communication mean that each person can tell their partner how they are feeling or thinking (this can be done verbally or in writing) and each person feels that they are being heard and understood. Many couples set aside a period of time each day to "reconnect" with one another and "check in" to see how each partner is feeling. It helps to use "I" statements when communicating with your partner to prevent defensiveness. For example, saying "I feel ____ when you do _____" is a much more effective way of telling your partner something than accusing him or demanding that he take responsibility for your feelings. Another strategy is to repeat back to your partner what has been said to make sure that you understand what he is saying. Misunderstandings and failure to clarify are often the cause of disagreements and arguments. Couples who work on maintaining effective communication strategies find that they are much better able to handle crises because they are able to work together to solve problems and support each other emotionally. If you and your partner have difficulty communicating in spite of your best efforts, or if you have difficulty resolving problems, you may need professional advice to help you find healthier and more flexible ways of dealing with stress and problems.

" In marriage, sometimes you give a little more; other days, you'll take a little more. And then if it becomes too unbalanced, I try to initiate a conversation about it. But it's hard to get him started to talk about it. Men run when we say, 'Can we talk?'"

One central issue in all marriages is that of sexual activity and sexuality. Human beings are sexual, and remain so throughout their adult lives. You likely look forward to establishing a sexual relationship that is pleasurable and fun for you and your partner. This sexual relationship usually develops over time as you become more comfortable communicating your likes and dislikes in general and your sexual preferences and needs in specific. Together you work out how often you want to have sex, and what kinds of sexual activity you are interested in. Communication with your partner is the key to having a sexual relationship that is pleasurable and exciting, and that meets your needs and fantasies. Many variables influence your sex life, including health and medical conditions; the stress of work and domestic responsibilities; and the emotional relationship between you and your partner. In addition, your sexual energy or libido can change over time, sometimes predictably and sometimes without warning, and it is important that you and your partner be able to communicate openly about what is happening between you sexually. If either of you is uncomfortable discussing sexual issues, you need to find some other way of communicating, such as putting your feelings in writing. In some cases, you may want to ask a third party, such as your health-care provider or therapist, to help you and your partner understand where you are sexually and what changes you would like to make in your sexual relationship.

SIX STRATEGIES FOR EFFECTIVE COMMUNICATION

🍂 Use "I" statements that avoid putting your partner on the defensive ("I feel _____ when you do _____").

🍂 Listen to what your partner is saying and then repeat it back to ensure you understand what is being said.

🍂 Be honest about your feelings and accept your partner's stated feelings. Feelings are never right or wrong, so do not try to talk someone out of how he or she feels, or imply those feelings are wrong or stupid.

🍂 Make time each day for "checking in" with one another to see how each partner is feeling and doing.

🍂 If verbal communication is difficult, try writing to one another to express your feelings and needs.

🍂 Never assume your partner knows your feelings or needs – unless you are living with a mind reader, you have the responsibility to tell your partner these things directly.

CONFRONTING THE THREAT OF INFIDELITY

One of the most common obstacles to the development of a healthy marriage is infidelity, when one or both partners have a relationship with someone outside the marriage. This relationship usually involves sexual activity, but it can also be a non-sexual but emotionally intense relationship. There are many reasons why someone would seek satisfaction outside the boundaries of the marital relationship. One common reason often given for infidelity is the sense that the person is not being heard or understood by his or her spouse. The person may feel that he or she is not being supported emotionally or that the partner does not care about his or her feelings or needs. Poor communication and an inability or unwillingness to confront and resolve marital disagreements can lead to infidelity. In addition, sexual problems in a marriage also contribute to unfaithfulness, when one or both partners are not satisfied with the frequency or quality of sexual intimacy.

Finding out that a spouse has been unfaithful is devastating to most people; such a revelation shatters faith in a partner, in marriage and in oneself. However, many marriages can and do survive infidelity. If you or your spouse has been unfaithful, you may be able to heal your relationship if you are willing to invest the time and energy necessary to resolve your problems. You can begin by making an inventory of your own strengths and weaknesses and the strengths and weaknesses of the marriage, and by committing yourselves to working on your problems directly instead of using an outside relationship to avoid dealing with issues in your marriage. Some couples can do this without professional help, but you may benefit from the help of a trained counselor or therapist. Infidelity shatters the basic tenets of respect and trust that are fundamental in a marriage, but it is possible to rebuild this foundation and to move forward together with a solid commitment from both partners.

CLIMBING YOUR MOUNTAIN

View life as a mountain climber would a large mountain.
The other side of the mountain is how you want your life to be in
the future. Visualize yourself in this beautiful field, and decide
what you want around you. If you want a husband, children,
grandchildren, extended family and friends, and a career, these
are all priorities to you. These are your goals in life, and each of
us visualizes different things we want in this field.

Now you must climb this mountain of life, which has
peaks and valleys, steep and challenging sections, with
constant variation. During your climb you must focus on the
field on the other side. If it is painful to continue or if you fall
backwards a few feet, decide if your field is worth it to you to
continue. If it is, you will find the inner strength to prevail
and push yourself on. Use your family support, community
resources and faith to guide and strengthen you on this
climb. When faced with a problem in life, look at it as a cliff
to ascend: study it, prepare to climb over and then give it all

*your effort possible. At the end of the day, when enjoying
everything around you in your field, you will be very happy.*

*If you do not have a real vision of yourself in this field, it
makes climbing life's mountain a greater struggle. With a clear
vision, I hope you find the climb full of excitement, challenge
and joy, as you know each step brings you closer to your dream.*

HOW TO HANDLE STRESS

- *Get regular exercise and eat well-balanced meals.*
- *Make time for fun and leisure activities.*
- *Plan ahead as much as possible.*
- *Communicate with your spouse and children about your
  needs and feelings. Don't hold things in until you explode.*
- *Use a written journal or a trusted friend or spouse to
  explore and process your stresses and your emotions.*
- *Laugh loudly and often.*
- *Use relaxation tapes, yoga, meditation, massage, muscle
  relaxation, guided imagery or other techniques daily.*

WHEN A MARRIAGE ENDS IN DIVORCE

Sometimes the differences between two people are so large and
so important, and the levels of trust, respect and love have deteriorated so much, that one or both partners decide to end the marriage. Deciding to divorce is never an easy decision, and the decision is usually reached after much time has passed and many efforts have been made to rectify the marital problems. If you or your
partner decide to end your marriage, you should know that this
time will be extremely stressful and difficult for you and your family. Divorce affects not only you and your partner but also your
children, your parents and extended families, your friends and your
associates. You and your family will have concerns and needs that

---

you have never faced before, and you will need to rely on the knowledge and strength of others as well as on yourself.

Many women fail to protect themselves legally when they are separating from or divorcing their spouses. It is imperative that you seek legal counsel in order to protect yourself and your children and to understand the legal and financial implications of a divorce. Regardless of how amicable the separation seems, many couples find that when they begin sorting out financial issues in a divorce, they are unable to agree and may even find that their relationship becomes hostile and uncooperative.

If you have children, you must be especially aware of what you say and how you behave following a separation. Children can suffer significant emotional damage by being caught in the middle of divorcing parents, or by being used as pawns or messengers by their parents, or because their needs are lost in the shuffle while the adults are busy tending to their own needs. Regardless of how angry you may be with your spouse, you and your children will adjust better if you control your anger and do not allow it to control you and your decisions. If you need assistance managing your emotions, do not rely on your children to be your confidants, but instead use trusted friends, family members or a professional counselor.

If you are going through a divorce, expect to feel different emotions that may be very intense and overwhelming. You may experience intense feelings of sadness and grief as you mourn the end of your marriage. You may lose confidence in yourself and your decision-making skills, and you may also feel lonely, angry, hurt, relieved and confused. While all of these feelings are normal, if you find that you are so overwhelmed emotionally that you are unable to work, care for your children or take care of yourself, you should seek professional help. As time passes, your emotional response to the divorce should change, and dealing with the changes in your life becomes easier. In order for this transformation to take place, however, you must be aware of your emotions and stress level and take care of yourself in healthy and appropriate ways. This means avoiding the abuse of alcohol or drugs, relying on friends and family for support when needed, protecting yourself legally and financially, and spending time doing things you enjoy. Many women find renewed strength and confidence in themselves following a divorce, and are able to rebuild their lives and move forward in a positive direction.

THE DEATH OF A SPOUSE

The death of a spouse is a tremendous challenge that can occur at any time in a marriage. Adjusting to the death of a loved one is never easy, and whether or not your spouse's death is expected, finding yourself alone is a difficult and painful experience. If you have lost a spouse, you need the comfort and support of family and friends as you grieve. Depending on your relationship with your spouse, the process of grieving may be very intense and very painful. If you have shared a significant portion of your life in an intimate relationship with someone, the period of bereavement can be rather long and may in fact go on until your own death, whether or not you remarry. None of us is ever fully prepared for the death of a spouse. While you both are living, it is important to communicate with each other regarding your wills, financial issues, legal and medical questions (such as whether or not to sign a living will) and funeral arrangements. This preparation at least alleviates some of the inevitable difficulties that arise when a spouse dies. Many people depend on family and friends, while others involve themselves in bereavement support groups or seek help from a professional counselor to assist them with their grief.

It is normal following the death of a spouse to have many confusing and intense emotions, and again, talking about your feelings can help you cope more effectively with this tremendous change in your life. Staying involved with others and with activities you enjoy also assists with the grieving process. There is no easy way to handle the death of a spouse, and each person grieves in her own way and in her own time. Don't expect more or less of yourself than you are able to handle. In time, your grief will subside and your life will proceed, although along a somewhat different course.

Parenting
PREPARING FOR THE CHALLENGE OF A LIFETIME

Of all the life changes that occur throughout our adult lives, perhaps none changes our lives so completely and so dramatically as having and raising children. While some couples decide when and how far apart to have their children, for many others, starting a family happens without much planning. Children are a source of tremendous pride and happiness, but they are also a tremendous responsibility and a source of stress. It is important to recognize the impact children have on your marriage, your emotions, your behavior, and all other facets of your life. Anticipating that your life will change will help you cope more effectively with the stresses and changes that children bring.

Children's needs change as they grow and develop, and it is a parent's job to anticipate these changes and respond to them in a positive and healthy way. Excellent books are available on the subject of child development, and many parents (particularly new ones) rely on these books, as well as other sources, for information about the developmental stages their child is going through. Friends, family, your child's caregivers or teachers, pediatricians and other health-care providers are additional sources of information about your child's development and developmental stages in general.

Many couples report that disagreement about parenting issues causes significant stress in their marriages. Children of all ages and developmental levels need parenting that is consistent and predictable. You and your partner may approach child-rearing with different expectations, philosophies and strategies; however, the more you work together to jointly parent your children, the healthier your partnership will be and the healthier your children will be. One way to help the two of you parent consistently is to talk about parenting issues prior to having children. This discussion should include topics such as the division of labor in child-rearing and the expectations each partner has about his or her own role and the role of the other. You also should discuss what types of punishments and rewards you will use (physical punishment, time out, etc.); your parenting goals and how best to achieve them, and each partner's feelings about children's roles and responsibilities in a family. It is also important for you both to examine your own childhood and your own parents' parenting styles, because these have a tremendous impact on the parenting style each partner brings to a new family. Adequate discussion and resolution of major parenting issues ahead of time reduce stress later on.

10 WAYS TO HELP ADOLESCENTS

❧ *Educate yourself about the developmental tasks of adolescence with books, online information services, seminars, etc.*

❧ *Try not to take everything your adolescent does or says personally.*

❧ *Work on keeping your emotions in check when talking with your adolescent.*

❧ *Recognize that your teenager will make some mistakes in judgment. Allow him or her to help decide what the consequences should be.*

❧ *Choose your battles. If your teenager is doing well overall but wants to experiment with hair dye, this battle may not be worth fighting. Decide what issues are important, state your position and stick with it.*

❧ *Be open to listening to your adolescent. You don't have to agree, but letting her be heard is often what she wants and needs most.*

❧ *Do not be afraid to set limits for your teenagers. No matter how responsible or mature they appear, they still need boundaries and guidance.*

❧ *Avoid lecturing – say what you have to say in one or two sentences and move on.*

❧ *Try not to bring up old issues or mistakes when dealing with current issues or mistakes – your teen may be trying to move on and prove he has changed, so give him this opportunity.*

❧ *Do not humiliate, shame or berate your teenager. Deal with her **behavior** and the impact of this behavior. Try not to do this in front of your child's peers.*

LEARNING THE SKILLS YOU NEED

Perhaps the most common parenting error is to assume the function of parents is to provide food, clothing and shelter, and that children will grow and develop without much guidance or parenting. This is simply not true, and research has consistently shown that children need their parents to serve as mediators and interpreters of the world, and they need their parents to provide love, nurturing, assurance and comfort.

As a parent, you are in the unique position of explaining and interpreting the world for your children, helping them understand not only how their world operates, but also what their world expects back from them. Children need firm and consistent limits, guidelines and rules to help them learn to control their impulses, become socialized and able to function well with others, and develop the self-confidence and skills to negotiate their environment when they are away from you. Children also need to know they are special and loved, and they are worthy and deserving of love and kindness from others. Your children deserve to grow up thinking they are special and knowing that regardless of everything else, you love them very much.

Many parents were raised in families where they themselves did not feel loved, or in families where they were not guided and disciplined appropriately. If you had such an experience, the task of parenting may be especially difficult for you, because you had no role models of healthy parents as a child. Regardless of how you were raised, you have the opportunity to parent your own children in a way that feels comfortable and healthy for you. If your own childhood was traumatic and you are not sure you know how to be a healthy parent, you may benefit from the assistance of a trained counselor, or from parenting classes or other educational or therapeutic opportunities.

FINDING TIME AND ACHIEVING BALANCE

In addition to the parenting skills noted previously, good parenting requires an investment of your time and your energy. Many women work outside the home either because they choose to or because they have to for financial reasons. When both parents work outside the home, children are often with other caregivers for a significant

> " *The most stressful time is around homework and dinner time. I have too much to do, my husband is usually not home yet, and I have to cope with three children."*

part of the day. Women who work outside the home often feel as though there are tremendous pressures on them to be "Superwomen," and feel they are responsible not only for their jobs, but also for the running of the household and the primary child - rearing responsibilities.

There must be a balance in everyone's life between work and play, and you owe it to yourself and your family to find time for the things you enjoy. Sometimes this means cutting back on time spent on household chores, or making financial choices that allow you to work fewer hours, but regardless of how you choose to organize your life, you must set your priorities and then work toward achieving your goals. Children and parents need time together for play, for fun and for sharing; adults need couple time together; and individuals need time for themselves. Each family must therefore find and negotiate ways of managing their time so that most of these needs can be met.

HOW TO MAKE THE MOST OF YOUR TIME

- 🐚 *List and prioritize your responsibilities. Delegate those you can, delete others.*

- 🐚 *Do not shortchange yourself – priority items must include things you do for yourself and your relationship.*

- 🐚 *When you have others helping you (spouse, children), accept they may do things differently from you and do not go back and re-do tasks they have completed. If something is not done well, have the person who did it go back and redo it; do not make this your responsibility.*

- 🐚 *Plan menus ahead of time and shop only for these menus. If you can, schedule time every week for cooking and freezing meals you can use throughout the week.*

♣ *Learn how to say "no" without guilt or indecision when asked to take on additional responsibilities.*

♣ *Beginning as early as you can, have your children assist in and take responsibility for certain household chores. This helps foster a sense of responsibility in them they carry into adulthood and it also helps you.*

ADJUSTING TO MOTHERHOOD

Becoming a mother radically changes the way a woman feels about herself and her world. So many things change with the birth or adoption of a child, and many women expect that things will be different when they become a mother; however, for others, the changes are unexpected and may cause stress or difficulty in adapting.

For women who give birth to a child, one of the most noticeable changes occurs in the body. There may be weight gain, changes in body dimensions, changes in breast size or shape, or just a sense that your body is different. There are things you can do to lose excess weight if you choose to, but there may not be anything you can do to alter other changes in your body after giving birth. Rather than bemoan these changes, accept them as the motherhood "badge" that they are. You may need to change your clothing styles or sizes to accommodate these changes and help you look and feel your best.

" After having children, I noticed my body changed. I started wearing a miracle bra, support panties, and control-top pantyhose."

Other changes may occur in your perception of yourself and your role in the world. Many women report that motherhood brings increased anxiety about both real and perceived hazards in their world that may affect their child. Things you previously took for granted may suddenly become precious commodities (such as time alone!). Again, it is important to learn to accept the changes in your life and embrace them, because these changes are part of becoming a parent. You may feel you are making a lot of sacrifices and giving up things you previously enjoyed, but at the same time, as you bond and connect with your child, you experience feelings of wonder and love that you may never have felt before. Many things in life involve compromise and trade-offs, and motherhood is no exception. Do not be surprised if you find yourself feeling differently about your job or career if you worked outside the home prior to motherhood. Many women realize after becoming mothers that their previous notions about returning to work may no longer be valid. Try and be flexible in your thinking and talk about these issues with your spouse in order to make decisions that are right for you and your family.

Many women also note their relationship with their partner changes following motherhood. You may feel differently about yourself as a sexual person, or you may feel that you are emotionally and physically drained, with little left over for your spouse. It is especially important that you and your partner work together to keep your relationship intimate, both physically and emotionally. Make time to spend together as a couple, whether you need to hire a babysitter or can take advantage of times when your child is asleep. If you are experiencing sexual difficulties, communicate with your partner about how you feel and together try to find a way to re-establish your intimacy. For first-time parents, the first year after a new baby joins the family can be a time of tremendous stress on the marriage, and it is important to keep the lines of communication open and to actively work on keeping your relationship healthy and loving.

> " After the baby was born, it took a few weeks or even months before I felt attractive enough or even the need to resume a sexual relationship with my husband."

ADDRESSING SPECIAL NEEDS

As if parenting were not stressful enough, certain circumstances can make it even more so. Some children have handicapping conditions, chronic health or medical problems, behavioral or emotional disorders, or other special needs. These have a direct impact on parenting and may cause additional physical, social, emotional or financial stress for a family. In such cases, you can significantly reduce your stress by learning as much as you can about your child's condition and needs. You can and should look for support and assistance from family and friends, health-care providers and community resources. If you believe you are the only one capable of taking care of your child's needs, you may never allow others the opportunity to help. You will have difficulty taking time for yourself to rejuvenate and replenish your energy, and you will ultimately be less able to care for your child's needs. An important first step in finding assistance may be talking with your pediatrician or contacting your local United Way agency to learn more about local resources available to you.

COPING WITH THE LOSS OF A CHILD

There are times when, due to an accident or a medical condition, a child dies. While this is not common, it does occur, and when it does, the stress that such a death causes is immense. Often parents blame themselves or each other in an attempt to find a cause for such a tragedy; however, blaming only causes more grief and pain. In the midst of their suffering, couples must work hard to share their grief and to depend on one another; otherwise, the tragedy of the child's death can easily create havoc in the strongest of marriages. In times of such tremendous stress, you need support, whether from friends, family, clergy or professional counselors. If you have lost a child, you may find community support groups helpful (particularly bereavement groups). Some grieving parents use their grief to work on rectifying social or medical problems for the public good, and they find some solace in this work. Every person mourns differently, and there is no right or wrong way to grieve the loss of a child. The passage of time makes the loss of a child somewhat easier to bear, but unfortunately, because of the intensity of our love for our children, the pain of loss is so great that it irrevocably changes the lives of the parents.

While the death of a child is an unusual way to lose a child, most parents' loss comes when their children grow up and leave home – either to go to college, to marry or to live independently. The feelings that accompany this period are sometimes referred to as the "empty-nest syndrome." When your child moves out, you may feel that your home is suddenly quiet and empty, and if you have relied on your child for companionship, you may feel lonely and saddened. At the same time, you may feel proud of your child's accomplishments or worried about the step toward independence your child has taken. In short, it is normal to have many different feelings as you adjust to the fact that your child is no longer living under your roof.

A marriage may feel the effects of the empty nest as well. If you and your spouse have spent the better part of your married lives concentrating on raising children, you may have neglected parts of your marriage. When the children leave home, you may find yourselves in the position of having to readjust to being alone with each other, without the children to serve as buffers or to run interference. In order to minimize the stress from this situation, recognize what is happening and take steps to renew the feelings of intimacy and connectedness. Even better, if you are reading this chapter before you become a parent or before your children leave home, you and your partner can realize the importance of making your relationship a priority and help ease the eventual transition back to just the two of you at home.

> " I felt depressed and alone when my children left. I had to find new interests and hobbies to keep me busy and happy."

If you are a single parent, you may have particular difficulty when children leave home because you are then truly alone. Plan ahead for this transition; find activities and people that you enjoy.

You also need to acknowledge that as difficult as it is when children leave home, the ultimate goal of parenting is to send your children into the world armed with the skills and knowledge they need to be healthy and productive adults. If you have done this, you have succeeded at one of life's most challenging tasks.

The Aging Process

As we mature through adulthood, we experience many changes in our life circumstances, our attitudes and beliefs, and our physical capabilities. There is no way to defy the aging process, but our attitude and our knowledge about aging are the keys to helping us age gracefully and accept the changes that occur. Usually the physical component that most clearly and dramatically signifies the aging process for a woman is menopause. While going through menopause may seem scary or overwhelming, you should prepare yourself for the changes that will occur in your body (reading the "Menopause" chapter in this book is a good way to begin). Knowing what is happening can help you feel more in control and can prevent a natural and normal physical process from creating emotional distress. Cultivate an open, trusting relationship with your doctor or healthcare provider so you feel comfortable asking questions and gathering the information you need. Women who accept and understand the natural process of aging have a much easier time making the transition into their later years than women who resist accepting what is normal and expected.

Our society places a premium on youth; however, with age come wisdom and experience and the opportunity to share these with others. No matter what messages you may pick up from advertising or the movies, do not buy into the fallacy that once you have lost your youthful appearance or the capacity for reproduction, you are no longer a valued or valuable member of your community. This kind of thinking can lead to depression, bitterness and anger, which can

> " I don't like the fact that my body is no longer slim and youthful. And I don't like it that when I look in the mirror, I look older. Of course, if you want to look at the positives, I'm a lot better off than a lot of people; I eat right and exercise, and I take care of myself. I keep aware of my body so if anything goes wrong, I get it checked out."

create psychological and physical difficulties. Throughout our lives, we have the capacity to love and help others and to work toward personal goals. Unfortunately, many older adults focus on what they can no longer do, instead of focusing on the capabilities they still have and the contributions they can still make, both to their families and to their communities. As you grow older, you can provide much-needed expertise to members of your family; you can volunteer your time and experience in your community; you can hold a job and be active in political or social organizations. Growing older does not mean that your life stops, it means that your life changes. Once again, accepting the changes and finding new challenges and opportunities helps you stay healthy, both psychologically and physically.

"We do a little bit more traveling now than we used to do. I have the ability to pick up and go with my husband on a business trip."

The deterioration of physical health can be an obstacle to your reaching your full potential as a mature adult. As they age, people experience a range of physical problems from hearing and vision losses to circulatory or cardiac conditions. You cannot predict what your health will be like as you age, but certain factors, including genetics, nutrition, and fitness, can affect it. If you have chronic health problems early in your life, these may also affect your health as an older person. Most of the medical and physical changes that occur as we age will happen gradually. You may find yourself tiring more quickly or find that it becomes more difficult to engage in activities with the ease of the past. Be sure to have regular visits with your health-care provider, and to exercise regularly and eat nutritious foods. The aches and pains or creaks and groans associated with aging do not mean you have to stop doing things you enjoy; they just mean you need to pay attention to the signals your body is sending. Avoid those things that are health hazards (alcohol, tobacco and poor nutrition) and keep yourself involved in activities and relationships that are positive, enjoyable and helpful.

In spite of your best efforts, at some point in your later years, you may find your health and medical condition has deteriorated to a point where you need assistance. It is not easy to lose physical functioning or capabilities, or to become dependent on others for your care. These changes may be accompanied by feelings of helplessness, sadness, frustration or anger. Recognize your feelings about your loss of health, and be honest in sharing your feelings with others. Psychologists and other mental-health professionals have known for years that talking about unpleasant feelings with a supportive person can greatly alleviate the negative impact of such feelings, and can allow a person the opportunity to explore and resolve these feelings. While talking about your feelings will not change your physical health, it will improve your outlook and your attitude – an important part of doing everything you can to keep yourself as healthy as possible. Communicating your feelings to friends, family and caregivers also helps them understand not only how you are feeling, but also what they can do to help make this period of your life as good as it can be.

You can also prepare yourself and your family for the possibility your health may deteriorate by making decisions regarding your future medical care, your financial arrangements, your will and your funeral or burial arrangements while you are in good health. While these decisions may be difficult to make, doing so ensures that your wishes are respected in the event you are unable to communicate them. You also spare your family and loved ones the difficulty of deciding what would be in your best interest if you become unable to do so.

Facing the Changes Ahead

Changes and stresses occur throughout adulthood. While some of these changes happen only to women, others happen regardless of gender. Remember: the more you expect change, the better equipped you will be to handle not only the changes themselves, but the accompanying stresses, in healthy ways. You do not have to handle difficult times or circumstances by yourself, and although it may be hard, it is important to rely on others when you need to. Asking for assistance is not a sign of weakness, but rather a sign of strength and health, even if it sometimes does not feel that way. You have an obligation to yourself and to the friends and family who care about you to take care of yourself both physically and emotionally. As we live our lives, and as we face life's changes, we continue to learn new things about others and ourselves. The way we choose to handle and manage life's stresses and changes has a tremendous impact on our health as well as our happiness.

WHAT YOU CAN DO NOW TO PREPARE FOR AGING

🐾 *Learn about Living Wills.*

🐾 *Prepare a Last Will and Testament and include your wishes about funeral and burial as well as disposition of your assets.*

🐾 *Maintain good nutrition and a regular exercise program (consult with your doctor about this).*

🐾 *Consider barrier-free design when buying or building a home.*

🐾 *Talk with a financial planner specifically about strategies for paying for any care you might need as you age.*

🐾 *Talk with family members about your plans and get their input, particularly if there is a chance you will be depending on them for assistance of any kind.*

Additional Resources
Books
FAMILIES

- **The Seven Habits of Highly Effective Families,**
  Stephen R. Covey, Golden Books, 1997.

- **The Shelter of Each Other: Rebuilding Our Families,**
  Mary Bray Pipher, Ph.D., Ballantine Books, 1997.

- **The Intentional Family,** *William J. Doherty, Ph.D.,*
  Addison-Wesley, 1997.

- **Reviving Ophelia: Saving the Selves of Adolescent Girls,**
  Mary Pipher, Ph.D., Ballantine Books, 1994.

DEATH/BEREAVEMENT ISSUES

- **How To Survive the Loss of a Parent,** *Lois F. Akner, C.S.W.*
  William Morrow, 1993.

- **Motherless Daughters**, *Hope Edelman*, Dell Publishing, 1994.

- **The Mourning Handbook**, *Helen Fitzgerald,*
  Simon and Schuster, 1994.

- **When Your Spouse Dies,** *Cathleen Curry,*
  Ave Maria Press, 1995.

- **Dying Well,** *Ira Byock, M.D.,* Riverhead Books, 1997.

- **The Worst Loss: How Families Heal From the Death of a
  Child,** *Barbara Rosof,* Henry Holt and Co., 1994.

LIFE CHANGES

- **Passages,** *Gail Sheehy,* Bantam Books, 1976.

- **New Passages,** *Gail Sheehy,* Ballantine Books, 1995.

MARRIAGE

- **His Needs, Her Needs: Building An Affair-Proof Marriage,** *Willard F. Harley, Jr.,* Fleming H. Revel, 1994.

- **A Good Marriage,** *Judith Wallerstein,* Warner Books, 1996.

- **Love, Honor and Negotiate,** *Betty Carter, MSW and Joan K. Peters,* Pocket Books, 1996.

- **Love is a Verb,** *Bill O'Hanlon and Pat Hudson,* W.W. Norton, 1995.

- **Love is Never Enough,** *Aaron T. Beck, M.D.,* HarperPerennial, 1988.

- **Adultery, The Forgiveable Sin,** *Bonnie Eaker Weil, Ph.D.,* Hastings House, 1994.

- **Fighting for Your Marriage,** *Howard Markman, Scott Stanley and Susan L. Blumberg,* Jossey Bass, 1994.

- **After the Affair,** *Janis Abrahms Spring, Ph.D.,* HarperCollins, 1996.

SEPARATION AND DIVORCE

- **The Single Again Handbook,** *Thomas Jones,* Thomas Nelson Publishers, 1993.

- **Marital Separation,** *Robert S. Weiss,* Basic Books, 1975.

- **Our Turn: Women Who Triumph in the Face of Divorce,** *Christopher L. Hayes, Ph.D., Deborah Anderson and Melinda Blau,* Pocket Books, 1993.

- **A Guide to Divorce Mediation,** *Gary J. Friedman, J.D.,* Workman Publishing, 1993.

- **Divorced Families,** *Constance R. Ahrons and Roy H. Rodgers,* W.W. Norton, 1987.

- **The Boys and Girls Book About Divorce,** *Richard A. Gardner, M.D.,* Bantam Books, 1970.

- **The Parents Book About Divorce,** *Richard A. Gardner, M.D.,* Bantam Books, 1970.

- **Second Chances: Men, Women, and Children A Decade After Divorce,** *Judith Wallerstein and Sandra Blakeselee,* Houghton Mifflin, 1990.

Organizations

- **Stress Release Health Enterprises**
  Shirley Babior, L.C.S.W.
  Center for Anxiety and Stress Treatment
  4225 Executive Square, Suite 1110
  La Jolla, CA 92037

Internet Resources

- **http://www.divorce-online.com/**
  Divorce Online provides free articles and information on the financial, legal, psychological, real-estate and other aspects of divorce. Additionally, you can turn to the professional referral section of Divorce Online to locate professional assistance near you.

- **http://www.psych.med.umich.edu/web/aacap/factsFam/grief.htm**
  This site helps adults understand better how a child views death and how you can help a child through a difficult experience.

- **http://www.psych.med.umich.edu/web/aacap/factsFam/ divorce.htm**
  This site explains how children experience divorce and gives ways to help them understand the changes occurring in their family.

CHAPTER THREE

NUTRITION AND WEIGHT LOSS

Eating & Moving for Life

Food is more than fuel for our bodies; it is nourishment for the soul. It is comfort, it is celebration, it is memory. At times – and for some women more than others – it is also the enemy. This chapter tells you what you need to know about this formidable friend and foe. You will learn what nutrients you need to be healthy and how to get them; you also will learn just what you have to do to lose weight and keep it off. In addition, you will learn how to recognize the signs of common eating disorders and what to do if you or someone you know is struggling with one.

A woman's focus on diet and nutrition probably starts during adolescence, when so many buy in to the myth of the perfect body. As we discuss in Chapter One "Adolescence," how much you weigh and how you look are largely determined by your genes. Another important point that bears repeating is that you are special for many reasons that have nothing to do with how much you weigh. Please read the "Adolescence" chapter regardless of your current age; it has some very important advice about how to value yourself.

Although your genes determine your body type to some degree, you should form your dietary habits based on an understanding of good nutrition. Your daily intake of nutrition in the form of food, liquids and

> " *I went on my first diet at about 15. I was overweight as a child. I got lots of teasing, people calling me fat.*"

supplements has an enormous effect on your lifetime well-being. Over-indulging occasionally can be fine, but habitual overeating (bringing in more calories than you need) increases your weight and dramatically increases your likelihood of developing cardiovascular disease, cancer, diabetes mellitus and osteoporosis. Twenty percent of women between the ages of 20 and 29 are overweight, and that percentage increases with age: More than half of women age 50 to 59 are overweight. You can calculate your ideal weight in pounds with the following formula:

100 + (4 x [height in inches - 60]).

If you are more than 20 percent over this weight, you should seri-ously evaluate your diet according to the information in this chapter. For help, consider consulting a dietitian to better understand your needs. If you have a large frame or are very muscular, you should adjust this ideal weight up by 10 to 20 percent.

" I've gained 20 pounds in the last year. I probably think about food all the time. My family and I grew up loving food."

How to Do the Calorie Countdown

Before we get into an overview of nu-trition, you first need an understanding of how we measure the energy stored within food. A **calorie** is that unit of en-ergy. When we consume calories as food, our bodies either use them as the fuel for body functions or store them as fat or muscle. Most Americans do not know how many calories they should take in during a day to meet their energy needs. Many of us consider ourselves to be on a low-calorie diet, but when we are asked how many calories we need to maintain our weight, we can only guess. Variations in your daily activities change your caloric needs. If you do nothing but rest all day, you require fewer calories to maintain your weight. To calculate your daily needs, perhaps it is best to begin with the caloric needs of the body at rest, add the caloric needs of daily activities and then add the caloric needs of activities related to fitness. Once you know this, increasing or decreasing this number of daily calories allows you to gain or lose weight as appropriate.

HOW TO CALCULATE
CALORIES NEEDED AT REST

The Harris-Benedict equation gives an approximation of calories needed per day just to maintain your weight. This equation calculates the daily calories needed for a person who is inactive and resting only. Activities such as computer work or aerobics are added to this total to find the calories that you need daily.

To figure the calories an average female **at total rest** requires to maintain energy needs, take 655 + (4.4 x weight in pounds) + (0.67 x height in inches) - (4.7 x age).

For example:

WEIGHT	HEIGHT	AGE	REQUIRED CALORIES
120 lbs.	66"(5'6")	40	1,039
135	66	40	1,105
150	66	40	1,171
180	66	40	1,303

This equation lets you compensate for being older or taller when finding your resting caloric needs. The same woman at the same weight requires about 200 fewer calories at age 85 than at 45. Basically, we know that most women need somewhere between 1,100 and 1,500 calories per day to sustain their bodies at rest.

Remember, the Harris-Benedict equation is for when you are at rest. If you take care of children, run a 10K race or even just work at your desk, you are burning calories beyond the resting calories calculated.

How Many Calories You Burn...

In a 30-Minute Period		In a 10-Minute Period	
Walking	165	Carpet Sweeping	32
Aerobic Stepping	360	General Cleaning/Dusting	40
Cycling (10mph)	150	Scrubbing Floors	73
Basketball	250	Painting Inside	23
Swimming	250	Painting Outdoors	52
Cross-Country Hiking	250	Raking	37

(Averages for 150-pound person)

HOW TO FIGURE EXERCISE INTO THE EQUATION

" I try to get regular exercise. I like walking rather than getting on the floor and doing all that strenuous stuff. I walk about four times a week."

We need exercise not only to maintain or lose weight but also to keep our bodies in good working condition. Moderate exercise has been shown to reduce the number of deaths from obesity, high blood pressure, diabetes and heart disease. Twelve percent of deaths in the United States may be due to diseases associated with the lack of exercise.

Currently, experts recommend that you accumulate 30 minutes of moderately intense physical activity every day or at least every other day. But we often become discouraged because we cannot set aside that block of time. The experts recommend that you walk a couple of miles, swim, golf, perform home repairs, or garden to accumulate your 30 minutes. Calorically speaking, more vigorous exercises burn more calories in the same time period than less vigorous exercise. Remember, when you increase the total energy you use in physical exercise, you reduce your risk of heart disease.

To get the maximum cardiovascular benefit, you should reach and sustain your target heart range for 20 minutes daily. To find your target heart rate, you may use this equation:

Target heart rate = (220 - age) x 75% to 85%.

SO WHAT SHOULD I EAT?

Now that you know how many calories you need to maintain your weight, you next need to know which foods should make up this ideal number. For the most part, experts agree that these calories should be made up of 50 percent carbohydrates, 30 percent fat and 20 percent protein. Each of these categories is necessary. For instance, an extremely low-fat diet may result in a scaly skin rash because of essential fatty-acid deficiency. Low-protein diets do not provide your body with enough energy, so your muscle tissue is broken down for energy. This results in your feeling weak and tired. Carbohydrates provide the bulk of your body's fuel. Limiting carbohydrates is a good way to reduce calories without affecting overall health. Food labels include information such as the percent of daily calories from fat, protein or carbohydrates and can help you plan your diet. It is easy to calculate calories by finding the grams of fat, carbohydrates or protein in a meal. To calculate calories of a serving:

> 1 gram fat = 9 calories
> 1 gram carbohydrate = 4 calories
> 1 gram protein = 4 calories

START WITH THE RDA

Malnutrition is rare in the United States and mostly seen in poor women of childbearing age. However, many women are deficient in protein and several essential vitamins. Below is a list of the recommended daily requirements for women. If you are pregnant or attempting to become pregnant or are breastfeeding, you should pay particular attention to the increased needs for protein, vitamin A, vitamin C and folic acid.

The chart on page 64 covers the important vitamins and minerals needed for a healthy diet. The best way to ensure that these vitamins are included in today's eat-on-the-run society is to combine supplementation and eating from the food pyramid (page 65). A balanced diet includes:

" I eat breakfast, toast. For lunch, leftovers. For dinner, it's usually a two-course meal, meat and vegetables or a vegetarian dinner with bread. Between meals, I eat candy, cookies, crackers, usually not anything terribly healthy."

> ♣ 6 to 11 servings of breads *(pastas, cereal, rice)*
> ♣ 2 to 4 fruit servings
> ♣ 3 to 5 servings of vegetables
> ♣ 2 to 3 servings of meat *(poultry, fish, beef and protein-rich meat alternatives like beans, eggs and nuts)*
> ♣ 2 to 3 servings of milk, yogurt and cheese and
> ♣ only sparing use of fats, oils and sweets

Vitamins and Minerals

	Age in Years				Physiologic Status		
Nutrient	15-18	19-24	25-50	51+	Pregnant	Lactating 1st 6 mo	Lactating 2nd 6 mo
Protein, g	44	46	50	50	60	65	62
Vitamin A, mcg	800	800	800	800	800	1,300	1,200
Vitamin D,mcg	10	10	5	5	10	10	10
Vitamin E, mg	8	8	8	8	10	12	11
Vitamin K, mcg	55	60	65	65	65	65	65
Vitamin C, mg	60	60	60	60	70	95	90
Thiamin, mg	1.1	1.1	1.1	1	1.5	1.6	1.6
Riboflavin, mg	1.3	1.3	1.3	1.2	1.6	1.8	1.7
Niacin, mg	15	15	15	13	17	20	20
Vitamin B6, mcg	1.5	1.6	1.6	1.6	2.2	2.1	2.1
Folate, mcg	180	180	180	180	400	280	260
Vitamin B12, mcg	2	2	2	2	2.2	2.6	2.6
Calcium, mg	1,200	1,200	800	800	1,200	1,200	1,200
Phosphorus, mg	1,200	1,200	800	800	1,200	1,200	1,200
Magnesium, mg	300	280	280	280	300	355	340
Iron, mg	15	15	15	10	30	15	15
Zinc, mg	12	12	12	12	15	19	16
Iodine, mcg	150	150	150	150	175	200	200
Selenium, mcg	50	55	55	55	65	75	75

Recommended Daily Dietary Allowances for Women, from the Food and Nutrition Board of the National Academy of Sciences/National Research Council.

(Key: g = grams; mcg = micrograms; mg = milligrams)

The labeling required on foods by the FDA gives you the number of servings and the percent daily requirements for a 2,000-calorie diet. The servings are smaller than you would think.

The typical American diet cannot supply a pregnant woman's increased need for iron, nor are your existing iron stores likely to be sufficient during this time; therefore, during pregnancy you should take a supplement of 30 to 60 mg of iron. You do not need the extra iron while breast-feeding, but it is advisable to continue taking the supplement for two to three months after your baby is born to replenish stores depleted by pregnancy.

THE FOOD PYRAMID

Fats, Oils & Sweets
USE SPARINGLY

KEY
☐ Fat (naturally occurring and added)
◩ Sugars (added)
These symbols show fats and added sugars in foods.

Milk, Yogurt &
Cheese Group
2-3 SERVINGS

Meat, Poultry, Fish, Dry Beans,
Eggs & Nuts Group
2-3 SERVINGS

Vegetable Group
3-5 SERVINGS

Fruit Group
2-4 SERVINGS

Bread, Cereal,
Rice & Pasta
Group
**6-11
SERVINGS**

The Food Pyramid, from the Department of Agriculture, Human Nutrition Information Service.

SUPPLEMENT TO FILL IN THE GAPS

Even if you follow the food pyramid, you probably do not get all of the nutrients you need. Most women are deficient in vitamins A and C, folic acid, iron and calcium. Deficiencies of these vitamins lead to serious health problems.

Vitamin A

Vitamin A is essential for proper vision and to have a healthy immune system. Any deficiency results in weakening of your immune system and increasingly poor vision. Too much vitamin A has serious consequences ranging from alopecia (hair loss) to liver damage.

Vitamin C

Your body cannot make vitamin C, so it must be provided in food. Vitamin C is necessary to maintain connective tissue, the tissue between your skin and muscles, and between your muscles and bone. With a deficiency of vitamin C, you also can develop scurvy, a condition where you have ulcers in your mouth and bleed into your skin. Scurvy was the condition sailors used to get when traveling over the ocean without fresh fruit.

Calcium

Calcium is found not only in milk products but also in sardines, salmon, and greens such as collards, kale, and turnip greens. Ninety-nine percent of the calcium in your body is found in your bones and teeth. The recommended daily intake of calcium for adults is 800 mg per day, with 1,200 mg per day recommended through age 24. If you are pregnant and lactating, you should get 1,200 to 1,500 mg per day. In addition to bone mineralization or strength, calcium also plays a role in your blood's ability to form clots and the normal activity of your glands and muscles.

Folic Acid

Folate, or folic acid, is present in many foods, including leafy vegetables, fruits, nuts and liver. Your body makes red blood cells with folate. Folate also lowers your risk of having a baby with a spinal-cord defect such as spina bifida, where there is an opening in the middle of the baby's spine.

Iron

Iron – found in meats, dried beans, liver, and peas – is used in the blood for oxygen delivery. Iron deficiency results in **anemia** (low blood count), and anemia makes you feel tired and have shortness of breath. Too much iron results in damage to your liver.

The average healthy woman obtains enough vitamins and minerals from her diet and vitamin supplementation. Care should be taken to avoid excessive use of vitamins and minerals, because they can cause harm. Pregnant women especially should avoid very high doses of over-the-counter vitamins. Too much vitamin A in early pregnancy can cause miscarriage or defects with the baby such as cleft palate (opening at the top of the mouth and lip) and heart abnormalities.

LOOK OUT FOR DEFICIENCIES

Factors that make you susceptible to nutritional problems include cigarette smoking, alcohol abuse, a strict vegetarian diet, chronic diseases and being elderly or an adolescent. Smokers need more vitamin C and zinc. Alcohol interferes with your body's uptake of vitamin A, thiamin, folic acid and zinc. If you have a chronic disease such as kidney disease, liver disease, heart disease or diabetes, you must make sure that you are getting enough food and energy. Often, liquid nutrition supplements such as Ensure or Boost are helpful in these situations. Teenagers and women up to 25 years old are building calcium stores that they will use later in life and need to add calcium supplements or additional milk sources to their diet. Vitamin D is also important in these years as it assists in calcium absorption. Vitamin D-enriched milk is a good source of both calcium and additional vitamin D. Supplementing calcium in postmenopausal women is just one way to prevent osteoporosis. Estrogen replacement therapy and weight training are also useful in this fight.

When the Condition is Constipation

If you have constipation, you can modify your diet to help get you to a normal routine of a bowel movement every day or two. You need to drink at least six to eight eight-ounce glasses of fluids per day. (Do not count alcoholic or caffeinated beverages toward this total.) You need to exercise by walking at least ½-mile per day. Eat fiber-rich foods, such as bran and whole grains (wheat, oats and rye). Include fruit, vegetables, beans, whole-grain cereals (such as oatmeal), pasta, nuts, popcorn and brown rice.

For a good natural recipe to be used if you have constipation, mix 1 cup of Miller's Bran, 1 cup of applesauce and ¼ cup of prune juice. Keep this in your refrigerator and replace it every week. Take 1 to 2 tablespoons daily for one week for best results. If needed, you may increase by 1 tablespoon per week. You may notice increased stool frequency, cramps and gas the first weeks, but this usually subsides after one month.

When You Want to Lose Weight
GET THE MEDICAL GO-AHEAD

The first step you should take in trying to lose weight is to visit your doctor and let him or her know that you are serious about wanting to lose weight. Your doctor will do a careful history and physical exam, and order a few labs to make sure you do not have a problem with your metabolism. If your thyroid gland is not working properly, you can diet all you want and still not lose weight.

GET MOVING

It is critical for you to understand that weight loss occurs when you take in the appropriate number of calories and also exercise regularly. We all know an obese person who does not eat very much. The problem is, this person has very little muscle mass. Muscle burns calories faster than fat, even when you are at rest. Therefore a muscular person loses more calories while sleeping at night than an obese person does. You must start an exercise program that provides a cardiovascular workout and also builds muscle mass.

GET TO KNOW YOUR WEAKNESSES

To get yourself into the right mindset to reduce your weight, take this quiz – and remember to be honest with yourself. Read the questions, observe yourself for a few days, then get your answers down on paper.

1. *At which meal or meals do I have the greatest appetite?*
2. *Do I frequently snack before or while preparing these meals?*
3. *What is my stress level at this time?*
4. *Do I eat sitting at the dining table?*
5. *Do I have second servings?*
6. *Do I clean my plate?*
7. *Do I consider food a reward?*
8. *Do I overeat on weekends or do I balance it with exercise?*
9. *What physical activities do I enjoy?*
10. *Who is responsible for my weight?*

Weight-loss programs are successful if you truly want more than anything to lose the weight. That means sacrificing; overcoming difficult situations; managing your stress, eating habits and relationships; and changing not only your body but changing your mind.

How to Set a Course for Change

KEEP A RECORD OF HOW MUCH YOU EAT

Your answers to the quiz give you the direction you need to change your habits. To further develop what you learned by taking the quiz, try keeping a food-and-exercise diary. This diary helps you to take stock of your current eating habits and optimize your diet. When everything is down on paper, you are forced to become honest with yourself about your daily food intake.

" My husband influences what I eat. I cook more meat and things for him. Children influence the way you cook, too, because they won't eat very many things."

Chart what you ate yesterday or the day before. Chart out last weekend. Be sure to write down every spoonful you can recall. Remember that only you will look at your pattern, so be honest. Estimate how much you ate and add up the calories. More than you thought? How much physical activity did you do on those days? Are weekends bad for you? How does your diet compare with the food pyramid? I know it is tedious, but take a look. How do your fat grams stack up? How about protein? It is very likely that you eat an adequate amount of breads and cereals, but not enough fruits, fresh vegetables, or protein. What about total calories? Add them up.

If you see that there are two or three times a day when you routinely snack, take a good look at what is happening. Is it crunch time with the kids, or is your work stress level at its highest? Perhaps you eat out of exhaustion or boredom. Identify your weaknesses, and teach yourself to react differently. Instead of reaching for food, walk to the other end of your building or your home or just stretch in place. If you really need a snack, reach for the low-fat granola bar instead of the potato chips or cake in the office kitchen. Limit yourself to eating at the table, not at the stove, spoon by spoon as you cook. Sit down, and always leave something on your plate; you are not in first grade anymore, and no one is watching to make sure you eat everything set

> " I eat some fruit and vegetables, not a lot. I like to eat candy, cookies, wine. I try to make healthy cookies, but no one eats them."

before you. Changing the way you think about food is the only way to change your body. You set the course.

WORK TOWARD A BALANCED LIFESTYLE

The best start is to get things back in balance. Beginning a diet and exercise diary gets you started. During this time, take multivitamins with iron to be sure you get enough calcium, vitamins A and C and folate. Allow yourself two small (4-ounce) servings of lean meat, eggs or poultry per day, providing only 30 percent of your calories from these food groups. Fruits, fresh vegetables and carbohydrates should make up the bulk of your diet. Watch for hidden fats in prepared foods, such as frozen dinners. Fruit, vegetable or carbohydrate snacks boost your energy and help you avoid binge-eating. If you normally have a snack just before a stressful time, train yourself to realize that you are feeling stress, not hunger. Hunger is managed with eating, while stress is managed by recognizing your sources of stress and learning to relax. Instead of snacking, walk away from temptation. If you do not exercise regularly, you may be surprised to discover that exercise can help you handle your stress while it burns calories and gives you something to do other than eating.

CALORIE COUNTING: DO THE MATH

Sooner or later, you will need to crunch some numbers in your quest to lose weight. To start, calculate your daily calorie intake and immediately reduce it by 10 to 20 percent. After a few weeks, calculate your resting caloric needs, using the Harris-Benedict equation you learned earlier in this chapter, and add in your activity level to see where you should be. If you want to lose weight, bring in fewer calories than needed for rest plus your activities. It is the only way to lose weight. Keep reducing your calories or increasing your activities to keep losing. It is easy to calculate calories by finding the grams of fat, carbohydrates or protein in a meal. Remember the following conversions:

1 gram fat = 9 calories
1 gram carbohydrate = 4 calories
1 gram protein = 4 calories

For example: If a serving is 10 grams of fat, 3 grams of protein and 5 grams of carbohydrate, this is 100 calories from fat, 12 calories from protein and 17 calories from carbohydrates, equaling a total of 129 calories. If you do not know the fat, protein or carbohydrate content of a serving, a simple pocket calorie-counter book found at the supermarket or bookstore can help for the most common foods.

WORK EXERCISE INTO YOUR SCHEDULE

Be patient and become a weekend warrior by getting most of the next week's exercise on the weekend, but watch that appetite. If you plan to exercise three times a week for one hour, get two of the workouts done on the weekend. It is much easier to squeeze one workout in during a busy work week than three. Plan ahead and make your exercise routine first on your list, not last.

DO NOT GO TOO FAR

If you cut your calories too much, you may end up defeating your purpose. Be careful not to go too far below your resting calorie needs or you will experience starvation syndrome. Starvation syndrome occurs when the body realizes it has too few calories to operate. The body reduces its metabolism or turns down its thermostat, so that it needs 25 to 35 percent fewer calories to survive. This makes weight loss more difficult. You should never go below 80 percent of the total of your basal needs plus the needs for your activity level. You can also

" Mealtime is pretty hectic. I work in the fast-food business, and I try to take to work what I eat for breakfast and lunch. I go to work at four in the morning, so by seven I'm eating. I try to take cereals and fruit a lot of the time, but when I get home I'm starving, so I eat whatever I can get my hands on."

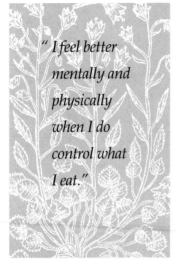

" I feel better
mentally and
physically
when I do
control what
I eat."

enter starvation syndrome if you are deficient in a particular vitamin or mineral.
So again, supplementing is recommended.

It is important to realize that women
are more likely to experience starvation
syndrome than men are. If you are dieting with a male partner, remember that
women are different and react differently
to this level of calorie-cutting. Men tend
to lose weight faster than women do,
mainly due to the larger muscle mass that
burns calories at a higher rate.

HANG IN THERE

There are no miracle cures or drugs to
solve the average American female's problems with her weight. You
have to be patient, keep good tabs on your eating habits, practice stress
management, exercise regularly and persevere. As a general rule, the
slower you lose the weight, the more likely you are to keep it off long-
term. Therefore, if your goal is to maintain a lower weight than you
currently are, you need to avoid weight-loss programs that offer quick
results and try to follow the instructions in this chapter. Try to limit
your caloric intake and walk ½ mile to 2 miles every day, and you will
lose all the weight you want. You do not need a treadmill, new clothes
or membership at a nice gym. If you have a treadmill, you should still
go outside for the walk. There is something special about getting
outside, listening to the wind and animals that is healthy both
physically and mentally. Simply go for your walks and in six
months you will be impressed with yourself. In one to two years,
you will be at the weight you want and stay there. Good luck
and enjoy yourself; you deserve it.

When You Have an Eating Disorder

There is a difference between wanting to lose weight and having an eating disorder. Most people at some time – or even most
times – want to lose a few pounds. The difference is that they do

not take measures to lose weight that are dangerous to their health. If you have an eating disorder, you are at significant risk of dying from the problem. You must take this problem seriously and let your family and physician know about it. If your doctor does not try to help you, find a new doctor.

The eating disorders **anorexia nervosa** (self-starvation) and **bulimia** (a disorder of binge-eating and then purging by vomiting or using laxatives) affect about 8 to 10 percent of the young female population. Unexplained weight loss or depression is usually the symptom that tips off a primary-care physician. But these disorders are complex and require an understanding of your physical, psychological and social situation so they can be appropriately diagnosed and treated. Anorexia and bulimia are now classified as psychiatric disorders, in contrast to obesity, which is classified as a physiological disorder.

ANOREXIA NERVOSA

Who Develops Anorexia?

Anorexia nervosa is a serious, sometimes fatal eating disorder where a person thinks she is fat when she is really painfully thin, and she deprives herself of food and develops rituals to control her appearance. Anorexia typically affects young, affluent, white females, although the same features are seen in other groups. Anorexia is seen in families where a heavy emphasis is placed on achievement and perfection. The child who later develops anorexia is often described as obedient, thoughtful and compliant – the "model child." This child is constantly seeking adult approval. She is rarely independent in her actions and does not display the typical rebellious attitudes of a teenager. It is not surprising that puberty is a distressing time for the child who becomes anorectic, with **menarche** (the start of menstruation), physical growth spurts, school activities and peer pressure encouraging separation and individuality from the family. When you have anorexia, you feel that eating is the one portion of life that you are able to control. You develop an image that you must be perfect to be worthy of love. The fear of becoming fat leads you to engage in a number of compulsive acts and rituals as you attempt to lose weight.

My Struggle With Anorexia

The diets would start off as counting calories, cutting back on calories and fat grams. Then it would snowball down to 500 calories a day. I knew the calories on every imaginable food. I wrote down anything that I ate, whether it was a slice of a banana or a cracker. I would write it down and tally it all up.

I was 30 when it happened. I had a lot of stresses in my life: my father had died, we had just moved – it was a major uprooting, moving from one city to another – and my husband was traveling a lot. What's important to understand about anorexia is that it's not a vanity thing, not about what you look like or what size clothes you wear, or getting compliments or getting attention. It's none of those things for me, at least. Everything else in my life seemed so out of control, and this eating was one thing I could control. It was definitely a control issue and a self-esteem issue.

I've always been a real perfectionist – always had to be best at this sport, really good at things at school – and I think for whatever reason I didn't feel good about myself. My body was something I could control, and a lot of times, I didn't feel worthy of having food.

I've had problems with depression and panic attacks. And that a lot of times goes hand-in-hand with eating disorders.

I did seek treatment; I ended up being hospitalized. Now I try to eat healthy three times a day. I was seeing a nutritionist for a long time and having to see my regular doctor to make sure everything was still stable, because anorexia could affect my heart or something like that. And I was in a support group for eating disorders once a week. I think it really did help. But now everything is fine with it. I found support with the group, my doctors and my family. It is difficult for my family to understand; they still say, 'Why?' 'What are you doing to yourself?' and all those things. Other people who have gone through it can understand it. That's why support groups are so important.

Now for breakfast I will have cereal, a glass of orange juice, a banana or some kind of fruit. Lunch, usually I will have some kind of sandwich, turkey and cheese or ham and cheese. I'll also have chips or potato salad or coleslaw, something on the side. Dinner – it depends; I cook for my little boy and my husband, chicken and two kinds of vegetables and potatoes. Basic dinner. I'm not at all into the calorie counting. I'm not counting at all anymore.

I get regular exercise, typically walking on the treadmill and doing some weights. For the most part, I like exercising. What I dislike is just getting motivated and actually going to do it. But once I'm doing it, I enjoy it. I exercise about three times a week.

I'm 33. I'm 5'7" and weigh 118 pounds. My ideal weight is where I'm at now, anywhere around 120 pounds. After that, I feel that my clothes are tight.

You must realize that it's not a vanity thing, and both women and men have problems with it. You do realize there's a problem, but you just put it in the back of your mind and you want it to end. You want it to stop, but you don't know how. And sometimes it takes something like a heart murmur and being so dehydrated and having nothing in you and having to be put in the intensive care unit to realize something is wrong.

How Anorexia Begins

The cultural ideal of the perfect woman's body has shifted in the last century away from plumpness, which represented wealth, to slimness, which represents assertiveness and success. Thinner women are seen as role models in the media, from television news personalities to actresses and beauty-pageant contestants. Social pressure from peers encourages teenagers to start dieting. These factors create an environment that pushes many young women toward anorexia.

No one is quite sure what the triggering mechanism for anorexia is. Suddenly, the idea of losing just 5 or 10 pounds does not seem like enough. Losing weight becomes an obsession. Then you begin starving yourself, often losing 60 to 80 pounds.

Biological factors make some women more susceptible to developing anorexia. Some researchers feel there may be a disorder of a portion of the brain called the hypothalamus, although this has never been proven. The hypothalamus controls body activities such as maintenance of water balance, regulation of body temperature, metabolism of food substrates and control of the secretions of other endocrine organs.

How to Recognize the Symptoms

When you have anorexia, you have an unusual preoccupation with food and may demonstrate bizarre food preferences. You truly struggle against hunger to achieve the weight loss you desire. You may prepare elaborate meals for friends, but eat little or nothing during the meals. You probably have a distorted view of how your body should look – the same weight that looks normal on a friend of your size makes you think you are grossly overweight when you look in the mirror. When you do lose weight, you feel that an emaciated state – often down to 70 or 80 pounds – looks about right. You may deny fatigue and hunger, and become obsessed with exercise, developing rigid training programs that burn many more calories than you consume.

With anorexia, you experience mood disturbances. It is not uncommon to be depressed and feel controlled by your environment. Your rigid personality leads you to view everything as either black or white.

Most of the physical symptoms of anorexia nervosa result from the starvation. You lose fat tissue, and your bones become more prominent. Your heart rate and body temperature may decrease. Your hair and nails may be brittle, and your skin may take on a yellow color. You may be unable to tolerate cold temperatures. You also may notice changes in your menstrual cycle or a lack of menstruation, infertility and a loss of sexual desire. Anorexia leads to such gastrointestinal complaints as bloating, constipation, nausea, vomiting and the feeling of fullness. Laboratory examination by a physician may reveal a decrease in your white blood-cell count, abnormal liver function tests, hypoglycemia (low blood sugar), low protein levels and low thyroid hormones.

How Anorexia is Treated

When you have anorexia nervosa, you need treatment by medical, psychiatric and nutritional experts.

Medical Treatment

Medical examination addresses any physical consequences of starvation, and evaluation by a gastrointestinal specialist investigates your many abdominal symptoms and rules out the possibility that other diseases are causing your weight loss.

Psychiatric Treatment

Individual psychotherapy can help you understand the disease and its effects. You need to develop a sense of autonomy and begin to take responsibility for your life and your treatment. You must grasp the reason you have fallen into a pattern of self-starvation. Psychotherapy revolves around your relationship with family and friends. If you have anorexia, your eating disorder is a major source of family stress. Psychotherapy encourages the family to work together for the well being of the anorectic individual and the family unit as a whole. Some behavior modification techniques may encourage short-term weight gain. In cases of severe depression, antidepressants are required. The success of treatment and the severity of symptoms may be assessed by using a scale known as EAT (Eating Attitudes Test).

Nutritional Treatment

Every woman with anorexia requires some dietary management. No matter what therapy is started, the most urgent concern is getting you to eat and gain weight. Mild weight loss (less than 15 percent of your original body weight) often responds to alterations in your eating patterns and choices. Moderate weight loss (15 to 30 percent of your weight) often requires the use of an oral nutritional supplement, such as Ensure or Boost. Severe malnutrition (30 percent or greater weight loss) may require hospitalization. If you are severely malnourished and are unwilling to eat, your treatment may require the use of a feeding tube into the stomach or the use of intravenous nutrition. Such treatment is described in a compelling way in Steven Levenkron's novel about a young woman's battle with anorexia, *The Best Little Girl in the World*. Rapid nutritional supplementation of the severely malnourished can have significant consequences, including heart failure and heart arrhythmias, and should only be done under the guidance of a physician and nutritionist.

How Likely Are You to Recover?

Treatment of anorexia takes patience. Short-term, you may respond to treatment with immediate weight gain. But immediate success does not always assure a permanent cure. Relapse is very common. Less than one-third of women who have anorexia regain a normal eating pattern. Therefore, you should continue therapy long-term. Six percent of women hospitalized for anorexia die, usually because of metabolic abnormalities (problems with the level of potassium or sodium in the blood). The best predictors of success with treatment relate not to immediate weight gain, but to the degree of social reintegration with family, friends and co-workers. In cases where no positive social relationship exists, the development of these relationships and this support system is the primary goal of therapy. If you are recovering from anorexia, please be sure to make the extra effort to integrate your friends and family into your daily activities. Make thinking about and talking with other people a major part of your routine.

WARNING SIGNS OF ANOREXIA

Watch for these warning signs in yourself, your children and your friends.

- ❧ *Refusal to maintain body weight*
- ❧ *Intense fear of gaining weight*
- ❧ *Sudden weight loss with no explanation*
- ❧ *Preoccupation with food and its consequences*
- ❧ *Undue preoccupation with body weight and shape*
- ❧ *Rigid exercise programs out of proportion to exercise needs*
- ❧ *Amenorrhea (lack of menstrual periods)*
- ❧ *Brittle hair and nails*
- ❧ *Unexplained, multiple gastrointestinal complaints*
- ❧ *Depression*

BULIMIA

Who Becomes Bulimic

Bulimia – derived from a Greek word meaning ox-eating – is manifested by episodes of overeating (bingeing) and then acts to undo the associated weight gain, such as self-induced vomiting, using laxatives and diuretics, fasting or driving yourself to extreme physical activity. Bulimia is almost exclusively a young woman's affliction. Bulimics can be underweight, overweight or normal weight, although overweight is more likely. Bulimics typically are extroverts who come from families where food and generous eating are a central part of every celebration.

How to Recognize the Symptoms

At the onset of bulimia, you make a conscious decision to diet. However, you lose control for forbidden foods and therefore have frequent episodes of binge-eating. Purging follows this binge-eating, setting up a binge-purge routine. Purging can be self-induced vomiting or use of laxatives. When you are bulimic, the social gratification you receive from eating is in direct contrast with your strong desire to be thin.

With bulimia, you binge and purge in secret – a pattern that accentuates feelings of frustration and isolation. You have no desire to discuss the problem with your physician. High-fat junk food is probably the food you are most likely to binge on. Later, the guilt of eating and associated nausea, headache or abdominal pain set up an episode of purging, generally with self-induced vomiting or laxatives. If you or a woman you care about frequently overeats and then wants to be alone after meals, you should watch for other warning signs of bulimia.

WARNING SIGNS OF BULIMIA

- 🐾 *Recurrent consumption of a large amount of food in a short period of time without weight gain*
- 🐾 *Lack of control of eating*
- 🐾 *Desire to be alone after eating*
- 🐾 *Undue attention to body weight and shape*
- 🐾 *Frequent use of cathartics or diuretics*
- 🐾 *Rigid exercise program out of proportion to exercise needs*
- 🐾 *Frequent vomiting spells without explanation*
- 🐾 *Multiple dental cavities and gum erosions*
- 🐾 *Frequent need for potassium supplementation*
- 🐾 *Depression*

What Somebody with Bulimia Looks Like

When you have bulimia, you generally look healthy. You may exhibit some antisocial activity, such as drug abuse or sexual promiscuity. You have a persistent concern with your body shape or weight. If you do go to see your physician, you probably do so because you have become depressed. Five percent of bulimics have attempted suicide prior to their diagnosis.

Still Bulimic 16 Years Later

Yes, I need to lose weight. I always try, but I am subservient to bulimia.

I didn't diet until I went away to college. I wanted to lose weight. No diet programs– nothing like that. I threw up, that's what I did.

I really wanted to be anorectic. I thought that was the hip thing to do. And I thought that if I starved myself, I would be skinny like everyone else. But I couldn't, so I punished myself by throwing up what I ate. At that time I didn't eat much more than a normal person would – maybe more junk food than I should have. Throwing up was hidden, so I would do it when I could. When I first started doing this, I was just out of high school and I had just graduated and it was summertime, and trying to teach myself to do this was really hard because it's not easy to make yourself throw up. I remember I was at my grandmother's house, and I would go into the bathroom and kind of hide and try. And then I wasn't really successful. It wasn't very easy. And then when I got home, I would wait until real late at night and try to throw up in the sink or in the bathroom or anywhere I could where nobody could hear it. Nobody knew at the beginning.

I am still bulimic. It's been going on for 16 years. I think my sisters suspected. I started between high school and college, and in college it really took off. When I was in college, I had the freedom to do what I wanted. I could hide in the bathroom stall, and nobody would ever know. And when I got home, I told my sisters. But they might have known before that.

I wanted to punish myself because I hated the way I looked and I wanted to lose weight.

I have been hospitalized twice. I have probably gone to eight or nine different psychologists, psychiatrists or nutritionists. Right now I have been seeing someone for a year. I have been on Prozac, and it didn't work. Support groups, I don't like, and I probably won't go again. I feel very uncomfortable there.

At my home, mealtimes are one big binge-fest. Not just mealtimes – anytime. My favorite food is peanut M&M's.

This is the part I want you to understand right now: my biggest hang-up with society and the way they look at eating disorders, is they tend to lump people into a category. 'They had a hard childhood' or 'they were beaten' or 'they had a weight issue' or something. And with me, even though some of those things still fit (I never had a bad childhood or anything like that, but weight was always an issue), it has changed so much from when I first started to now. Over the course of almost sixteen years, it has gone from one hideous stage to the next. I was last hospitalized six years ago, and I spent my own money to get over it, and that failed. I had decided at that time, "So be it. I am meant to live with this, and I have to get on with my life."

So I decided then if I had to throw up, I wasn't going to do it at work. It was too much for me to deal with. You know, I would put a little make-up on, but I would come back out of the bathroom looking like a wreck. So I couldn't do it anymore. So what I do now is I try. I always wake up in the morning thinking it's a new day and I'll try to have such-and-such for dinner and try to behave myself, but it doesn't work.

I try to have a muffin in the morning. However, my work time has changed and now I work from 9:30 to 6. So by the time I get to work, it's really too late to have breakfast, and I usually wind up having cookies or a bag of M&M's with peanuts. Lunchtime, if I have a friend to go out with, which is seldom, I may have a chicken salad. Otherwise, I will have a Coke, Icee or a Slurpee, a bag of M&M's, a box of animal crackers – anything junk food. Five years ago I could put away a pound of peanut M&M's a day because I could eat M&M's all day long and feel the need to binge and later on in the evening still throw it up. That is why I gained weight, because I would eat so much junk food during the day and only get to throw up at night. Plus my binges are huge now. I eat a lot at one sitting and take a long time.

I'm about 10 pounds away from my ideal weight. But I'm short. Ten pounds makes a difference in clothing for me. My clothing size is anywhere from 2 to 6. Most clothing I try to get in medium so I can wear most of it all the time. But now I'm in an up size, so everything feels tight.

I'm 33. I'm 5'1". I don't know how much I weigh; I don't step on scales anymore. I used to weigh myself 15, 20 times a day, but I don't go near them anymore. I think my weight is about 115 pounds. I think the ideal weight for me is 105 pounds. I don't count calories or fat grams. I don't have the control to worry about that. I used to exercise before, but now I don't have the time."

I get so offended by people, because we've been through hell with this. In fact a year ago, when I decided to get help it was because my husband had decided he couldn't take it anymore. It was driving him insane. Nothing has changed, but at least he is able to tolerate more now. I remember when we first told his mother or when she found out about it, the first thing she said was, "Just don't eat that much; quit eating. What's wrong with her? Why can't she do it?" But believe me, if I could I would.

And my psychologist right now is telling me that I'm doing better because I'm able to say no. I'm a real wimp because I do whatever anybody tells me. They love me at work because I work as many hours as they need me to, that sort of thing. I'm learning how to say no, and all that important stuff. What really has me stumped right now is, now that I can say no, and I have the ability to realize whatever I'm doing that makes that little trigger go off in me that makes me need to binge, why can't I stop it? I mean, I have to get better control of stuff. The only time I have ever been able to control it was when I was first in the hospital, both times for exactly a month. I lost weight there of course, about 20 pounds. I *just didn't eat anything. And when I went on vacation with my family – because there was so much going on, and we had so much fun, it was easy. And when they first put me on the Prozac, about 20 mg, it worked for about a week, and then it went back. And they increased it up to 80 mg and it wasn't doing anything. It was pointless for me to take it.*

I think the whole thing is very misunderstood. I would like to tell people why I can't do anything with them at night if they ask to go out, but I just have to say, "No, I can't." I would love to tell them that I have to go home and binge, but it's just not accepted. It's usually sneered at.

How Bulimia Affects the Body

There are many medical findings from bulimia. The salivary glands are enlarged, the teeth and gums may be eroded and the throat may be red and angry from the frequent episodes of vomiting. The knuckles may be bruised from rubbing against the teeth when trying to induce vomiting. Frequent vomiting may also cause extreme inflammation and irritation to the esophagus (esophagitis) and may cause vomiting of blood from tears in the lining of the esophagus during violent vomiting episodes (Mallory-Weiss tear). Frequent vomiting may also cause disturbances in blood electrolytes such as a low potassium or chloride level. These low electrolytes can cause symptoms of weakness, muscle cramping and even seizures. It may also result in abnormal heart rhythms. The frequent use of cathartics may cause damage to the colon, ultimately resulting in chronic constipation.

How Bulimia is Treated

The goal of treatment is to help you overcome your desire to overeat. You may be more willing to work with psychological treatments then someone with anorexia is.

There is a standardized questionnaire, known as the BITE

test (Bulimic Investigatory Test), that identifies whether you have bulimia, measures the severity of your symptoms and predicts the success of treatment. Behavioral techniques are frequently used for treatment and allow you to identify abnormal behavior and to eliminate it. Antidepressants are successful in decreasing the binge-eating. As with anorectics, developing a strong social structure allows you to have a solid support system that will encourage treatment success. Medical examination should also be performed to treat the physical consequences of frequent purging and to eliminate other disease, especially gastrointestinal disease, which may have caused or accentuated the frequent vomiting episodes.

What Should I Do?

Recognizing eating disorders requires the attention of your family, classmates, co-workers and medical personnel. These diseases are often ignored because of the difficulty and frustration in confronting an anorectic or bulimic. However, prompt treatment may not only reduce the physical and mental consequences of these diseases, but may also save your life.

If you think someone you know is bulimic, speak honestly to her about your concerns for her health. If she does not respond by seeking professional help, then talk to her parents, teachers, school counselors or physician.

Conclusion

Millions of copies of thousands of books are sold each year on the topic of weight loss. The popular press and media have added greatly to the fear of most American women that they are overweight by portraying the ideal figure as that of a twig. Our society is becoming progressively more superficial and trivial when we begin to think of our self-value in terms of pounds and inches. You are a special person because of who you are, not because you weigh a certain amount. We need to communicate to the media that we want them to stop holding the women of America hostage to this unrealistic weight expectation.

Use the information in the first part of this chapter to learn how to eat healthy and balanced meals. If you are more than 20 percent over your ideal weight, review the material about watching your calories and exercising regularly. While you do not need to be right at your ideal weight, you should try to avoid becoming obese due to the increased health risks.

If you or a friend has the characteristics of anorexia or bulimia, take this very seriously. These are not issues about diet and weight loss only. With these potentially fatal conditions, you must work with a health-care professional to get back on your way to enjoying life.

As with so many other things in life, our diet and exercise routines are never going to be perfect. We need to accept that we are human and stop mentally abusing ourselves. Work hard toward the goal of a proper diet and you will be impressed how often you succeed and how well you feel when you do.

Additional Resources
Books

- **The 1,200-Calorie-A-Day Menu Cookbook: Quick and Easy Recipes for Delicious Low-Fat Breakfasts, Lunches, Dinners, and Desserts,** *Nancy S. Hughes,* Contemporary Books, 1994.

- **1,001 Simple Ways to Lose Weight: Proven Tips for Losing Those Extra Pounds And Keeping Them Off,** *Gary L. Rempe,* Contemporary Books, 1997.

- **Aerobic Walking, the Weight-Loss Exercise: A Complete Program to Reduce Weight, Stress, and Hypertension,** *Mort Malkin,* John Wiley & Sons, 1995.

- **Anorexia & Bulimia: Your Questions Answered** *(Element Guide Series), Julia Buckroyd,* Element, 1996.

- **Anorexia Nervosa: A Survival Guide for Families, Friends and Sufferers,** *Janet Treasure,* Psychology Press, 1997.

- **The Deadly Diet: Recovering from Anorexia and Bulimia,** *Terrence J. Sandbeck, Ph.D.,* New Harbinger Publishers, 1993.

- **The Best Little Girl in the World,** *Steven Levenkron,* Contemporary Books, 1978 *(an eye-opening young-adult novel about anorexia by a psychotherapist who specializes in treating anorexia).*

Organizations

- **American Anorexia/Bulimia Society**
  293 Central Park West, Suite 1R
  New York, NY 10024
  (212) 501-8351

- **National Eating Disorders Organization**
  445 E. Greenville Rd.
  Washington, Ohio 43085
  (614) 436-1112
  (918) 481-4044

- **The Eating Disorders Association Resource Center**
  131 Leichhardt St, Suite 19, Level 4
  Spring Hill
  Brisbane QLD 4000
  Australia
  (07) 38316900

- **Eating Disorders Awareness and Prevention, Inc. (EDAP)**
  603 Stewart St, Suite 803
  Seattle, WA 98101
  (206) 382-3587

- **Overeaters Anonymous**
  6075 Zenith Ct. NE
  Rio Rancho, NM 87124
  (505) 891-4320

Internet Sites

- **http://vm.cfsan.fda.gov/~label.html**
  *This site gives the most up-to-date dietary guidelines released by the
  U.S. Food and Drug Administration's Center for Food Safety and
  Applied Nutrition. This is a very detailed and informative site that you
  should take the time to read. It helps the dieter understand food labels,
  how to lose weight safely and much more.*

- **http://www.cspinet.org**
  *This site, sponsored by the Center for Science in the Public Interest,
  offers articles from its popular Nutrition Action Health letter, a "Rate
  Your Diet" quiz, and links to other health and nutrition sites.*

CHAPTER FOUR

CONTRACEPTION

Selecting the Method For You

The phrase "there's a time and a place for everything" may have been developed to address how we all feel about pregnancy. While you probably want to be pregnant at some point in your life, there are many times you definitely do not. You may never want to be pregnant. The times to avoid pregnancy may include while you are dating a boyfriend, early on in a marriage, while you are completing your education or getting established in your career, when you have just had a child, or when you have completed your family and do not want any more children. These are all personal decisions, but you may fit into one or all of the above situations at some point in your life. Your choice for contraception could be different in each of these scenarios, so read this chapter carefully. With a thorough understanding of your options, you can find a birth control method that is best for you.

There are many forms of birth control available, with options for both men and women. Each form of contraception has its own risks and benefits. Choosing the right method for you involves many different factors. These factors include how effective the method is, how hard it is to use, other medical problems you have, whether you smoke, how old you are and how often you have sex. I will add to this list, the need to protect yourself from sexually transmitted diseases like AIDS.

There are many choices, and there is no one perfect option. What may work great for one person may be a miserable failure for another. You may have to try several methods to find the one that suits you and your partner the best.

How Pregnancy Occurs

So that you can understand how all the various forms of birth control work, let us first review how pregnancy occurs. Most young women begin having menstrual periods for the first time around the age of 11 or 12. Older women stop having periods when they go through menopause at around age 50. During the time in between (roughly age 11 through age 50), you are considered fertile – at risk for getting pregnant if you have unprotected intercourse. Most women have their periods once a month. The average time between the beginning of one period and the beginning of the next period is 28 days. This can vary from person to person by several days.

Your reproductive organs include the ovaries, fallopian tubes, uterus and vagina. The ovaries are responsible for producing an egg each month, with one egg made from either your right or left ovary each menstrual cycle. Which ovary produces the egg varies each month. The egg is released in a process called ovulation. This typically occurs in the middle of the cycle, between periods. The egg is then picked up by the fallopian tube and over a period of several days travels down the fallopian tube to the uterus, where the baby grows through the nine months of pregnancy from an embryo to a fetus. Fertilization – the joining of the egg and sperm – occurs in the fallopian tube. If the egg is not fertilized it is reabsorbed and disappears. Also, unless fertilization occurs, a menstrual period begins 14 days after ovulation. This 14-day interval occurs in almost every woman whether her periods are 26 days apart or 36 days apart. While the time from the start of your last period to ovulation is variable, the time from ovulation to the next period is set at 14 days.

When you have intercourse with a fertile man, during ejaculation sperm are deposited at the top of your vagina. The sperm swim into the uterus and out into the fallopian tubes. Studies have shown that sperm can get up into the fallopian tubes within minutes of being released. If an egg is present in the tube at this time, fertilization may occur. Sperm remain alive for three days after being released, and the egg survives for one day after ovulation. If fertilization occurs, egg and sperm form an embryo. The embryo grows and develops while in the fallopian tube for the first few days. The embryo is transported down into the uterus where it can then implant and grow. (If the embryo is stuck in the fallopian tube, an ectopic pregnancy occurs.) All the different methods of birth control stop or disrupt this process in some way.

What Are My Options?

The many different kinds of birth-control options can be placed into one of a few categories. After this overview, we will discuss each one in detail.

One option is **no contraception** at all. The chance of getting pregnant increases with younger age and decreases as you get older, especially after age forty. The chance also increases as the frequency of intercourse increases. On average, 85 percent of women having intercourse unprotected by birth control become pregnant within a year. It is a myth you cannot get pregnant if you do not have an orgasm!

There are **"barrier" methods** of contraception, where a physical barrier of some sort is placed between you and your partner to prevent the joining of sperm and egg. This category includes the male condom (rubber), the diaphragm, the cervical cap, and the new "female condom," the Reality. The IUD also falls into this category because in effect it blocks the egg and sperm from reaching each other.

There are **"hormonal" methods**, where your hormones are changed in order to prevent ovulation from occurring or to prevent the fertilized egg from implanting inside the uterus. These methods include the "pill," Norplant and Depo-Provera.

There are **"chemical" methods**, where a chemical substance is used to kill sperm or prevent fertilization. These chemical methods are commonly combined with a barrier method to increase their effectiveness. The chemical methods include spermicidal gels, creams and suppositories.

There are also **"social" methods** that include various actions that a couple may choose to take. These include some of the least effective as well as most effective forms of birth control. This category includes the withdrawal method and periodic abstinence, as well as total abstinence.

All of the above methods are considered reversible, in that the method can be discontinued when you desire to start trying to conceive. **Sterilization procedures** also are performed on both men and women. Sterilization methods are meant to be permanent and irreversible, and you should consider them only if you are certain you do not want any more children.

Social Methods of Birth Control
ABSTINENCE — JUST SAY "NO"

There is no better, safer way to prevent pregnancy than not having sex to begin with. It is easier to not start having intercourse than to start and then stop. You should never feel pressured into having sex with anyone at any time. It is never too late to say "No" or "Stop." You must realize that when you start having intercourse many other parts of your life become more complicated: your relationships with your partner, family and friends; your work (school or professional); and also how you feel about yourself. For a teenager, abstinence is wise because it allows you to mature physically and emotionally, without the complicating factor of a sexual relationship and its inherent risks, which include pregnancy and diseases. Once you are out of your teenage years, perhaps you feel ready for the complexity that sexual activity brings to a relationship, and you know you are no longer at risk for "teen pregnancy." There are still other benefits of abstinence that you may want to consider, as each person's situation is unique.

Try to avoid putting yourself in a situation that may lead to unwanted sex. Stay in groups with your friends, avoiding isolated areas even for a short time. If you find yourself in a situation that is getting "out of hand," get up and leave. Make your intentions and limits clear to your partner early on in a relationship. Say "No" when these limits are exceeded, and make it clear that if your partner persists you consider it rape. Remember that sexual intercourse is an act between two consenting adults. Make sure you give consent and plan accordingly.

By not having sex until you are prepared both physically and emotionally, you decrease your risk of unwanted pregnancy, sexually transmitted diseases, infertility and pelvic pain. Also, there is the issue of respect that must be considered when having intercourse – both your self-respect and your partner's respect for you. If you have intercourse freely, your partner is unable to respect you, because you have shown you do not respect yourself.

WITHDRAWAL

What Is It and How Does It Work?

"Withdrawal" is the oldest method of birth control. The idea is simple, but in practice it is difficult to perform. During intercourse, before your partner ejaculates, he removes his penis from your vagina. You then use masturbation or oral sex to accomplish orgasm. Timing is important with this technique to prevent spillage of sperm into the vagina. A small amount of sperm leaks from the penis before a full orgasm is reached, making pregnancy possible.

How Effective Is It?

The failure rate of this method is 20 percent, meaning one out of five couples using this method of contraception becomes pregnant each year. The failure rate is higher in younger couples than in older, more established couples, probably because in more established relationships both partners understand and have communicated the importance of withdrawing well before ejaculation occurs.

" A friend of mine who uses the withdrawal method says it works. Of course, she also conceived three children using it."

Who Should Use It?

Withdrawal is an excellent form of contraception if you are not actively trying to become pregnant, but would find pregnancy wonderful if it occurred.

Contraception: Selecting the Method for You

What Are Its Advantages and Disadvantages?

An advantage of the withdrawal method is that it can be used anytime and anywhere with no devices needed and no expense involved. Many couples do not like this technique, however, because intercourse is interrupted. The withdrawal method also does not protect against sexually transmitted diseases like AIDS, herpes, gonorrhea or chlamydia.

METHODS BASED ON PERIODIC ABSTINENCE

The rhythm method, the Billings method and the sympto-thermal method are all types of periodic abstinence. These "natural family planning" methods are among the oldest forms of birth control and still are widely used. They have varying degrees of success depending on the motivation of the couple. The idea behind this type of birth control is to avoid having unprotected intercourse during the time of your cycle when the egg is available for fertilization.

The Rhythm Method

The rhythm method involves avoiding intercourse in the middle of your cycle when the egg is released. In order for this method of birth control to be effective, you must have regular and predictable periods. If your periods are regular and predictable, the time of ovulation is 14 days before your period is predicted to start. For example, if you have a period every 30 days, you ovulate on the 16th day of the cycle, with day one being the first day of your menstrual bleeding. You avoid intercourse from five days before ovulation until four days after. This is because sperm survive in your cervical mucus for three days after intercourse. You may be able to tell when you ovulate by feeling a slight twinge of pain or pressure in your lower abdomen near this time. Unfortunately, the variation in normal cycles makes using this method unreliable. The rhythm method has a 20-percent failure rate and should also only be used by couples who would not mind if pregnancy occurred.

The Billings Method and the Sympto-Thermal Method

The Billings Method and the sympto-thermal method add another predictor of ovulation in addition to the timing issues discussed above with the rhythm method. Beginning four to five days before ovulation, the glands on the cervix produce more and more watery mucus. In both the Billings and sympto-thermal methods, you are taught to recognize this increase in vaginal moisture. The amount of this thin, watery mucus increases each day up until ovulation. At the time of ovulation, this mucus suddenly thickens and forms a "plug" in the cervix. Progesterone, produced by the ovary at ovulation, causes the cervical mucus to thicken. Prior to ovulation, a minimal amount of progesterone is produced; the cervical mucus is thin and watery, and sperm can easily swim through it on their journey to an egg. Once the cervical mucus plug forms after ovulation, sperm difficulty penetrating the cervical canal to get into the uterus and tubes. Remember the egg only stays alive for 24 hours once released. Therefore, if you can tell by the timing within your menstrual cycle, plus notice changes with your cervical mucus to tell when you are ovulating, you can avoid unprotected intercourse at this time. The sympto-thermal method adds another factor, the use of the basal body temperature to show when ovulation has occurred. You take your temperature, with a special thermometer each morning upon waking before you get out of bed and chart the results, which you can learn to interpret. Studies by the World Health Organization show that this form of birth control is effective if properly taught and followed, with a failure rate of 20 percent per year.

Certain religions that do not believe in artificial forms of birth control do allow and teach this method. The Catholic Church is one source of information, and most parishes have at least one couple who helps teach this method to new members and newlyweds.

Advantages of this form of birth control include that it is cheap and has no known side effects. A disadvantage is that it is not as effective as other options. If pregnancy would be dangerous to your health, you should consider other options. Also, this method does not offer protection from sexually transmitted infections.

Hormonal Methods of Birth Control
THE "PILL"

What Is It?

The birth-control pill is an oral contraceptive – one you take by mouth. This method of birth control is by far the most commonly used. The "pill" is actually a combination of two different female hormones, estrogen and progesterone. More than 25 different combinations are available, and several different manufacturers produce them. Your heath-care provider can help you select one that should work well for you. No one pill is ideal for everyone. There are so many different ones because each person is different; while one pill may have no side effects and be great for you, it may not agree with someone else. Some women need to try a few different ones before finding one without significant side effects.

How Does It Work?

The pills work by preventing ovulation – the release of an egg from the ovary. They also make the lining of the uterus thinner, making implantation difficult if conception occurs, and the cervical mucus thicker, which prevents sperm from getting up into the fallopian tubes.

The pills must be taken in a specific order to be effective. A typical pack has 28 pills, both active pills that have hormones in them as well as other pills that have no hormones in them. With a 28-day pill pack, you take a hormonally active pill once a day for three weeks and an inactive pill every day for a week (except with Micronor, where all 28 pills are active). The pills without the hormones are used as a reminder to help keep the specific order going. Your menstrual period usually occurs during the week these inactive pills are taken.

There also are packs with only 21 pills in them. The hormonally active pills are the same, but the 21-day pill packs do not have inactive pills. Most women who have been on the pills a long time can remember to start a new pack after a period and therefore do not take the inactive pills. If you have never taken birth-control pills before, most health-care providers usually prescribe a 28-day pill pack to make sure you get into the habit of taking a pill every day.

How Effective Is This Method?

If taken correctly, oral contraceptives are 96-percent effective. The effectiveness decreases if pills are missed. There are also medications that interfere with the effectiveness of the pills, so ask your health-care provider if you need to use a backup method of birth control if you are started on a new medication. Even some common antibiotics interfere with the birth-control pill. As a general rule, if you are not sure what to do, do not take chances and use a backup method, such as condoms.

" I used the pill. That was my choice so I wouldn't get pregnant, but I also did it so I would have regular periods."

How Do I Use It?

The pills are started in one of two ways, depending on the manufacturer. Most pills are started the Sunday after a period starts. If your period starts on a Wednesday, four days later you start your pills. If you start your pills in this fashion, use a backup method of birth control (foam and condoms) for the first month. The birth-control pills do not prevent ovulation that first cycle. After the first cycle they are effective. The advantage of starting the pills the Sunday after your period is that you start your pills at the beginning of a new week, and most women find this easier to remember than in the middle of a busy week. Also, if you start on a Sunday, you have your period during the middle of the week and not on the weekends. The other way of starting the pills is to start them the day your period begins. With this method, if your period starts on a Wednesday, you would start your pills that day. The advantage of this method is that you do not need to use a backup method of birth control that first cycle.

Most health-care providers recommend you take the pill around the same time each day. Try to link taking the pill to some other daily activity, such as brushing your teeth, waking up or going to bed. Most women seem to have fewer side effects if they take the pill before they go to bed. One trick is to put your toothbrush on top of your pill pack as a reminder. Another is to put a "P" on your mirror in the bathroom.

What Happens If I Forget?

Most women on birth-control pills remember to take them regularly, but nobody is perfect. Occasionally you may forget to take your pill. Which pill you forget to take and when you remember to take it affect what you should do next. If you are ever in doubt, keep taking your pills but use a backup method of birth control until you start a new pack. If you miss one of the inactive pills in the pack, you do not need to use a backup method of birth control. If you miss an "active" pill at night but remember to take it first thing in the morning, you are still protected. If you are late in taking your pill you may experience some spotting. If you forget the pill for 24 hours, you should take the pill, you forgot as well as your scheduled pill, that day – two pills in one day. Most drug companies state that you should still be protected; however, I suggest you use a backup method of birth control for the next week just to be sure. If you miss two pills in a row, take two pills a day until you are back on schedule, but use a backup method of birth control the rest of the cycle until you start a new pack of pills. If you miss three or more pills in a row, stop that pack and start with a new one the next Sunday. Use a backup method of birth control until you have been on the new pack for a full month. If you keep missing pills, you need to discuss other options of birth control with your health-care provider.

> " The pill was the most popular thing, but it didn't work for me because I had problems remembering to take it. "

What Are the Advantages of This Method?

The pill has become the most popular form of birth control because it is so effective and easy to take. When you are in the mood to make love with your partner, you do not have to stop and use a barrier method. The pill also tends to make periods lighter and decrease the amount of cramping that occurs. If fact, many women are on pills because they feel better on them.

What Are the Side Effects?

There are side effects that can occur with the pill. Most of these are not serious and tend to go away the longer you use the pills. Common problems include bleeding in the middle of the cycle (breakthrough bleeding), which occurs in about 30 percent of women who start on the pill. This bleeding may be spotting, or like a period. It should resolve on its own within three cycles. If it persists, speak with your provider about changing the type of pill you are on.

Other common side effects include nausea and breast tenderness. Again, these tend to resolve after a month or two of pill use. Other changes that can occur include missed periods, headaches, hair loss, and weight changes. Women are very concerned about the possibility of weight gain on the pills. With the new low-dose pills, very little change in weight occurs. About one-third of women gain a small amount of weight, one-third stay the same weight and one-third lose weight. Most studies show the average weight gain is no more then five pounds.

Fluid retention and an increase in blood pressure can occur. Also, you may have problems with using contact lenses. Some women also notice a pigmentation change on their faces that may persist even once the pills are stopped. If you have any of these problems, discuss them with your health-care provider. Most providers make an appointment to see you back a few months after you start on the pills to check your blood pressure and discuss any side effects.

There are serious side effects that can occur with the pills, including stroke and heart attack, which can lead to permanent disability or death. These are very rare. The chance of a serious side effect increases as you get older or if you have other health problems, such as high blood pressure or diabetes, or if you are a smoker. Most healthcare providers take a careful history and discuss your risks with the pills. If you are a smoker and over age 35, you are not a candidate for using the birth-control pill. Pill use is also associated with an increased risk of gallbladder stones and liver tumors. The liver tumors are benign (not cancerous), but they can rupture and cause death from internal bleeding. Luckily these tumors are very rare. If you are a non-smoker and in good health, your chance of death from using birth control pills is less then the chance of death due to a pregnancy. An advantage of the pills is that they decrease the risk of ovarian tumors, anemia and abnormal bleeding.

Who Should Not Take the Pill?

In addition to smokers over 35, some other people should not take birth-control pills at all. This group includes women who might be pregnant. If there is any chance you might be pregnant, check a pregnancy test and contact your health-care provider for instructions. Also, you should not take pills if you have ever had a stroke or heart attack, or if you have a history of blood clots in the legs, lungs or eyes. You also should not use pills if you have a history of liver disease or tumors.

What Else Should I Know?

There is still debate as to whether or not pills increase the risk of various cancers. Most studies have not shown an increased risk of developing breast cancer or cervical cancer due to the pills. There are several studies that have shown a decreased risk of ovarian cancer and cancer of the uterus.

While birth-control pills do a wonderful job in preventing pregnancy, they offer no protection from sexually transmitted diseases. It is important to remember you should use the pills only to prevent pregnancy and add condoms to help prevent sexually transmitted diseases like AIDS, hepatitis, herpes, gonorrhea and chlamydia. AIDS and hepatitis are life-threatening illnesses, and pelvic infections due to gonorrhea and chlamydia can cause permanent damage to the fallopian tubes, leading to infertility. (You can read more about these conditions in Chapter Six, "Pelvic Infections and STDs.")

Most birth-control pills cost about $20 to $30 per pack, and some are covered under prescription plans. There are also some generic pills available that cost about half as much.

THE "MINI-PILL"

What Is It?

The "mini-pill" is an oral contraceptive that only has one hormone (progesterone) instead of the two (estrogen and progesterone) normally found in birth-control pills. Micronor and Nor-Q-Day are common ones prescribed. The mini-pill is very effective when taken correctly, and the side effects and contraindications are similar to those for regular pills.

CONTRAINDICATION

A situation where a certain drug or treatment would not be appropriate; a reason you should not use a certain drug or treatment.

When Should I Use the Mini-Pill?

Because there is no estrogen in the mini-pill, it is used when estrogen is contraindicated. One of the most common times when estrogen is not appropriate is during breast-feeding. Estrogen in regular birth-control pills decreases breast-milk production, and birth-control pills containing estrogen should not be used during breast-feeding. Since the mini-pill has no estrogen, it can be used safely during breast-feeding.

How Do I Use This Method?

You take the mini-pill differently than regular birth-control pills. You take a mini-pill every day, and every pill is hormonally active. There is no "week off." Expect not to have a period while breast-feeding and using this pill. Once you stop breast-feeding, the mini-pill causes irregular or continuous bleeding. Therefore, once you stop breast-feeding, most health-care providers switch you to regular pills. Of course this is not mandatory, and you may elect to continue on the mini-pill alone.

Which Pill Is Best For Me?

As we discussed at the beginning of this chapter, finding the best pill for you may require trying several different ones. However, there are times when you can start with certain pills based on your needs. If you are a smoker under the age of 35, or a non-smoker over the age of 35, you should be on a pill with very low estrogen. Two excellent options are Alesse and Loestrin. If you have concerns about weight gain, acne or hair loss, the pill Desogen is ideal. If cost is a major concern, the pill Ortho-Novum 1/35 is available as a generic and is much less expensive.

DEPO-PROVERA

What Is It?

The Depo-Provera injection is one of the most effective types of reversible contraceptives available. You get this progesterone hormone shot every 12 weeks in the upper arm or buttocks. You go in for the first shot during the first few days of a menstrual cycle to ensure you do not receive Depo-Provera while pregnant. The cost per shot is about the same as a three-month supply of pills.

After the first shot, you should use condoms for the first month, but after each subsequent shot you do not need to do this. When you get the shot on schedule every three months, Depo-Provera is 99-percent effective. If you are more than two weeks late for your injection, you are not protected from getting pregnant. In this situation, get the injection and use condoms for the next month. The great advantage of this method is that you only need to remember to come in for a shot once every three months – four times a year. It does not require you to do anything at the time of intercourse, unlike the condom and diaphragm.

How Does It Work?

Depo-Provera works similar to birth-control pills by preventing ovulation, thickening the cervical mucus and thinning the lining of the uterus.

Who Can Use It?

Almost anybody can use Depo-Provera. Women who cannot take estrogen use it. It is ideal if you are breast-feeding; however, it is usually started at six weeks postpartum.

The best candidate for Depo-Provera is a young woman who is unable to remember to take a birth-control pill every day or is not assertive enough to demand that her partner use a condom every time they have intercourse. If you have had one or more unwanted pregnancies, I strongly encourage you to consider this form of contraception. While there are some side effects with Depo-Provera, you must compare them to the emotional pain and suffering you experience from an abortion or unplanned pregnancy. I have cared for many women over the years and have seen too many go through tremendous pain after deciding to have an abortion. Please avoid this difficult decision by using the best type of birth control for you. If you have a hard time remembering to use a pill every day or do not feel strong enough to insist on the use of condoms, Depo-Provera is right for you.

Who Should Not Use It?

You should not use Depo-Provera if you might be pregnant, or if you have abnormal bleeding without a known reason. You also should not use it if you have had a stroke, heart attack, breast cancer or blood clots in the legs. Similar to birth-control pills, Depo-Provera is not recommended if you have a history of liver disease.

What Are the Side Effects?

There are side effects to Depo-Provera. The most common is a change in the menstrual period. Most women experience a change in their periods. You should expect to have irregular bleeding for the first three to six months after starting on Depo-Provera injections.

Within those six months, most women stop having periods, which is one of the benefits for women with painful periods. This method of birth control is ideal if you have uterine fibroids, endometriosis, painful periods or pain with intercourse. With each of these problems, estrogen is felt to be the stimulant of pain. When you take Depo-Provera, there is much less estrogen in your system compared with a normal cycle or with birth-control pills.

> " *I didn't want to have to remember about taking anything, so I went with the Depo-Provera shot every three months."*

Other side effects you may have include headaches, bloating, depression, irritability and weight gain. You do not gain more weight if you do not eat more food, but this medication may make you want to eat more. Therefore, if you use Depo-Provera, make sure you do not increase your food intake and try to get regular exercise. If you are prone to these problems, discuss them with your provider before starting on Depo-Provera. You may also notice a decrease in your sex drive and occasional hot flashes. All these side effects are reversible and go away if no more shots are given. It can take up to 12 months to have your periods return to normal from the time of your last shot. I suggest you stop taking the shots six months before you plan to start trying to get pregnant. Prior use of Depo-Provera does not interfere with your ability to be pregnant; there is no increased risk of infertility.

What Else Should I Know?

Other considerations in deciding to use Depo-Provera include that some studies that suggest a very slight increase risk of bone loss, which could lead to bone fractures later in life. There does not appear to be an increased risk overall of breast, ovarian, uterine or cervical cancer. Similar to birth-control pills, Depo-Provera may decrease the risk of uterine cancer and ovarian cysts.

Lastly, Depo-Provera is not effective in preventing the spread of sexually transmitted diseases like AIDS, gonorrhea and chlamydia. You should always think about preventing the risk of these infections with the use of condoms.

NORPLANT

What Is It?

The Norplant system is a relatively new, reversible method of birth control. It is also highly effective, with a failure rate of less than 1 percent. Six small capsules, each about an inch long, are inserted under the skin on the inside of your arm. Once in place, these capsules provide continuous protection from pregnancy for five years. After five years, they need to be replaced. The old capsules need to be removed and new ones inserted. The capsules are made of Silastic (a soft silicone rubber material). Each one is filled with a hormone called **levonorgestrel**. Levonorgestrel is a progesterone commonly used in birth-control pills. The progesterone is slowly released in tiny amounts from the capsules over five years.

How Does It Work?

Norplant works in a fashion similar to Depo-Provera and birth-control pills: It prevents ovulation, thickens the cervical mucus and thins the lining of the uterus.

How Is It Inserted?

The capsules are placed in your arm at your doctor's office or clinic. A local anesthetic such as lidocaine is used to numb the area before the implants are inserted. Once the lidocaine is placed under your skin, the procedure is painless. The capsules are placed in a fanned-out arrangement just under the skin. You can feel them under your skin, but they are painless once in place.

What Are The Risks?

The risks of insertion include infection, bleeding, damage to a nerve in the arm, bruising and pain. Infection around the site of insertion is possible, but your provider uses a sterile technique to avoid this problem. A moderate amount of bruising occurs, and to minimize this your arm is wrapped tightly over the implants for 24 hours. Serious side effects from insertion, such as nerve damage or serious bleeding, are rare.

Who Should Use This Method?

Norplant is a good option for women who are looking for a long-term contraceptive that is highly effective. It is particularly good for women who cannot remember to take a pill regularly. It is safe to use while breast-feeding.

Who Should Not Use It?

You should not use Norplant if you have a history of liver tumors, breast cancer or blood clots in your legs, lungs or eyes. It should not be placed if you might be pregnant or if you have abnormal, unexplained bleeding. These contraindications are similar to those for other hormonal methods of birth control. Specific for Norplant, however, the capsules should not be placed if you have a history of increased intracranial pressure (a rare condition known as pseudotumor cerebri).

What Are the Side Effects?

Most women with the Norplant system do very well without serious side effects. Common problems include abnormal spotting and bleeding or no periods at all. These menstrual abnormalities tend to resolve on their own over six months to a year. Other common complaints include headaches, dizziness and nausea.

What About Removal?

The Norplant capsules are removed at the end of five years, or anytime you want to start trying to get pregnant. After removal of the capsules, the effects disappear within a few weeks, and pregnancy can occur soon thereafter.

The biggest problem to date with the capsules is the difficulty in removal. After several years, the capsules are scarred in and sometimes are difficult to remove. Prior to removal, the skin around the end of the capsules is injected with a local anesthetic like lidocaine. A ½-inch incision is made, and the capsules are removed one at a time. Sometimes the capsules may move under the skin with time, and a second or third incision is needed to remove them all.

You may develop skin changes over the capsules that may be permanent, and the scarring that the capsules cause may also cause cosmetic changes. There have been several lawsuits related to patients not being told of these risks ahead of time. Your local newspaper may contain ads asking women with Norplants in place to call a lawyer who will sue their doctors. With this type of "ambulance chasing" by the lawyers, many doctors have stopped offering this option of safe and effective birth control.

What Else Should I Know?

The cost of the Norplant system is one of the highest up front. The typical charge to place the capsules is usually between $300 and $600. However, remember the capsules are effective for five years. They are cheaper than birth-control pills if used for more than three years.

Lastly, while the Norplant capsules are highly effective in preventing pregnancy, they do not offer any protection against sexually transmitted diseases like AIDS, gonorrhea or chlamydia.

Barrier Methods of Contraception

Barrier methods of contraception are so named because a physical barrier is placed between you and your partner to prevent his sperm from getting to your egg. There are several different options in this category, each with its own advantages and disadvantages. Most of these methods are not used alone, but are combined with a chemical spermicide. The spermicide kills sperm and increases the effectiveness of the barrier method.

THE IUD (INTRAUTERINE DEVICE)

What Is It?

The IUD is another highly effective method of birth control that has been available for many years. Two different IUDs are available in the United States today. Several years ago there were many more, but due to liability risks most of these are no longer available. It is important for you to realize that the IUD of today is not the same as the IUD of 20 years ago, when there were serious problems with infection. If you meet certain criteria for IUD use, your risk of infection over the years from using an IUD is no higher than that of a woman not using an IUD.

IUDs are made out of a soft, flexible plastic. The Paraguard Copper-T is shaped like the letter "T" and is wrapped with copper around the stems. Two nylon strings extend from the end of the IUD. When the IUD is in place, these strings come out of the cervix and curl up in the upper vagina. There is only an inch of this string at the very top of the vagina, which neither you nor your partner should be able to feel during intercourse. The string is soft and the size of very thin thread.

How Does It Work?

The copper helps prevent sperm from getting through the uterus and into the fallopian tube where fertilization occurs. It also prevents the sperm from fertilizing the egg if they come into contact with each other. If fertilization does occur, the IUD prevents the egg from implanting. The main action of the IUD is to prevent fertilization from occurring, not to prevent a fertilized egg from implanting. This action is very similar to that of the birth-control pill. With the pill, the egg is prevented from being released, while with the IUD, the sperm are prevented from getting into the fallopian tubes. With both methods, if fertilization occurs, the lining of the uterus has been altered to make implantation difficult.

How Is It Inserted?

The IUD is inserted into your uterus in an office or clinic setting. It is placed during a period or the week after a period to prevent accidental insertion during pregnancy. Also, during this time your cervix opens up a little and makes insertion easier. The insertion process causes some cramping that lasts a few hours. Once in place, the IUD begins working immediately. It is 99-percent effective in preventing pregnancy, and it does not require daily attention. Most providers recommend you check the position of the IUD by feeling if the string is still at the cervix after your period. If you do not feel the IUD string, use condoms until you see your physician. You should see your provider within three months of insertion to check the IUD and then annually thereafter.

Once in place, the IUD is effective and has been approved by the Food and Drug Administration for use up to 10 years. At 10 years, the IUD needs to be removed and replaced. It can be removed anytime before, and fertility returns within two months. While using the IUD, you should not be able to feel something inside yourself without doing an exam with your finger to feel the string. The IUD does not interfere with your sex drive (common problem with the pills or Depo-Provera) or your ability to have an orgasm.

" I've had an IUD for more than a year now. I have no fear of scar tissue or infertility problems anymore because I don't want any more kids. It is easy, convenient and gives great freedom."

What Are the Risks?

Risks with the IUD include perforation of the uterus with the IUD during insertion, which is very rare. Your uterus could expel the IUD; if so, a new one would need to be placed. The IUD may also move inside the uterus and be difficult to remove. To remove the IUD, the strings are grasped and the IUD is gently pulled out. If the IUD string retracts into your uterus or if the IUD is stuck to the wall of the uterus, the IUD is removed during an outpatient procedure called hysteroscopy. With hysteroscopy an instrument is placed through your cervix and into the uterine cavity. The IUD is located and removed with this instrument. This is rarely needed for IUDs that have been in place less than 10 years. The normal experience is to feel minimal pressure while the IUD is removed in the office in two seconds.

The risk that causes greatest concern with the IUD is that of infection. There is a risk of infection during insertion. In order to minimize this risk, your physician sterilizes your cervix with Betadine and keeps everything sterile during insertion. Many physicians also give you an antibiotic to take around this time. I prescribe Doxycycline 100mg twice a day for three days after an IUD is placed. If you are in a mutually monogamous relationship, your risk of obtaining an infection over the following 10 years is no greater than that of a woman not using an IUD.

Who Should Use It?

The ideal time to use the IUD is when you have had all the children you plan to have, but do not want to do anything permanent like a tubal ligation or vasectomy. It is also good is you plan to wait at least two years between having children, especially if you do not like the way you feel while on birth-control pills.

Who Should Not Use This Method?

You should not use an IUD if you are not in a long-term, monogamous relationship like marriage. If you are dating, practicing serial monogamy (having sex with only one partner for a period of time, but then possibly having another partner in several months), or have had a prior sexually transmitted disease like gonorrhea or chlamydia, the IUD is not a safe method of birth control for you. You should not use the Copper-T IUD if you are allergic to copper.

What Are the Advantages?

Ninety percent of women who try the IUD like it and stick with it. Unlike pills, the IUD has no hormonal effects – such as decreased sex drive and vaginal dryness – to interfere with enjoyment of intercourse. The cost is one of the lowest if you use it for more than two years. Because of the up-front cost of the IUD and insertion ($200 to 400), it is not cost-effective to use for less than two years.

What Are the Side Effects?

The most common complaints related to the IUD are a slight increase in bleeding and cramping with periods. If you have a history of difficult periods when not on birth-control pills, do not switch to the IUD. If you use the IUD, expect your periods to be slightly heavier and more painful. For the first two months after insertion, you may feel constant mild pain. I recommend 800mg of Motrin every six hours for three days after insertion and for the first three days of your next two menstrual cycles to prevent this problem. Thereafter, the pain seems to be minimal for most women. Increased bleeding and cramping are the two most common reasons women have the IUD removed. Having stressed the negative side effects, it is important to again remind you that 90 percent of women using the IUD are very happy and continue it long-term.

What is Different About the Progesterone IUD?

Another type of IUD is the Progestasert. This is the same as the Copper-T IUD; however, instead of copper wire, the IUD contains progesterone. The effect of this IUD is similar to other progesterone-containing methods. The progesterone has a local effect in the uterus, thickening the cervical mucus and thinning the lining of the uterus. This IUD has all the same risks and contraindications as the Copper-T, except for the copper allergy. The other important difference is that this IUD needs to be replaced every year, which makes it less cost-effective. The Progestasert, however, is good for women who have heavy bleeding already but want to use an IUD. The thinning effect on the lining of the uterus decreases the amount of bleeding and cramping that occur.

What Else Should I Know?

Both of these IUDs can be used to provide emergency contraception if they are inserted within seven days of a high-risk situation, such as a broken condom or unprotected intercourse.

IUDs do not protect you from getting sexually transmitted diseases like AIDS, herpes, gonorrhea or chlamydia.

CONDOMS FOR MEN AND WOMEN

The most popular barrier method is the male condom. It is available at any drugstore and can be purchased without a prescription. Condoms are made out of various materials, latex being the most common. They come in different colors and shapes, and they all work and are used the same.

The male condom is placed over your partner's erect penis just before intercourse. You must insist he put it on before he enters you, because sperm leak from the penis before he begins to feel ready to ejaculate. During ejaculation, sperm are trapped in the end of the condom, preventing them from entering your vagina. After ejaculation, the condom is removed and discarded. It cannot be reused. Your partner must stop intercourse after ejaculation, since his penis softens after he ejaculates, and some sperm could escape from around the base of the penis or the condom could fall off in the top of your vagina.

Unfortunately, condoms may leak or break, leading to pregnancy and exposure to sexually transmitted diseases. For this reason, it is recommended that a spermicidal gel or cream be used in addition to the condom. Some condoms come pre-lubricated with a spermicide.

The condom is the only method of birth control that is useful in reducing the spread of sexually transmitted diseases such as AIDS, herpes, hepatitis, gonorrhea and chlamydia. There is evidence that spermicides containing nonoxynol-9 also protect against transmission of the AIDS virus.

> " The reason I didn't want to use condoms anymore was because I was starting to get irritated by them. Even when we used the gel and stuff, after so many minutes, it would start itching me. We tried all different brands. I think I was allergic to something, like the latex."

There is also now a new female condom called the "Reality" condom. This polyurethane sheath is designed with one closed end and flexible rings at the other end. You insert the closed end in your vagina, leaving the outer ring on the outside, and lubricate the condom with an enclosed lubricant. During intercourse, the penis is placed into the sheath; your partner should come out of the sheath after ejaculation, before his penis becomes soft. You then remove and discard the sheath. It should not be reused. The Reality condom costs $2 to $3 per condom. Because it is made of polyurethane, people who have latex allergies can use it. Some people complain about a "rustling" sound the condom makes when it is first placed. Using the lubricant on both sides of the condom can decrease this.

A disadvantage of both the male and female condoms is that their use requires some planning. They need to be purchased and available. Time must be taken out during a romantic event to stop and place the condom. Condoms also decrease the sensation that both you and your partner feel during intercourse and may lead to decreased enjoyment. They do help with a common problem many men have with intercourse – premature ejaculation. Using condoms may help you to enjoy intercourse longer, allowing lovemaking to be more mutually pleasurable and a stronger bonding event. Another benefit that we have constantly pointed out is that condoms help reduce the spread of sexually transmitted diseases. This is not a minor issue with the current epidemic of infections at all levels of society.

" I used the diaphragm in between pregnancies. I did not want the pill but was not ready for an IUD."

THE DIAPHRAGM AND CERVICAL CAP

Other options in the category of barrier methods are the diaphragm and cervical cap. The diaphragm is the more popular and commonly prescribed of the two.

The diaphragm is a shallow rubber cup that fits into your vagina and covers the cervix. The cervical cap is a smaller cup that fits directly over the cervix. The cervical cap is harder to place. The diaphragm and cervical cap come in different sizes and need to be fitted to you in order to be effective. Fitting of a diaphragm is performed in the office or clinic. Your provider makes sure the diaphragm prescribed is the correct size to prevent sperm from getting to the cervix. You receive instructions on use and care of the diaphragm at this time.

Diaphragms and cervical caps must be used with spermicidal gel. Without the gel, these devices are not very effective. This gel is placed around the edge of the device as well as within it. When properly inserted, these devices hold a "pool" of spermicide against the cervix. They not only act as a physical barrier but as a chemical barrier to the sperm. You place the diaphragm or cap before starting intercourse and leave it in place for at least six hours afterward. You can leave it in overnight, but to prevent infection you should then remove it, clean it with soap and water, and store it. These devices do allow skin-to-skin contact between you and your partner during intercourse and therefore do not decrease sensation as much as condoms do. If you have intercourse several times in one episode, you should not remove the device, but you should place additional spermicidal gel in your vagina. These devices are relatively inexpensive ($30 to $40) and with proper care may last years.

> " We use condoms because I'm breast-feeding and don't want to take any hormones. But they really do get in the way. I'm so tempted to skip it. But then my husband asks if I'm ready for another baby. Talk about a reality check!"

Failures of diaphragms and cervical caps are due to movement of the device off the cervix, allowing sperm to get up inside the cervical mucus. The failure rate with the diaphragm and cervical cap is 20 percent. They are ideal for couples who do not mind if they do get pregnant. If you strongly desire to avoid pregnancy, use one of the other options discussed in this chapter, such as Depo-Provera, the birth-control pill or the IUD. There are, however, no known adverse effects from the spermicides should pregnancy result. These devices do provide some protection against sexually transmitted diseases, but not nearly as much as the condoms. Many people combine the use of a diaphragm with a condom to prevent sexually transmitted infections and to increase their effectiveness.

Chemical Methods of Contraception

Many different products are available over the counter for use as chemical spermicides. Most of these contain the spermicide nonoxynol-9 and provide a moderate degree of protection from pregnancy, with failure rates of 20 percent. The spermicides should be combined with the use of a condom to increase their effectiveness.

Spermicides come in many forms; there are contraceptive jellies, creams, films and suppositories. The choice of which one to use is a matter of personal preference. The contraceptive gels and creams are placed into the vagina immediately before intercourse, using an applicator that comes with them. With each episode of intercourse, another applicator of cream or gel is first placed into the vagina. The contraceptive film also goes into your vagina immediately before intercourse. It "melts" and releases the spermicide within the film to provide protection. Contraceptive suppositories are popular because they are less messy and do not require an applicator. (An applicator is available if desired.) You unwrap a suppository and place it in the top of the vagina. You should then lie down and delay sex for at least 10 minutes to allow the suppository to "melt" and release the spermicide. The suppositories should be placed immediately before intercourse.

The advantage of these products is that they are quick and easy to use. They are also available without a prescription, and parental consent is not needed to purchase them. These products can easily be carried in a purse, glove compartment or pocket. Also, you can use a spermicide even if a man refuses to use a condom.

On the minus side, some couples do not like the mess that spermicides cause. Also, some women are allergic to them and can't use them. You may feel a mild burning with their use (this is not necessarily an allergic response).

These chemical methods of contraception do not protect against sexually transmitted diseases. There are some reports that the spermicide (nonoxynol-9) found in most of these products might help inactivate the AIDS virus. This action, however, should not be relied upon.

Sterilization Procedures

Sterilization procedures are an excellent option if you never want to be pregnant again. If you have any doubt about having more children, do not have one of these procedures done. Sterilization procedures are meant to be permanent and should be considered irreversible.

VASECTOMY

Sterilization procedures can be performed on you or your partner. In men the operation is known as a vasectomy. The tubes (vas deferens) that carry sperm from the testicles are cut and tied, effectively preventing the sperm from being released during orgasm. An urologist is the type of surgeon who performs vasectomies. They are performed under local anesthesia in the doctor's office, or in an outpatient surgical facility. Men typically are in mild to moderate pain for a few days afterward. Vasectomy procedures do not interfere with your partner's sensation during orgasm. The semen that is released during orgasm is mainly made up of secretions from the prostate gland, and only a small amount of the volume produced is the actual sperm. These prostatic secretions are produced beyond the point where the tubes are tied, so the ejaculate appears the same as before the vasectomy. When you look at the ejaculate under a microscope, it contains no sperm. After your partner has a vasectomy, you should use a backup method of contraception until his ejaculate has been tested and proved to be without sperm.

" The vasectomy procedure took 20 minutes. I was sitting in the office reading an article, and my husband was through before I finished the article. He thought it was fine, and he told other people there was nothing to it."

The failure rate with a vasectomy is 1 in 500. There is the concern that having a vasectomy increases the risk a man will develop prostatic cancer. This has been well studied and the consensus is that there is minimal to no increased risk.

TUBAL LIGATION

What Is It?

In women these procedures are known as tubal ligations. Most women refer to these operations as "having my tubes tied." There are a lot of different ways these procedures can be done, but they all involve surgical blockage of the fallopian tubes in some way.

The tubes can be cut and tied, burned (cauterized), clipped, banded or removed. No matter the method, the idea is to prevent the sperm and the egg from reaching each other.

How Is It Performed?

In women, a tubal ligation is performed by many different techniques. When first developed, the procedure was performed under general anesthesia in the operating room. The fallopian tube on each side is grasped in the middle and cut and the ends tied. There are lots of variations of this "classic" operation. The most common involves removing a piece of the fallopian tube – creating a gap – in addition to tying the ends. This procedure was performed through a relatively small incision (1 to 2 inches long) just above the pubic hairline. This classic procedure is commonly performed today on postpartum mothers who request permanent sterilization immediately after the birth of a baby. Postpartum, the incision is made just under the umbilicus (belly button) and is less than 1 inch.

Over the past 15 years, the use of a **laparoscope** to perform tubal ligations has become common. A laparoscope is a slender metal telescope that is placed into the abdomen through a small incision in your belly button. This procedure is also done under general anesthesia in the operating room. Once the laparoscope is in the abdomen, the doctor can either burn (cauterize) the fallopian tubes, put clips on the tubes or put small, rubber band-like rings on the tubes. All of these methods permanently damage the tube and seal it off in the middle. These procedures take about 20 minutes to perform and are done on an outpatient basis. You go home the same day and are back to normal function in a few days. These procedures are effective immediately.

What Are the Risks?

Because these procedures involve surgery, there are surgical and anesthesia risks involved. These risks should be discussed with your provider. The risks include – but are not limited to – bleeding, infection, and damage to the bowel, bladder, ureters, pelvic nerves and blood vessels. With any surgery, there is also a slight chance of stroke, heart attack or death. All of these risks are very rare, as this procedure is done routinely by most obstetricians and gynecologists. Make sure to discuss these risks with your doctor prior to having any surgery.

What Else Should I Know?

When performed correctly, these procedures provide the greatest protection from pregnancy short of having a hysterectomy. There is a 1-in-300 chance the tubal ligation will not work forever. Failures occur for several reasons: because you were already pregnant when the surgery was performed, because the tubes repair themselves or because the wrong structure was tied off within your abdomen. The surgery is scheduled for the early part of your menstrual cycle, before ovulation, to prevent operating on you if you might already be pregnant.

If a pregnancy occurs after a tubal ligation, there is an increased risk of implantation in the fallopian tube. This is known as an **ectopic pregnancy**. Ectopic pregnancies are very dangerous because the fallopian tube can rupture and lead to severe internal hemorrhage. Untreated, ectopic pregnancy can be life-threatening. If you think you are pregnant after having a tubal ligation, seek medical attention immediately.

There is evidence that having a tubal ligation lowers your risk of ever developing ovarian cancer by 70 percent. One theory on how this occurs is that a tubal ligation prevents toxins in the vagina from getting through the fallopian tubes and onto the capsule of the ovary. When the ovarian capsule repairs itself after ovulation each month, toxins on the capsule may increase your chance of developing cancer. While this explanation is only a theory, it would account for the greatly reduced incidence of ovarian cancer in women who have had tubal ligations.

What If I Want Another Baby?

Even though these sterilization procedures are meant to be permanent and irreversible, sometimes a situation occurs where a couple would like to have their fertility restored. Common situations include remarriage or the death of a child. A **tubal reanastomosis** is a microsurgical procedure that puts the tubes back together again. A specially trained gynecologist performs reanastomosis in a woman, and a urologist does the procedure in a man. The success rate of a tubal reanastomosis depends on the type of sterilization procedure that was done originally and how much undamaged tube is still present. The laparoscopic "clip" procedure has the highest success rate at reversal.

Again, due to the risk, cost and difficulty of reversal, sterilization procedures should only be considered if you never want to be pregnant again.

Emergency Contraception

Most sexually active women have experienced a "high-risk" situation where the chance of an unwanted pregnancy is increased. These situations include a broken condom, an unplanned and unprotected sexual experience, a slipped diaphragm or a sexual assault. In either case, pregnancy is usually preventable if an emergency contraceptive is prescribed within 72 hours (three days). There are two options; one is to use multiple birth-control pills and the other is to use an intrauterine device (IUD).

MULTIPLE BIRTH-CONTROL PILLS

The Food and Drug Administration has not approved any one pill for the purpose of emergency contraception. However, in February of 1997, the FDA published a notice that it was ready to accept applications from drug manufacturers for the emergency use of birth-control pills. It is expected that in 1998 or 1999, new products will be available by prescription for this use. While a morning-after pill does not have FDA approval, physicians have used various pills for this purpose for decades. Many treatments used in medicine are not FDA-approved, but this does not mean they are not effective, safe or appropriate.

If you notify your healthcare provider about a "high-risk" situation, he or she can prescribe eight regular birth-control pills for you to take in one day. You take four pills at one time and another four pills 12 hours later. The type of birth-control pills used this way contains a progesterone called **levonorgestrel**.

Another option is to use a stronger pill, Ovral. With this pill, you take two at one time and two 12 hours later. Some of the new ultra-low dose pills, like Alesse, require a dose of five pills at one time and five pills 12 hours later. These options are available to you to protect yourself from pregnancy if you have unprotected intercourse. Please speak with your physician as soon as possible after having intercourse. Just after the unwanted exposure occurs, use a douche and call your doctor either that day or the next day if the encounter occurs at night.

Nausea is common with taking multiple pills at one time, and many providers also prescribe an anti-nausea medication. Nausea is more common with the pill Ovral, even though only two are taken at a time.

There are no absolute contraindications to the use of the pills in this manner. Even if you would not be a candidate for taking birth-control pills long-term, you can use emergency contraception rather than risk pregnancy. Due to the short duration of use of these pills, the risk is reduced.

Emergency contraception is not 100-percent effective. Your chance of becoming pregnant if you use the morning-after pill within 72 hours of exposure is 1 percent. Studies have shown that using emergency contraception decreases the risk of pregnancy 75 percent over what would occur without emergency contraception. If this treatment is used over and over during the course of a year, the risk of pregnancy is 36 percent – much less effective than birth-control pills taken in a routine fashion. Therefore, the morning-after pill should only be used for those rare times when another method failed (broken condom) or no protection was used. Because of the higher doses of hormones prescribed, there may be adverse effects on a baby if pregnancy should occur. Discuss this with your provider.

THE IUD

The other option for emergency contraception is to have an IUD placed. This is more expensive, but the IUD can be left in place for long-term contraception. Also, the IUD can be placed and be effective even up to seven days after the "high-risk" situation. The birth-control pill option must be used within 72 hours to be effective. The risks and benefits of using the IUD in this fashion are the same for its normal use, which is covered earlier in this chapter.

Decisions, Decisions

The method of birth control you choose depends on many factors. You must first determine how strongly you feel about avoiding pregnancy. If the desire is very strong, please consider not having intercourse or using one of the most effective methods that we discussed in this chapter. Try to keep in mind your priorities regarding your desire to not be pregnant when you experience a minor side effect.

Other considerations when choosing a birth-control method include the ease of use, effectiveness, interference with sexual enjoyment, costs, risks and benefits. No one type of birth control is ideal for everyone. Throughout your life, you may use many different methods as your social, medical and economic situations change.

❧ *If you are looking for permanent sterilization and no longer desire pregnancy, consider a tubal ligation. It is the most effective, and long-term, least expensive.*

❧ *If you are looking for highly effective, but reversible birth control, consider birth-control pills, Depo-Provera, Norplant or an IUD.*

❧ *If you need protection from sexually transmitted diseases or are concerned about getting AIDS, use a condom and a contraceptive spermicide in addition to any other method.*

❧ *If you would like to delay pregnancy, but if pregnancy occurred it would not be detrimental, consider a diaphragm, condom, cervical cap, natural family planning, spermicidal product or withdrawal.*

The key to successful contraception is to communicate with your health-care provider your priorities and desires. Talk about what has worked for you in the past and what has caused you problems. If you have a concern, most likely your provider can modify the form of contraception without decreasing your protection from pregnancy or your enjoyment of intercourse.

Additional Resources

Books

- **Contraception: A Guide to Birth-Control Methods,** *Vern L. Bullough and Bonnie Bullough,* Prometheus Books, 1997.

- **The Whole Truth About Contraception: A Decision-Making Guide for Teenagers to Middle-Agers,** *Beverly Winikoff et al.,* National Academy Press, 1997.

- **Advocating for Self: Women's Decisions Concerning Contraception,** *Peggy Matteson,* Haworth Press, 1995.

- **Barrier Contraceptives: Current Status & Future Prospects,** *Christine K. Mauck,* Wiley-Liss, 1994.

- **The Birth Control Book: A Complete Guide to Your Contraceptive Options,** *Samuel A. Pasquale and Jennifer Cadoff,* Ballantine Books, 1996.

- **A Clinical Guide for Contraception,** *Leon Speroff and Philip D. Darney,* Williams and Wilkins, 1997.

Organizations

- **Couple to Couple League**
  P.O. Box 111184
  Cincinnati, OH 45211
  (513) 471-2000
  E-mail: ccli@ccli.org
  http://www.ccli.org/
  The largest natural family planning group in the United States, the CCL teaches the sympto-thermal method of natural family planning. CCL publishes a book and materials catalog, trains volunteer teaching couples and offers a home-study course.

- **Association of Reproductive Health Professionals**
  2401 Pennsylvania Avenue N.W.
  Suite 350
  Washington, DC 20037-1718
  (202) 466-3825
  Fax: (202) 466-3826
  E-mail: ARHP@aol.com
  http://www.arhp.org
  Founded in 1963, ARHP has a mission to educate health-care profes-
  sionals and the public on family planning, conception and other
  reproductive-health issues.

- **American College of Obstetricians and Gynecologists**
  409 12th Street, S.W.
  P.O. Box 96920
  Washington, DC 20090-6920
  http://www.acog.com/
  The organization that certifies obstetricians and gynecologists also
  maintains a web site with a catalog of patient-education materials.

Internet Sites

- **http://opr.princeton.edu/ec/ec.html**
  The Emergency Contraception website, operated by the office of
  Population Research at Princeton University, offers information, a
  directory of providers, new items about emergency contraception and a
  list of scholarly and government publications on the subject.

- **http://gynpages.com/ultimate/index.html**
  This site, "Ann Rose's Ultimate Birth-Control Links," includes
  information about several contraceptive options including abstinence,
  cervical cap, male and female condoms, the contraceptive sponge,
  diaphragm, emergency contraception, hormonal implants and
  hormonal injections.

- **http://plannedparenthood.org**
  The site of Planned Parenthood offers information about birth-control options and women's health.

- **http://www.fhi.org/fp/fpfaq/index.html**
  Family Health International, a group that "works to improve reproductive health around the world," presents answers to frequently asked questions on contraception, including information on postpartum IUD insertion and the correct way to use progestin-only pills (mini-pills).

- **http://www.ama-assn.org/special/contra/library/library.htm**
  The library of the Contraception Information Center, presented by the Journal of the American Medical Association, reviews the major contraception articles published in the literature and related reading from AMA scientific journals and other publishers. The site also includes an education support center, a "Best of the Net" collection of Web links, a treatment center and a newsline.

CHAPTER FIVE

PMS, DIFFICULT PERIODS
&
PELVIC PAIN

Finding the Cause - Getting Relief

F ew things in the world are as equally dreaded and desired as a woman's menstrual cycle. While as a young woman you probably want your periods to start to prove that you are "normal," as a mature woman nearing menopause you no doubt anticipate the end of monthly bleeding while perhaps having mixed emotions about the impending loss of your fertility. In between these life stages, you may dread the discomfort and inconvenience of your period at the same time you look for reassurance that you are not pregnant.

The amount of bleeding with a period and the degree of pain associated with the menstrual cycle vary among women. Most women notice some variation within their own cycles. A cycle is normal if it lasts from 26 to 34 days, and your bleeding is anywhere from spotting to active bleeding requiring you to change a tampon or pad every four hours. If your bleeding requires you to change every two hours or if you pass clots, I suggest you visit your physician. The pain of your period may be minimal and of no consequence, or it may be so severe that you feel irritable, unable to work or even go out of your room. How much pain is too much? That is

> *" The pain draws all the energy from me. The only thing I can think of is getting rid of it. It keeps me from focusing on anything. It seems to me that the pain is getting worse with the passing years."*

hard to say. While there is no objective measure, I feel that when your pain is having a negative impact on the quality of your life every month, you should speak to your physician.

For many women, the time before the start of each period is just as bad or worse than the period itself. If you have PMS (premenstrual syndrome), you and your family may dread this time more than any other time of the month. After reading this chapter, please have your family also read it to better understand what PMS is about and how to manage it.

> "It sometimes feels as though my cycles rule my life. I sometimes wonder if I'll be able to have children. I don't understand the pain."

When you experience painful periods or other pelvic pain, you may be concerned about whether or not you have a problem with your uterus or ovaries. Specifically, your concerns may include having cancer, not being able to have children, needing major surgery or having to live with this pain the rest of your life.

Pelvic pain can disrupt the quality of your life very easily. I am amazed at how many of the women in my practice try to live with pain every day, expecting themselves to carry on in life as if there were no problem. I strongly encourage you not to do so, because your behavior has to be affected by daily pain. Your temper gets shorter with yourself, your children, your co-workers and your partner. You may notice that you no longer want to have intercourse if it is painful, leading your partner to complain of not "feeling loved" by you anymore. The impact of pelvic pain can be serious, so do not take this problem lightly. You may slowly find yourself enjoying each day less and less, possibly sinking into a true depression. Life is too short and precious to live with pain needlessly. If you have pelvic pain or painful periods, please visit your physician for a complete exam. There is a solution with most causes of pain and you should not have to "just live with it."

This chapter presents information about female anatomy, a normal menstrual cycle, the main sources of pelvic pain and painful periods.

The chapter also explains your treatment options and reviews the typical evaluation you receive from a caregiver who is trying to determine the cause of your pain. First, though, I want to discuss the problem of premenstrual syndrome.

PMS: Real or Imaginary?
WHAT THE PROBLEM IS

Last week your child spilled milk on your blouse, your husband told you the Visa bill was twice the normal amount and a telephone solicitor called just as your family was sitting down for dinner. You were calm and collected when managing these situations. This week, the week before your period, you have yelled at your child for not eating all of her food and your husband for not keeping his clothes picked up, and you just called the telephone solicitor names you would be embarrassed to hear.

The first thing you must know is that PMS is real, and not just in your head. If you are affected, PMS typically occurs during your 30s and 40s, especially if you have small children and are working at the same time. If you have PMS, you probably feel in control all month except the week or two before you period. As your period approaches, you become very irritable and quick to anger, and you may lash out at your family, friends and co-workers. Your fuse is very short, and you get your feelings hurt and cry very easily. This is PMS.

Your menstrual cycle is like a frozen lake, with thin ice in the middle. The area of thin ice is the two weeks before your period – PMS time. My goal in this part of the chapter is to help you identify this area of thin ice and teach you how to cross it gently. If you had to

" I have pain and mood changes with my period. I am irritable, nauseous. I have heavy, extreme pain – sometimes like stabbing in my abdomen – impatience, headaches and exhaustion. The pain does interfere with things. During the first two days I have to take off of class or work. Although I hate to move, exercise helps. I also cope with major Advil, a hot water bottle and a dark room."

walk across thin ice, you would not put 50 pounds in your backpack and run full speed. Instead, you would remove all extra weight and gently walk across. I want you to know how to lighten the weight and walk gently.

With the stress of life, especially the constant demands of small children, the level of serotonin in your brain is lowered. When your brain levels of serotonin decline, you are less able to handle even small stresses. You become angry, cry easily and feel depressed. The difference between PMS and depression is that with PMS you only feel this way the week or two before your period. As your menses start, you feel the tension flow out of your body with the blood. You are usually fine the first two weeks after your period, but then the PMS starts once again.

With PMS you feel tense internally, and your family, friends and co-workers learn to avoid you during this time. There is great potential for damage to your relationships with all three groups if you do not address this problem. Your husband may feel he can do nothing right for two weeks. He avoids you and is hurt by your behavior. Over time he gets tired of the emotional roller coaster and begins to seek more distance from you. This only leads to problems. If you have PMS, you owe it not only to yourself, but also to your children and husband, to learn how to manage this problem. Include them in the process by educating them about what you are reading now.

" About one week before my period, I just feel tired, very irritable and sometimes angry. Things just get to me."

HOW YOU CAN ALLEVIATE THE SYMPTOMS

Before treating PMS, I like to rule out other problems such as depression and thyroid disorders. Depression is ruled out if you have no complaints any other time of the month except the week or two before your period. With blood tests, we can be sure your thyroid gland is working properly.

There are three areas to consider when treating PMS: diet, stress management and medication.

Dietary Changes

The most important thing for you to know today is that caffeine has to go out of your diet. Taking caffeine with PMS is like trying to put out a fire with gasoline. Caffeine takes a fuse that is normally three feet long and cuts it down to three inches. Keep this in mind when you get mad. Ask yourself: Did my family do something wrong, or is my fuse too short? Make your coffee half caffeinated and half decaffeinated for two weeks, then switch to all decaffeinated. All sodas should be decaffeinated for the entire family, and everyone will feel better. With your diet you also need to make sure you eat a full meal three times a day and two small snacks. Do not try to skip meals during the two weeks before your period (or any other time for that matter).

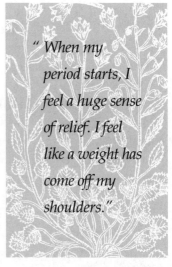

" When my period starts, I feel a huge sense of relief. I feel like a weight has come off my shoulders."

Stress Reduction

Stress management is critical in treating PMS. Stress lowers the level of serotonin in your brain, making PMS much worse. If you manage stress better, your brain produces more serotonin and you feel much better. You should not try to live without stress, but learn how to manage it.

The first thing you can do is to make the entire family aware of when you are premenstrual. This helps them not feel so personally attacked if you seem angry. During this time you must avoid taking on extra responsibilities, such as planning a party at your home or accepting extra loads at work. You must find five to 10 minutes in the morning to sit alone and do nothing. Do not read the paper or talk to anyone. If possible you should sit outside and just listen to the birds or the wind in the trees.

Each week you need to have one day where you have two hours

to yourself. This is time without your children or partner. You could go into the bedroom, lock the door, have a warm bath and read a novel. This is your night to not do the bedtime routine with the children. You should also provide this personal time for your partner at some point in the week.

Finally, find one evening a week when you and your partner have time to be alone. This can be a "date night" where you go to a movie or dinner, or simply go for a walk. If you are unable to manage your stress alone, do not hesitate to call a psychologist for help. With stress management, your body is able to maintain a healthy level of serotonin and you feel much better.

" Taking the vitamins, evening primrose oil and Saint John's wort, I just feel less irritable and a little more happy, not so down."

Non-Prescription Treatments

For medical management of PMS, try Optivite multivitamins (mainly for the Vitamin B$_6$), evening primrose oil, and Saint John's wort. These are all non-prescription items you can use without going to see your doctor. You take one of each of these every day of the month, except the eight days before your period, when you take two to four a day.

Prescription Drugs

If these over-the-counter medications do not work, I strongly encourage you to use the antidepressant Prozac for three to four months. This medication, like Saint John's wort, works by increasing the level of serotonin in the brain. Prozac helps you through the first few months while you remove caffeine from your diet and learn stress-management skills. It takes three weeks for Prozac to work, so do not give up too soon. After Prozac has increased the level of serotonin and you feel better, your stress management and avoidance of caffeine keep the levels elevated so you can stop taking the medicine. You will learn that at certain times in your life you are better able to handle stress. You may need to repeat the treatment of Prozac at different times.

One of the greatest mistakes you can make in life is to ignore PMS. It can not only make you feel terrible, but also ruin your relationship with your loved ones. PMS is very real and very treatable. Speak with your provider and seek help from a psychologist as soon as you realize you have PMS. If your family members are telling you they notice a dramatic change in your behavior, do not argue with them. Believe them, see your physician and start reading everything you can about PMS. By avoiding caffeine, managing your stress and possibly taking a short course of Prozac, you and your family can enjoy having the old you back.

Having covered PMS, let us now turn our attention to causes of pain originate in your pelvis. We first review your anatomy and how a period occurs. Before starting this discussion, I want to stress that there are times when the cause of your pain is not detectable. You may have very painful periods and yet have normal results to all the tests you undergo. Please try to be patient with your physician as he or she tries to help you as fast as possible without doing anything that impairs your ability to have children.

Pelvic Anatomy: What Is There and Where

Your pelvis is the floor of your abdominal cavity. It contains your bladder, uterus and ovaries, and is covered by multiple loops of bowel. A good way to imagine the shape of your pelvis is to think of it as a bowl sitting at the bottom of a paper grocery bag.

Toward the front of your pelvis is your bladder, which is like a water balloon that rests just under the pubic bone. The bladder stores urine, the liquid waste produced in the kidneys, and contracts to help expel it as you urinate. The back of the bladder sits on top of the uterus, or womb. A muscular organ normally the size and shape of a large pear, the uterus can expand to several times its normal size during pregnancy. The uterus is in the middle of the pelvis and connects to the top of the vagina, or birth canal, at the cervix – the area that is tested with a Pap smear. The cervix, the entrance to the uterus, is normally closed, but it can open just enough to allow the passage of menstrual blood or as much as 10 centimeters to allow a baby to be born.

Two tubes, about the size of your little finger, are attached to the upper sides of the uterus. The free ends of these fallopian tubes rest over the ovaries, which are on the right and left sides of the pelvis. The ovaries store your lifetime supply of eggs until they mature and are released, about one a month, from the time you begin your period until your reproductive years cease at menopause.

Behind the uterus, tubes and ovaries is the large intestine, the end of your body's digestive tract. The portion of the large intestine that rests behind the uterus is the sigmoid colon, which holds your body's solid waste matter until you have a bowel movement.

Along the sides of the pelvis, tubes called ureters transport urine from your kidneys to your bladder. (The kidneys are in the mid-portion of the abdomen toward your back, not in the pelvis.)

The very back part of the pelvis is made of muscle and bone. There are many joints in the pelvis, since this area is where the forces of your upper body and lower body meet. There also are many muscles, which allow movement of your legs and hips.

How the Menstrual Cycle Works

Although the organs involved in menstruation are located in your pelvis, the process doesn't originate there. Your brain controls your menstrual cycle. The brain sends follicle stimulating hormone (FSH) and luteinizing hormone (LH) to the ovaries to encourage the production of estrogen and progesterone. Both estrogen and progesterone travel from the ovaries through the bloodstream to the uterus. The lining of the uterus responds by developing a menstrual lining.

In the first half of your cycle, estrogen is the predominant hormone. Estrogen builds a thick endometrial lining in the uterus, preparing the uterus to receive a fertilized egg if you get pregnant. Near the middle of your cycle, you ovulate, or release the egg from the ovary; then progesterone becomes the predominant hormone. If the egg is fertilized and you become pregnant that cycle, progesterone helps support a new embryo as it becomes established in the endometrial lining of the uterus. If you are not pregnant, the progesterone level declines and you shed the thickened endometrial lining as a menstrual cycle. This is when you have your period.

What Causes Pelvic Pain and How it is Treated

Now that we have reviewed menstruation and which organs are in your pelvis, we can discuss how each organ can contribute to pelvic pain or difficult periods. The **uterus** is the source of pain with endometriosis, fibroids, cancer, pelvic relaxation and adenomyosis. Each of these can cause you to have severe pain with your periods. The **ovaries** cause pain with cysts, tumors, torsion and *Mittelschmerz*. The **intestinal tract** can create pelvic pain through irritable bowel syndrome, Crohn's disease, ulcerative colitis, appendicitis, diverticulitis and colon cancer. The **urinary tract** may cause problems in the pelvis with a bladder infection or renal stone, and possible **musculoskeletal problems** in the pelvis include pain in the hip joint and lower back. These causes of pain are presented in a table below and then thoroughly reviewed. When you finish this chapter, you should appreciate why your caregiver may not be able to tell why you have pain at your first visit. Finding the cause of pelvic pain may take several tests, which is why I review the typical evaluation performed on a woman with pelvic pain at the end of this chapter.

CAUSES OF PELVIC PAIN

Uterine	*Endometriosis, fibroids, cancer, pelvic relaxation, adenomyosis, pregnancy*
Ovarian	*Infection, cysts, tumors, torsion Mittelschmerz*
Intestinal	*Irritable bowel syndrome, Crohn's disease, ulcerative colitis, appendicitis, diverticulitis, colon cancer*
Urologic	*Bladder infection, kidney stone*
Musculoskeletal	*Hip joint, lower back joint*
Psychological	*Relationship conflicts, history of rape, incest, mental abuse*

> " All the way through high school and college, it was so obvious when I was on my period, because my first day I was in bed and it was like I had the flu every month. After the first day, I could get up and do stuff, I just wasn't as active."

When the Uterus Causes Your Pain

Whenever you have pain in the lower abdomen or painful periods, the uterus is the first organ of concern. The uterus is a source of pain if there is endometriosis, fibroids, cancer, pelvic relaxation or adenomyosis.

ENDOMETRIOSIS

The lining of the uterus, called endometrium, is shed in your monthly menstrual period. This lining normally passes out through your cervix and vagina in a normal cycle. If a portion of the lining passes through your fallopian tubes, this tissue can become established anywhere in your pelvis. It produces spots on your ovary, bowel, bladder or fallopian tubes. These spots of endometrium within your pelvis are called endometriosis. Each month, as hormones from the ovaries stimulate the endometrial lining within your uterus to thicken, these same hormones stimulate this lining that is now in your pelvis. Thus a small amount of bleeding occurs within your pelvis each month. The internal bleeding and inflammation create a great deal of pain in the pelvis during the menstrual cycle.

The body tries to contain endometriosis by forming scar tissue over these sites. Scar tissue over the ovaries results in pain throughout the month, and a great deal of pain with intercourse during deep penetration. Scar tissue over the bowel creates pain with bowel movements, just as pain over the bladder results when endometriosis is on the outside of the bladder.

Your doctor can diagnose endometriosis only by looking within your pelvis during a procedure called laparoscopy. During this outpatient procedure, the doctor makes a small incision in your belly button and inserts a viewing device called a laparoscope. Endometriosis appears as small brown lesions in your pelvis. The doctor then uses a laser in the laparoscope to ablate, or evaporate, any lesions of endometriosis that are visible.

If your symptoms recur after ablation, hormone therapy is an alternative to surgery. Hormones are given in the form of birth-control pills taken continuously (without allowing a break for menstrual bleeding to occur), Depo-Provera or Depo-Lupron. Depo-Provera is an injection given every two to three months for an indefinite time, and Depo-Lupron is an injection given every month for a maximum of six months. The pills and Depo-Provera have more progesterone than estrogen, resulting in suppression of endometriosis. The Depo-Lupron creates a state similar to menopause, with the decline in estrogen production, and that is why you can only take it for six months. With these hormonal treatments, the goal is to suppress abnormal endometrial tissue and eradicate the lesions forever. With the loss of estrogen stimulation, endometriosis regresses.

Scarring from endometriosis can occur between your uterus and the bottom of the pelvis, creating a "tilted" or "stuck" uterus. Infertility results if the scarring is on the fallopian tubes. If you become pregnant and your uterus is scarred down, you can expect to have moderate pain in the first trimester while the uterus grows out of the pelvis and into the abdominal cavity. After pregnancy, since the scar tissue has been disrupted, you may find that the pain has resolved. It is unknown if pregnancy itself causes endometriosis to grow or regress.

The pain of endometriosis is treated with medications such as Motrin or Anaprox. I encourage you to avoid narcotics, as they are addictive. If you cannot control the pain without narcotics, you need to consider surgery to ablate endometriosis. If endometriosis

" The pain is extreme, more cramping and more piercing, like a knife."

" To find out what I had, they did a vaginal sonogram and then a laparoscopy. The laparoscopy was a breeze. It was outpatient. I did feel really good for about six months. And then the endometriosis was back."

continues to recur, and you have had all the children you plan to have, consider surgical removal of your uterus and ovaries. When your ovaries are removed, you lose the source of estrogen that stimulates endometriosis, and it should go away. With time you can take low doses of estrogen as hormone replacement therapy with very little risk of stimulating a recurrence of the endometriosis and pelvic pain.

FIBROID TUMORS

" The pain was to the point where I could barely even walk. I had surgery to have the fibroid removed. It was big. It got to be bigger than a grapefruit. And it caused me a lot of pain while I was pregnant and afterward. The doctor told me that if I get pregnant again, I wouldn't be able to have a normal labor; I would need a c-section."

Fibroid tumors in your uterus can also cause pelvic pain and painful periods. A fibroid is a benign, or non-cancerous, tumor of the uterus. The tumors vary in size from a pea to a cantaloupe, with golf-ball size being average, and a woman usually has several within the muscle of her uterus. These tumors occur more frequently in the African-American population. Fibroids are not caused by anything you do or eat.

Fibroids are diagnosed with an exam in the office and frequently confirmed by ultrasound. If fibroids are not causing pain, nothing has to be done about them. However, typical problems encountered with fibroids include pelvic pain, painful periods, heavy or irregular periods, pressure on your bladder or rectum, and infertility or recurrent miscarriages. The treatment of fibroids is a hysterectomy if you have completed your childbearing. If you wish to have children and have problems with fibroids, the tumors are surgically removed from within the muscle of the uterus. Depending on their size and location, fibroids are removed through your cervix with a hysteroscope, through your umbilicus with a laparoscope or – most commonly – through a regular incision in your lower abdomen.

CANCER OF THE UTERUS

The most serious cause of pelvic pain that comes from the uterus is cancer. Most women with uterine cancer are over age 50; it rarely occurs before age 35 or 40. Postmenopausal bleeding is the most common symptom; in a woman still having periods, cancer presents with heavier periods or bleeding between two periods. If you are over age 35 and have an enlarged uterus with pain or abnormal bleeding, you can expect to have your physician perform an endometrial biopsy. This simple office procedure has replaced the D & C, dilation and curettage, as most doctors' diagnostic method of choice. If cancer is found, you need a hysterectomy and the removal of your ovaries and a sampling of many lymph nodes within your pelvis and abdomen. Some women with uterine cancer are treated with radiation therapy in place of or in addition to the hysterectomy. Your physician will discuss this in detail if you need to consider radiation treatment.

Risk factors for developing uterine cancer include obesity, entering menopause after age 52, never having given birth, and being exposed to **unopposed estrogen**. You are exposed to unopposed estrogen if you take estrogen (Premarin) for hormone replacement therapy without also taking progesterone. Another way you are exposed to estrogen without progesterone is to not have periods for months at a time (although this does not apply to when you are breast-feeding). In this situation your ovary is making estrogen, but without ovulation you do not make progesterone. The lack of progesterone prevents you from having a normal menstrual cycle and also exposes you to unopposed estrogen. This is why it is important to speak with your physician if you go more than two months without a period on a regular basis. Taking birth-control pills reduces your risk of uterine cancer by 50 percent. The strong progesterone component of the pills helps prevent the estrogen from stimulating the development of cancer.

PELVIC RELAXATION

Pelvic pain also results from pelvic relaxation. With this condition, damage has occurred to the support of the bladder, uterus and rectum, and these organs begin to fall out the vaginal opening. Supporting ligaments are trying to keep them up in the pelvis, but they are being strained and pulled. These ligaments attach to the lower back, and therefore most pain from pelvic relaxation is in the lower back and pelvis. Pressure on the pelvic organs is much greater when you are standing or lifting something heavy. You may even notice a mass protruding from your vagina when you strain. The pain from pelvic relaxation is much worse in the evening than in the morning.

This condition is diagnosed by an exam of your vagina while standing or bearing down as if to have a bowel movement. Surgery may be required to return your vaginal supports to their appropriate state, or your physician may recommend the use of a pessary. A **pessary** is a small device placed within the vagina to hold your organs up in their proper place.

You can help prevent pelvic relaxation by avoiding excessive force within your abdomen. This force is created with heavy lifting, chronic coughing and chronic constipation. One very preventable cause of pelvic relaxation is the chronic cough that results from smoking. If you are a smoker, seriously consider stopping for this and other reasons, and ask your doctor for helpful ideas to make quitting less stressful.

ADENOMYOSIS

Another cause of pelvic pain from the uterus is adenomyosis. With adenomyosis, the endometrial lining grows into the muscle of the uterus. Each month during menstruation, you bleed into the muscle, creating very painful periods. Adenomyosis is almost always seen in women who have given birth. During pregnancy, the endometrium enlarges tremendously. After birth the uterus shrinks to nearly the size it was before pregnancy, and the endometrium collapses like an accordion. If indentations of endometrium are caught in the muscle of the uterus while it is returning to its normal size, adenomyosis results. If your caregiver suspects you have this condition, you first are treated with birth-control pills, Depo-Provera or pain medication. If these do not provide enough relief and you have completed your family, you should consider a hysterectomy. There is no way to diagnose this condition other than through hysterectomy. Unfortunately, you are not sure you have adenomyosis before the surgery, because the pain is similar to that felt with the other causes we are discussing in this chapter. Only after looking for other causes of pelvic pain do I offer a hysterectomy with the anticipation that adenomyosis is the problem.

PREGNANCY

The last uterine source of pelvic pain is pregnancy. In the first trimester of pregnancy, the embryo imbeds itself into the uterus. This implantation causes moderate cramping and occasional bleeding. During the first trimester of pregnancy, as the uterus is outgrowing the pelvis and moving into the abdomen, you feel pressure and pain in your pelvis.

In addition, when pregnancy ends in a miscarriage, strong pelvic cramping occurs while the uterus is trying to remove the pregnancy tissue.

As an aside: another pregnancy-related cause of pain is the serious condition of ectopic pregnancy, where the embryo stays in the fallopian tube. There is not enough room in the fallopian tube, so the tube swells and may rupture. This is a life-threatening event, so please tell your physician about pelvic pain if you could be pregnant.

The presence of pain during pregnancy causes a great deal of anxiety, because the causes are so variable and the outcome is so important. This is why it is very important to have an established relationship with a doctor you like and trust before you become pregnant.

When the Ovaries Cause Your Pain

Whenever you have pain in your lower abdomen, your physician is working to make sure an ovary is not the cause. Common tests include cultures of the cervix to look for an infection that could have invaded the ovary, and ultrasound to determine if there is a cyst or mass on the ovary. Pelvic pain that comes from the ovaries feels sharp and is usually off to one side of the lower abdomen. It is normal to fear cancer, but pain is an infrequent complaint with ovarian cancer. Also, if you are under age 50, your chance of having ovarian cancer is only 7 in 100,000.

INFECTION

One of the leading causes of pelvic pain in younger women is infection. Bacteria travels from the vagina, through the cervix, uterus and fallopian tubes to land on the ovaries. An infection of the ovary causes tremendous pain and results in the formation of an abscess if not rapidly treated. The two most common causes of infection in the pelvis are chlamydia and gonorrhea. These sexually transmitted diseases can cause serious damage to the pelvic organs. If an abscess forms, you may have to have your ovaries and uterus removed to save your life. For a young woman without children, that would be a great loss. Using condoms during intercourse and minimizing the number of lifetime sexual partners reduces your risk for infection of the ovaries. An infection is diagnosed by taking a culture from your cervix. If you have an infection, you are given antibiotics either through your veins or by mouth. Only if you have an abscess and antibiotics do not work is a hysterectomy needed. For a complete discussion of pelvic infections, look through the chapter on pelvic infections and sexually transmitted diseases.

CYSTS AND OTHER TUMORS

If a mass is found on the ovary, an ultrasound is done to see if it is solid or cystic (fluid-filled). Both of these are referred to as tumors. Both kinds of tumors – cysts and solid masses – can be cancerous, but a solid mass is more concerning. You form a cyst every month before ovulation. It should be small (less than one inch) and not persist over three months. If ultrasound reveals the mass to be solid, you should have it surgically removed at that point. If it is cystic, a repeat exam in two months is appropriate. If the mass persists, or if it is greater than 10 centimeters at first evaluation, it should be removed.

Cysts formed in the ovary around a developing egg during a menstrual cycle are usually about one centimeter. Occasionally the ovary does not release the egg, and the small cyst becomes much larger, growing as big as nine centimeters (four inches) in diameter. The cyst creates a moderate amount of pain that is constant and usually isolated over the ovary with the cyst. Your menstrual cycle starts late during one of these episodes. Intercourse is very painful when there is a large cyst in one ovary.

Ovarian cysts are diagnosed with a pelvic exam or an ultrasound evaluation, and the exam is repeated two months later. If the cyst resulted from the ovary's failure to release an egg, the cyst is usually gone in two months. If it is still present at the repeat exam, the cyst should be surgically removed to make sure there is not a malignant tumor. Many caregivers place women on birth-control pills while waiting for cysts to resolve, but this treatment has been found to have minimal beneficial effect. If you are taking infertility drugs, you have an increased chance of forming very large cysts within the ovary that should resolve on their own over two months. The cysts found with **polycystic ovarian syndrome** are very small and rarely make the ovary larger than normal.

A tumor also can develop in the ovary just like in any other part of the body, creating pelvic pain. The tumor may be noted during a regular exam or when you go in for an evaluation of pain. Most tumors of the ovary in a woman younger than 50 are benign, while the risk of cancer is much higher if you are over 50. Every woman with a tumor of the ovary is rightfully concerned about having cancer, but the risk of this is very small if you are under age 50. The topic of ovarian cancer is discussed more in the chapter on cancer screening, but we will review some issues now.

CANCER OF THE OVARY

Ovarian cancer occurs in women over age 65 in the majority of cases, but can happen to a women in her 20s or 30s. The risk of having ovarian cancer increases for women who start periods at a young age or have menopause after age 52. The risk is greater for white women than for African-Americans. Your risk is decreased if you have used birth-control pills or had a tubal ligation. The longer you ovulate, the greater your risk of having ovarian cancer. By suppressing ovulation, as with birth-control pills, you lower your risk.

The first symptom of ovarian cancer is usually abdominal bloating and feeling full very quickly during a meal. A pelvic mass is an unusual and late finding. The bloating and fullness result from the spread of cancer cells throughout the abdominal cavity. The bowels become surrounded, and there is mild obstruction of the intestinal tract. If you are over age 50 and have abdominal swelling and difficulty eating, please see your physician immediately for an evaluation.

TORSION

If you have a cyst of the ovary that is smaller than five inches, it is left alone and observed. This wait-and-see attitude is very appropriate, as so many of these cysts never cause a problem. Many women have small cysts of the ovary, and it would be a mistake to remove all of them through surgery. However, these smaller cysts of the ovary can twist on themselves, a condition called **torsion**. When an ovary undergoes torsion, blood is forced into the ovary and is unable to leave. Rapid swelling of the ovary occurs, and you experience intense, sudden pelvic pain. If an ultrasound evaluation suggests you are experiencing ovarian torsion, you are given pain medication and observed for changes. If the ovary does not untwist, it must be surgically removed. Occasionally, the ovary can be untwisted and saved, but this decision is a difficult one your gynecologist has to make after looking at the condition of the ovary.

OVULATION

Pain associated with ovulation is one of the most routine sources of mild to moderate pelvic pain. Fourteen days before your menstrual bleeding begins, you ovulate. Ovulation involves the rupture of the small cyst within the ovary, which contains the egg. As the egg breaks through this covering membrane of the ovary, you experience a sharp pain known as ovulation pain or *Mittelschmerz*. There is no test to diagnose *Mittelschmerz*, but the regular occurrence of pelvic pain that lasts only one day and occurs 14 days before your menstrual flow is strong evidence. When you feel this pain starting, the best treatment is to take mild pain medication, such as Advil, Motrin or Aleve.

When Your Intestines Cause Pelvic Pain

Your intestines rest within the pelvis and can be the source of pelvic pain. The intestinal causes of pelvic pain include irritable bowel syndrome, Crohn's disease, ulcerative colitis, appendicitis, diverticulitis and colon cancer. These conditions should have no impact on your menstrual cycle. Therefore pelvic pain that changes according to the stage of your menstrual cycle is probably not related to your intestinal tract.

IRRITABLE BOWEL SYNDROME, CROHN'S DISEASE AND ULCERATIVE COLITIS

With irritable bowel syndrome, Crohn's disease and ulcerative colitis, pelvic pain is associated with changes in your bowel habits. You have intermittent constipation and diarrhea during the times of pelvic pain. The diarrhea may be mucous-like. These episodes of cramping pain and abnormal bowel function go on for many months, if not years, for most women who suffer from these problems. With irritable bowel syndrome there is an abnormality of the intestinal motility, or wave-like motions within the intestines that help move food through the bowel. Crohn's disease and ulcerative colitis are inflammatory problems of the intestines, with Crohn's disease affecting the small and large intestines, and ulcerative colitis affecting the end of the large intestine near the rectum. The causes of the inflammation are not always known, but infections and inheritance are two possible factors.

" I suffered from irritable bowel syndrome for several years, and the cramping and diarrhea were misery. It got to where I was afraid to eat at all. Now I function much better by getting lots of fiber in my diet, avoiding certain foods that really bothered me, and handling some stressful situations in a healthier way."

APPENDICITIS

Your appendix is a three-inch tubular protrusion off the large intestine, where the large and small intestines join. Sometimes, waste matter can become trapped here, and the appendix becomes swollen and inflamed. If you have severe abdominal pain on your lower right side, tenderness when this area is touched or examined (especially when the pressure is released), nausea with or without vomiting, and an elevated white blood cell count, your physician is very concerned about appendicitis. The appendix can rupture if not removed. The final diagnosis is made by a surgeon when looking at the appendix through a small incision in your abdomen in the operating room.

You may have the classic symptoms of appendicitis and be taken to the operating room, only to find that your appendix is normal. (However, in this situation, the surgeon is likely to remove your appendix anyway, since it serves no function and could possibly become a problem later.) Other problems that can resemble appendicitis include a kidney stone, an ovarian cyst or abscess, or torsion of the ovary.

> " I cannot eat any nuts, popcorn or anything with seeds in it, but I can do without those if I don't have pain. The pain was so awful. I was afraid I was going to die. Then I was afraid I wasn't going to die."

DIVERTICULITIS

Normally, the large intestine is a smooth tube, but sometimes small pouches, called diverticuli, are created. They tend to occur in women over age 40 who have had a problem with chronic constipation. These pouches become obstructed much like the appendix, resulting in painful inflammation and a condition called diverticulitis. Pain associated with diverticuli is usually localized to the left lower abdomen, and you may have a fever. Your physician looks into your intestinal tract with a colonoscope or sigmoidoscope to make the diagnosis. Treatment for a mild case involves rest at home, a liquid diet and oral antibiotics. Once the inflammation has decreased, you are advanced to a high-fiber diet. Occasionally, the inflammation and pain do not improve, or you develop an obstruction, fistula or bleeding, requiring surgical removal of that portion of the bowel.

COLON CANCER

Colon cancer is one of the most serious possible causes of pelvic pain. This cancer is among the top three causes of cancer deaths among women, behind lung cancer and breast cancer. Most women with colon cancer are older than 50. If you have colon cancer, your bowel movements become smaller, like a pencil, and frequently contain blood. That is why after age 40 you should have an annual check-up with a rectal exam. The stool is tested at that time for microscopic evidence of blood. If blood is noted, your large intestines are evaluated with a colonoscope or barium enema. As part of routine screening you should have a flexible sigmoidoscopy (exam of the large intestine with a fiberoptic scope) every three to five years after age 50.

With colon cancer, surgical removal of the cancerous portion of the bowel is required. Please remember that this is the least likely cause of pelvic pain, but one of the most serious, so it will be screened for during your exam. Your risk of developing colon cancer is increased if you eat a diet low in fiber and high in fat.

When the Urinary Tract Causes Pelvic Pain

Your bladder rests behind the pubic bone and on top of the lower portion of the uterus and upper vagina. Pain in the pelvis can occur with a bladder infection or kidney stone. The two have different causes, and the pain is slightly different.

BLADDER INFECTION

When you have a bladder infection, the pain is usually in the lower abdomen, toward the front. Other than pain, you feel burning with urination (dysuria), a need to urinate frequently and a sense that you still need to urinate just after voiding. Bladder infections occur very rarely for most women, while others have one every month. You may notice these infections after intercourse. During intercourse, the penis tends to push bacteria found in the vagina into the bladder, which is normally sterile. In order to minimize your chance of having a bladder infection, urinate soon after intercourse. If you are prone to recurrent infections, try to increase the amount of cranberry juice you normally drink. Cranberry juice increases the bladder's resistance to bacteria. If you have a very difficult case, your physician may have you take a low-dose antibiotic every day or at least whenever you have intercourse.

Evaluating your urine with a microscope provides the diagnosis. If there is an abundance of bacteria and white blood cells, sometimes with red blood cells present, you have a bladder infection. For most infections, this check under the microscope is all your caregiver needs to start you on antibiotics. If you have recurrent infections, your physician will identify the name of the bacteria causing your infection so as to prescribe the most effective antibiotic. To obtain this information, your urine is collected with a catheter, and the lab does a culture and sensitivity. This testing is more expensive than just looking under the microscope, which is why it is not done for every woman thought to have a bladder infection.

The treatment of a bladder infection is with the most effective, best-tolerated and least expensive antibiotic. If you are not allergic to sulfa drugs, Septra is an ideal choice. Other options include Keflex, Amoxicillin and Macrodantin. A stronger drug is Floxin, but it is also more expensive, which is why I reserve this medication for resistant or severe infections. For pain relief while waiting for the antibiotics to work, you may take Pyridium. This medication turns your urine orange, but it gives rapid relief from the pain. If your infection travels from the bladder into your kidneys, you develop pain in the middle of your back, nausea and a fever. In this situation, you probably need to be admitted to a hospital for treatment with higher doses of antibiotic in an intravenous line (IV).

> " I've had 20 years of bladder infections. It's chronic. The pain sometimes feels like a thousand needles piercing the skin. Sometimes my bladder feels like it's turning into a fist. It is real, real tight and it starts to spasm."

You can see how a bladder infection can be a very simple issue or a very serious condition. As a result, you may find that your caregiver does not want to just call in a prescription for antibiotics. I hope you now understand how making the correct diagnosis and giving the appropriate antibiotic is sometimes impossible over the telephone.

" I'd rather have my twins come out at the same time than have another one of those. The pain was a very hard pain, kind of throbbing. It's a doubling-over pain, worse than labor."

KIDNEY STONES

These stones, made of calcium deposits, form in the kidney and flow with urine toward the bladder. The ureters – muscular tubes the diameter of a straw – carry urine from the kidneys to the bladder. The muscular contractions of the ureters help move urine into the bladder. As a stone passes from the relatively large kidney into the narrow ureter, the stone becomes stuck and obstructs urine flow. The ureter tries to force urine past the stone with strong, rhythmic contractions. If the stone is large enough, urine does not pass, regardless of how strongly the ureter contracts. The portion of the ureter behind the stone swells, causing very intense pain that radiates down your leg. The pain comes in waves with each contraction of the ureter, and it is unaffected by your moving. Women who have had children compare this pain to the pain of labor.

If you suddenly have severe pain that is on one side of your pelvis and radiates down your leg, you need to see your physician. Your urine is tested for the presence of blood and to make sure you do not have a bladder infection. Then an X-ray with dye, which collects in the kidney, is done to look for an obstruction in the ureter.

Once the diagnosis of a stone is made, the management can vary. If you have mild pain that can be controlled with oral pain medication, you are sent home to drink plenty of fluids. With time, you may pass the stone during urination. You can strain your urine with a filter, but this is not required, as you will know if you passed the stone by the resolution of the pain. The stone may look like a small rock or gravel. If you are in severe pain, you are admitted to the hospital to receive pain medication and fluids through an intravenous line.

Rarely, the obstruction is so severe that the urine backing up in the kidney must be drained by passing a catheter through your back and into the kidney. A specialist called a urologist tries to break up these difficult-to-treat stones by passing a catheter through your bladder and into the ureter from below the stone. With either a basket to grab the stone or a laser or sound wave to break up the stone, you should be able to get quick relief. There is nothing you can do to avoid getting stones.

When Pain Comes from Your Muscles, Bones and Joints

Pelvic pain of musculoskeletal origin in a premenopausal woman is usually from the lower back joints, while in a post-menopausal woman, it is frequently from the hip joint. The lower back joint, which joins the pelvic bones to the spinal column, is the sacroiliac, or SI, joint. Pain at the SI joint occurs with poor posture, or lifting and bending at the waist instead of the knees. This pain is felt in the small of the back, and is worse with excessive movement, while pain from the hip joint is felt deep in the upper hip. Many women not using estrogen replacement therapy are at risk of having a fracture of the hip joint, which causes severe pain in the pelvic region.

The diagnosis of pain related to the joints is by physical exam and X-ray. Pain that is worse when you sit cross-legged on the floor suggests a problem in the SI joint. X-rays detect evidence of bone spurs, collapsed discs between vertebrae, or fractures of the hip joint. If you have a fracture, you are sent to an orthopedic surgeon for further evaluation and treatment, which may include surgery to place a pin in the hip joint. While this surgery is effective in relieving the pain for most women, any surgery at this age that involves decreasing your ability to walk around for a while, carries significant risk of life-threatening complications such as a pulmonary embolus (a clot that goes to the lungs).

If there is strain of the hip joints without fracture, the X-ray will be normal. At this point, treatment consists of avoiding unnecessary strain while also increasing the muscle strength around the joints, and taking non-steroidal pain medication such as Motrin. If the pain persists, I suggest you see a chiropractor or message therapist. Massage and chiropractic treatments provide tremendous benefits to many women who have pain from unaligned bones or muscle spasms.

When You Have Pelvic Pain for Psychological Reasons

While the topic of psychological causes of pelvic pain has been left for last, this is one of the most common problems. The physical conditions are addressed first, because we all want there to be a "real problem" to explain our pain. The truth is that psychological pain is as real as any other pain, if not worse. In many situations there is a combination of the two, with the psychological problem making the physical condition much more debilitating.

In relation to pelvic pain, the most important psychological issues involve some type of sexual trauma. This trauma could have been a date rape, incest or mental abuse as it relates to your early sexual development. If you have had a traumatic experience or feeling that centered on your vagina or pelvis, it is not unusual later in life for your brain to tell your body that this area is still in pain. If you have had a bad experience in the past, please relate this to your physician when you talk about your pelvic pain. This information does not preclude a careful evaluation for other causes of pelvic pain, but it does allow your caregiver to address this history as a potential contributor to the pain.

Another important consideration is your relationship with your partner. If you are unhappy with your relationship with your partner, you may have subconsciously developed pelvic pain in order to avoid sexual contact. Your pain may resolve through marital counseling, not major studies or surgery. This is a difficult issue to consider when you are feeling "real pain," but there may be no difference between this pain and the pain felt with endometriosis as far as your brain can tell. As you can see, it is imperative that you have a strong relationship and trust in your physician in order to open up and consider these possibilities. Remember, if your doctor suggests these possible causes of pain to you, he or she is truly trying to sort out the cause of your pain and relieve it in the most efficient method – not trying to tell you it is "just in your head."

How Your Doctor Finds the Source of Pelvic Pain

When you go to your doctor for an evaluation of pelvic pain, realize the diagnosis may be made quickly and easily, or it may require several tests and be more difficult to pin down. To start, your physician takes a careful history and performs a physical exam to help guide the decision for additional tests. Your urine is analyzed to rule out pregnancy, bladder infection and kidney stones. If there is no blood in your urine, you are unlikely to have a kidney stone. If a mass is noted during a pelvic exam, you undergo further evaluation with an ultrasound to look for masses of the ovary and uterus.

If no etiology, or cause of the problem, is noted at this point, medication is used to see if the pain resolves with time. You may receive antibiotics, such as Doxycycline or Floxin; hormonal treatments, including birth-control pills or Depo-Provera injections; or pain medications, including Motrin, Aleve and Anaprox. Narcotic medications are avoided because they are habit-forming, and if the pain is that severe, additional testing is appropriate.

If medicine has been unsuccessful at eliminating your pelvic pain, it is time to perform additional tests. A diagnostic laparoscopy is done to rule out endometriosis. The intestinal tract may be evaluated with a colonoscopy, sigmiodoscopy or a barium enema. X-rays could be needed to evaluate the bones in the pelvic region. At some point during this evaluation, consideration must be given to a psychiatric consultation, as some pelvic pain is a physical manifestation of a psychiatric disorder.

How You Can Take Part in Resolving Your Pain

If you have pelvic pain, I hope this chapter helps you understand some of the possible causes. In particular, I want you to know why certain tests are needed before your physician can tell you what is causing the pain. In some situations, a minor test such as a urine analysis is done to identify a bladder infection. In other situations, such as endometriosis, a major procedure such as laparoscopy is required before a diagnosis is made. Still in others, a simple discussion about past events or current social problems is all that is needed.

HOW TO HELP YOUR DOCTOR HELP YOU

❧ Prepare answers to these questions before you see your doctor:

Where does the pain occur?

When in your menstrual cycle do you have pain?

What makes the pain worse?

What makes the pain better?

Is the pain related to meals, urination, bowel movements, or intercourse?

❧ Be honest and trust your doctor with sensitive information about any relationship conflicts.

❧ Inform your doctor about any prior sexual abuse, even if you do not think there is any chance this pain is related; this information is important in caring for you in many aspects of your life.

It is very important to tell your doctor everything about your pain, such as when it started, what makes it better or worse, if it changes with your menstrual cycle, and have your bowel functions changed. Please be patient if your physician needs time to do certain tests before telling you exactly why you are having pain. When you understand the information in this chapter, you can be a more active member of your health-care team. I feel this information can help you through a difficult process and make that team more effective.

Additional Resources
Books

- **Alternatives for Women with Endometriosis:
A Guide by Women for Women,** *Ruth Carol (Editor),*
Third Side Press, 1994.

- **Endometriosis : Current Understanding and Management,**
Robert Shaw (Editor), Blackwell Science Inc., 1996.

- **The Endometriosis Sourcebook: The Definitive Guide to
Current Treatment Options, the Latest Research, Common
Myths about the Disease, & Coping Strategies – Both Physical
& Emotional,** *Mary Lou Ballweg,* Contemporary Books, 1995.

- **Uterine Fibroids: What Every Woman Needs to Know,**
Nelson H. Stringer, Physicians & Scientists Publishing, 1996.

- **Crohn's Disease & Ulcerative Colitis,** *Fred Saibil,*
Firefly Books, 1997.

- **Good Food for Bad Stomachs,** *Henry D. Janowitz,*
Oxford University Press, 1997.

Organizations

- **International Headquarters Endometriosis Association**
8585 N. 76th Place
Milwaukee, Wisconsin 53223
(800) 992-3636
(US, Puerto Rico, & the Virgin Islands, and the Bahamas)
(800) 426-2END *(Canada)*

- **Crohn's & Colitis Foundation of America, Inc.**
  National Headquarters
  386 Park Avenue South, 17th Floor
  New York, NY 10016-8804
  (212) 685-3440
  (800) 932-2423
  Fax: (212) 779-4098
  E-mail: info@ccfa.org

Internet Sites

- **http://www.ivf.com/endoassn.html**
  This site, sponsored by the International Headquarters Endometriosis Association, gives information about the condition and about joining the association.

- **http://www.acog.com/from_home/publications/**
  womans_health/wh6-17-6.htm
  This site about fibroids is presented by the president of the American College of Obstetrics and Gynecology.

- **http://members.aol.com/jokersaf/IBD_Home.htm**
  This site is a support group of people with Crohn's disease and ulcerative colitis, with links to conventional treatments and holistic options.

CHAPTER SIX

PELVIC INFECTIONS & STDs

Protecting Yourself With the Facts

ll you have to do is turn on the television to be confronted with the reality of pelvic infection. A supermodel touts the latest, quickest cure for vaginal yeast. Actors from the top medical dramas encourage viewers to "be safe" and "be smart" about sexual activity. A drug company brings information about the newest treatment for herpes straight to the consumer. While these ads may make you giggle, squirm and sometimes change the channel, they do bring home a serious point: Every woman can be exposed to a pelvic infection at some point in her life. According to *The Hidden Epidemic: Confronting Sexually Transmitted Disease* (National Academy Press, 1996), more than 12 million people in the United States contract an infection during sexual activity each year. Most women get at least one yeast infection or other non-sexually transmitted vaginal infection in their lifetime.

Regardless of the source, most infections cause a great deal of stress. They also can cause discomfort, though not always; the most common complaints are vaginal discharge, pelvic pain, itching, and nausea and vomiting. If you get a pelvic infection, you need to know why you are having these problems, how you were exposed, and what you should do to get relief.

The goal of this chapter is to provide information useful to women of all ages and at all stages of life, with an aim toward preventing these infections. This information is especially crucial for adolescents and other young adults, as it can help you make better decisions when faced with new and stressful demands.

This chapter divides infections into two groups: those related to sexual exposure (AIDS, gonorrhea, chlamydia, syphilis, herpes, hepatitis, condyloma, molluscum contagiosum, pubic crabs and trichomonas) and those unrelated to intercourse (yeast infections and bacterial vaginosis). For each group, you will learn how you become infected as well as how to prevent yourself from becoming infected. Also, you will read about the usual complaints associated with each infection, its treatment and any long-term effects the infection can have on your life.

Many of these infections cause similar symptoms in a woman. A heavy vaginal discharge, for example, may be from yeast, trichomonas, gonorrhea or chlamydia. Obviously, the implications are very different depending on the source of the discharge. Therefore, the chapter also features a chart that outlines many of the "chief complaints" that often lead a woman to visit her health-care provider, and the various infections that can cause each complaint or problem. You also learn which tests are typically run for each complaint, with a focus on why each test is needed.

How Your Age Influences Your Risk of Becoming Infected

A woman's age has a large impact on her chance of getting an infection. If a 13-year-old and a 30-year-old woman have sex with the same man, the 13-year-old is three times more likely to walk away from the experience with an infection. The vagina develops a protective lining as it matures. A very young woman who has intercourse with an infected man does not have this protective lining; therefore, her chance of contracting a disease is much greater. No one knows for certain when this protective lining has matured, but most gynecologists feel it is present by about age 18.

Do not infer that a more mature age protects you from sexually transmitted diseases. Instead, if you are a young woman, you should make an informed decision about sexual activity. When a man wants you to have intercourse, you must realize that the implications are much more severe for you than for him. It is rare for a man to become severely ill with most sexually transmitted diseases (AIDS and hepatitis being exceptions). However, a woman can become very sick from nearly all of these infections. The reason for the greater risk for a women when exposed to infections is related to a major difference between the anatomy of a man and a woman.

Unlike a woman's system, a man's reproductive system is not connected to his abdominal cavity. The abdominal space – where your bowels lie – is sterile, and not equipped to fight infections. An infection in the abdomen progresses rapidly to an abscess, which is a mass of pus. An abscess in the abdomen makes you septic, and this condition can kill you.

If a man has intercourse with a woman and catches an infection, the infection typically remains in his testicles. He may have no complaints or pain. Occasionally, men develop drainage from the penis or have a great deal of pain with urination. However, many men do not realize they have infections and do not know they can infect their new partners.

A woman's anatomy, on the other hand, connects the outside world to her abdominal cavity. For example, sperm travel from the vagina, through the cervix and into the uterus. From the uterus, sperm pass through the fallopian tubes to the abdominal cavity, where the ovaries are located. Just as sperm can travel through this system into this sterile space in the abdomen, bacteria and various infections also can enter. Once bacteria have reached the abdominal cavity, there is little defense to prevent a severe infection. An infection in your abdomen damages your fallopian tubes, the passages through which eggs travel to your uterus. The tubes develop scar tissue, resulting in chronic pelvic pain and infertility. You could have problems conceiving because the scar tissue often prevents eggs from entering the fallopian tubes. If the egg and sperm do join, the pregnancy is at high risk of getting stuck in the tube instead of implanting in the uterus, resulting in an ectopic, or tubal, pregnancy. Obviously, a baby cannot grow to term in a space as small as your fallopian tube, and the tube is at risk of rupturing. Ectopic pregnancy is fatal for the baby and very serious for the mother. Surgery is often needed to remove the pregnancy and sometimes the tube itself, further hindering your chance of becoming pregnant in the future.

Protecting Yourself From Sexually Transmitted Diseases

The best and most obvious form of protection from sexually transmitted diseases is to not have intercourse. The next best protection is to have a mutually monogamous relationship – one where both you and your partner have sex only with each other, for life. Many people practice a variation on this ideal, called serial monogamy. Serial monogamy means having sex with only one partner, but that your partner may be a different person each year, month, week or day. If you are involved in serial monogamy, the issue of protection is vital to your long-term health. By having a large number of partners throughout your life, you increase your cumulative risk of contracting an infection.

Love or Sex: How Can You Tell the Difference?

There are many ways you can express love and affection for a partner other than through sex. Love is a feeling felt in your heart and soul – it is not generated through sex. But many people confuse love with passion. A person can strongly desire to have sex with another person, feeling great passion, and still feel no love for that person at all. Young women need to understand this difference between making love to a lifelong partner, and simply engaging in the act of sex for the passion itself. When a young man requests, demands or pleads for sex, before you even think of accepting, you should consider his motives. A man who loves a woman should not ask her to have sex just to satisfy his passion. Both the man and the woman who would have sex in such a situation have shown lack of respect or reverence for their partners, themselves and even for the act of making love.

The traditional conflict has a man pursuing a woman for sex to fulfill his need for sexual satisfaction. In the more "modern" scenario, a woman has casual sex with a man to satisfy her passion. This second image is being presented in many women's magazines as an example of how today's mature woman should think, but the risk involved is enormous. As long as this storyline keeps magazine sales high, I can assure you that the line will not change. I wish the same amount of space were devoted to how to develop a strong and loving relationship without sex. If this were the main focus of establishing a relationship, we would see a much lower rate of divorce in America.

A condom is by far the best method you can use to keep yourself free of sexually transmitted diseases. Condoms provide sexually active women with the best protection available from the AIDS virus, gonorrhea, chlamydia, syphilis, herpes, hepatitis, condyloma, molluscum contagiosum and trichomonas. Condoms do not provide complete protection, but they lower your risk of becoming infected. For condoms to work effectively, your partner must wear one each and every time you have sex. Also, the condom must be on your partner's penis before he enters your vagina. Once he has ejaculated, he must come out of the vagina and remove the condom. If the condom is left on after ejaculation, and you continue to have sex, your partner's penis will soften, which allows sperm to leak from the condom into the vagina. When sperm reach your vagina, you are at risk for all the sexually transmitted diseases, as well as for getting pregnant.

Other than abstinence or condoms, there are no other effective methods of protection from sexually transmitted diseases. However, the most common method of protection used by couples today is a hope and a prayer. Every clinic and doctors' office has seen its share of infected young women who have relied on this method and been disappointed. If you have unprotected sex with anyone other than your lifelong partner, you are being very naive to think you will not get an infection. It is, however, human nature to believe these things only happen to other people. This thought process, plus the usual stress of a relationship, lead many couples into having unprotected intercourse. If you happen to have unprotected intercourse, please do not let it be your normal routine, as the more you are exposed to an infected person, the greater your risk of also becoming infected.

Sexually Transmitted Infections

The infections obtained through sexual intercourse are the most dangerous and damaging to a woman's body. These include the AIDS virus, gonorrhea, chlamydia, syphilis, herpes, hepatitis, condyloma, molluscum contagiosum, pubic crabs and trichomonas. Below we will review how you become infected, the symptoms, normal tests available, treatment options and long-term effects from each of these infections. If you have any concern that you have been exposed to a partner with one of these infections, speak with your health-care provider. With certain infections, you may receive treatment just on the chance you could have the disease.

HIV AND AIDS

How You Become Infected

The AIDS virus is this generation's form of the plague. Acquired Immune Deficiency Syndrome is the disease, and it is caused by the Human Immunodeficiency Virus (HIV), also referred to as the human T-cell lymphotropic virus (HTLV). This deadly virus is passed from one individual to another through various means. One of the most common ways to contract the AIDS virus is sharing needles with IV drug users. Since most people do not use IV drugs, we might all feel safe. However, normal sexual activity is becoming a more frequent means of getting infected with HIV.

With intercourse, infected fluid comes in contact with the other person's skin. If your skin has any openings – such as cuts, sores or even microscopic tears – you are at high risk of getting HIV. The infection has spread very rapidly among the male homosexual population, perhaps due to the fact that the skin often tears slightly during anal-receptive intercourse. Infected fluid (in this case, semen) easily gets into the bloodstream through these tears in the anal tissue. Once HIV is in another person's bloodstream, there is a very high chance that person will be infected and die.

There is also a risk of contracting HIV through heterosexual inter-course. If you have a small tear in your vaginal or anal skin and have intercourse with an infected man, there is a strong chance you will become infected. If a man has a sore or tear on his penis and has intercourse with an infected woman, there is a strong chance he will become infected. Women have a greater chance of having skin breakdown through the act of intercourse. Women, therefore, are at greater risk than men of contracting HIV with sex. Most men contract HIV through homosexual activity, due to the greater fre-quency of skin breakdown with anal sex. Men can contract HIV through sex with an infected woman, but this is not the most com-mon way. Women, on the other hand, are frequently contracting HIV through intercourse with infected men.

There has been great fear that people are contracting HIV through blood transfusions. This did occur with alarming frequency in the 1980s, when the virus was first identified. However, the risk today is extremely low. The risk of contracting HIV from one unit of blood is less than 1 in 50,000. Since there is now a test for the AIDS virus, all donated blood is carefully tested to make sure the blood is safe.

Pregnancy and HIV

Another way of passing the AIDS virus to another person is through pregnancy. If you have a baby while infected with HIV, there is a 30- to 50-percent chance that your baby will be infected at birth, depending on your T-4 lymphocyte count. (The lower your T-4 count, the greater the risk for transmission of the virus to your baby.) Since most children who get AIDS from their mothers die from the infection, women are being screened for HIV when they become pregnant.

If you are HIV-positive, your baby will be tested at birth. Because some of your antibodies are present in the baby's blood, a positive test result does not necessarily mean your baby has HIV. The test is re-peated in six months, at which time all of your blood antibodies are gone from the baby. If HIV antibodies are still present, this means the baby has the AIDS virus. Of all babies who test positive at birth, only half are found to have the virus at six months. The method of delivery of your baby, vaginal versus cesarean section, is not influenced by your HIV status. If you are HIV-positive, though, during labor your physician will not place a scalp electrode (an instrument that sticks to the baby's scalp to monitor the heart beat) on your baby. The electrode punctures the top layer of skin, increasing the risk of transmitting the virus to your baby.

If you are found to have the infection, you can take medications to lower the chance that your baby will become infected. Treatment with AZT (zidovudine) lowers the rate of transmission by 27 percent.

If you are HIV-positive and not pregnant, I strongly encourage you to consider having a tubal ligation (the surgery to get your "tubes tied") and avoiding the risk to a baby. If you do get pregnant, you can have an abortion, or you can take AZT to lower the risk of transmission to the baby. I know this information adds to your pains and concerns if you are HIV-positive, but as I have said throughout the rest of this book, I strongly feel that with good information you can lower your stress by making better decisions.

Before making any decision, please consult with your doctor, as this area of medicine is rapidly advancing, and your options may improve.

Symptoms and Treatment

HIV attacks a person's immune system. The immune system involves your white blood cells, which fight off infections. If you have HIV, you slowly lose your ability to defend against infections. You initially have swollen lymph nodes, weight loss and diarrhea. With progression, you develop yeast infections of the mouth and vagina, and then pneumonia. In time, you begin to get very ill and slowly die. There is no cure for AIDS. While antibiotics work well against bacteria, they are ineffective against viral infections. However, many medications are being given to slow the rate of progression. Medication to treat viral infections (HIV, hepatitis, herpes, venereal warts, the common cold, etc.) are in the early stages of development, and some long-term cures are anticipated soon.

Testing

The test for HIV is a blood test. If the preliminary result is positive, another more advanced test is done to make sure you have the virus that causes HIV. Every couple considering having a child should have an HIV test before they get pregnant. If either one is found to have the HIV virus, they need to reconsider the option of getting pregnant.

Reducing Your Risk

The best way to avoid contracting HIV is to abstain from intercourse. If you are going to be sexually active, use good judgment in choosing a partner. If your potential partner has a history of IV drug use, homosexuality or sexual promiscuity, have him get tested for the AIDS virus before starting a sexual relationship. Even if you think the man is a "good" person, you still need to use a condom. The condom is the only method of protection available that decreases your risk of contracting this virus. Condoms do not totally remove the risk, but they do provide significant protection.

GONORRHEA

Gonorrhea is one of the most common sexually transmitted diseases seen in the physician's office. This infection is transmitted through sexual contact. The younger you are, the more likely you are to become infected when having intercourse with an infected man. Men may have this infection and have no complaints. They will therefore give gonorrhea to all their subsequent partners without knowing how much damage will occur to the women.

Symptoms

If you become infected with gonorrhea, you have a vaginal discharge and pelvic pain. If the infection is limited to the cervix or uterus, the pain may only be moderate. If the gonorrhea has progressed to the fallopian tubes and on into the abdominal cavity, a life-threatening infection may result. Your body's defense is to wall off the infection in a ball of infected material or pus, creating an abscess. The abscess frequently surrounds the fallopian tube and ovary, and is therefore called a tubo-ovarian abscess or TOA. If an abscess is not treated, it may burst, releasing infected material throughout the abdominal cavity and making you septic. Once septic, even with the best antibiotics, you may need to have your uterus and ovaries removed in an attempt to save your life. If you are a 20-year-old with no children, you can end up paying a high price for making a bad decision about sex.

Testing

The test for gonorrhea is a cervical culture. This very simple test feels similar to a Pap smear. Results are back from the lab in two days. If you are having pain and your physician is concerned you may have gonorrhea, you will be treated before the culture results are known. Waiting two days without treatment is too dangerous if you are infected. If you are concerned you may have been exposed to a partner with gonorrhea but have no pain, then waiting for the test result is reasonable.

Treatment

Treatment for gonorrhea is with antibiotics. The most frequently used antibiotic is Rocephin, an injection given just once. Alternatively, you may be given penicillin or doxycycline. If you have gonorrhea, you are usually treated for chlamydia at the same time. These two infections occur together in many women.

Reducing Your Risk

Condoms provide a good measure of protection from gonorrhea. Just as with the AIDS virus, condoms do not completely remove the risk of getting a gonorrheal infection. But condoms do provide significantly more protection than a spermicidal gel, diaphragm or nothing at all.

The Lasting Consequences

The long-term effects of a gonorrheal infection come from the damage done to the fallopian tubes. Damaged fallopian tubes increase your risk of infertility and ectopic pregnancy. In addition, a prior gonorrheal infection may lead to a lifelong problem with pelvic pain. This pain may be mild or severe, and intercourse or the menstrual cycle may aggravate it. Obviously, gonorrhea is a serious and common sexually transmitted disease. You need to consider every sex partner as potentially infected. Use your best judgment in determining how to avoid ever becoming infected with gonorrhea.

CHLAMYDIA

Infection with chlamydia can be just as severe and just as life-threatening as infection with gonorrhea. The difference is that with chlamydia, you are more likely to have no complaints or symptoms. The problem with having an infection with no symptoms is that you can infect other people by accident. Also, your body becomes damaged if the infection goes untreated.

The Lasting Consequences

With chlamydia, scarring occurs slowly around the fallopian tubes, resulting in infertility or ectopic pregnancy. Since you may have chlamydia without knowing it, the amount of damage to the tubes may be extensive and permanent.

Symptoms, Testing and Treatment

If you do have symptoms with a chlamydial infection, they include a vaginal discharge, pelvic pain, pain with intercourse and painful periods. The test for chlamydia involves obtaining a culture of the cervix, just as with gonorrhea. Results are available in one to two days. Treatment is with antibiotics. The most commonly used antibiotic is doxycycline, given as a pill twice a day for seven days. Other options include Zithromax, erythromycin and ciprofloxacin.

Reducing Your Risk

The best method of protection against chlamydial infection is to use a condom. As with other infections, condoms do not provide complete protection against an infected partner. Also, they must be used from the start to the end of sexual activity.

SYPHILIS

Syphilis is less common today than many other sexually transmitted diseases. It is transmitted through unprotected intercourse and is carried in the bloodstream.

Symptoms

If you are infected, you initially have a sore on your labia that is painless, round and about the size of a nickel. There are swollen lymph nodes in your groin that are also not painful.

Syphilis occurs in several stages. The above problems develop first, but the infection can then go into hiding within the body. Syphilis creates a diffuse rash on the palms of your hands during this hiding time. With time the infection can reappear in the brain, or any other part of the body. When the infection is in the brain, you can become insane. During the late 1800s, most major cities in Europe had institutions full of people who had become insane from syphilis.

Testing

Currently the test for syphilis is a blood test. If the initial test is positive, another, more specific test is done to make sure you have syphilis. This infection is frequently seen in people with AIDS. Therefore, if you have the HIV virus, you should be tested for syphilis, and vice-versa.

Treatment

Syphilis is treated with antibiotics. For an infection that has been present less than a year, a single dose of penicillin is given as an injection. If the infection has been present more than a year, or if you do not know when infection occurred, the injection is given each week for three weeks. Alternative treatments include doxycycline and erythromycin.

HERPES

Herpes is a virus transmitted through sexual activity. During the 1970s and 1980s, herpes was the most feared sexually transmitted disease, because there is no cure. With the discovery of AIDS, herpes has taken a less prominent place in the minds of sexually active women, but the disease is no less serious.

Symptoms

The initial infection with herpes involves a patch of small blisters on the vulva (opening of the vagina). These patches are very painful, and they last for three to five days. Then the blisters open, leaving painful sores for another five days. After the initial infection, recurrent episodes similar to the first can occur at any time.

The frequency of recurrences or repeat outbreaks varies greatly from woman to woman. Some lucky individuals never have another outbreak, while others have outbreaks every month. Most women with herpes have episodes every three to six months. Stress affects the frequency of outbreaks. Certain illnesses also lead to more frequent episodes, with the AIDS virus being one of the more serious.

Herpes and Pregnancy

Herpes presents some risk in pregnancy. If you have an outbreak of herpes when you go into labor, you are at high risk of passing the infection on to the baby. The risk is much greater if you deliver the baby through your birth canal (vagina); therefore, a cesarean section is done to protect the baby.

Testing and Treatment

A culture of the blisters on the vulva makes the diagnosis of herpes. The test requires two to three days to get a result. Treatment is given before the culture returns based on the classic blisters seen on the vulva. An antiviral medication called acyclovir is given five times per day for five days. Acyclovir shortens the length of time the painful blisters are present, but it does not cure the infection. There is no cure for a herpes infection. A new treatment for herpes is Valtrex, which has the advantage over acyclovir of being taken twice per day instead of five times per day. If you are having very frequent recurrences, you may be given a low dose of acyclovir or Valtrex every day to prolong the time between outbreaks. These drugs may be used safely during pregnancy.

In addition, treatment is available to decrease the amount of pain you have during a herpes outbreak. The easiest to use is a lidocaine ointment applied to the vulva or labia every two to three hours.

How to Reduce Your Risk

Protection against herpes infection is obtained through the use of condoms. A partner with herpes can still pass the virus to you even if no blisters are present; likewise, if you have herpes, you can infect someone else even if you are free of symptoms. If you are infected, it is important to let your partner know. That way both of you will be sure a condom is being used. However, remember that many individuals are embarrassed to tell you they have a sexually transmitted disease. They therefore expose you to the risk of obtaining a life-long problem if you do not demand the use of a condom every time you have intercourse.

HEPATITIS B

Hepatitis B is a viral infection obtained through unprotected sexual activity. This viral infection attacks the liver, causing temporary or permanent damage. The liver is an organ in the upper right part of your abdomen, the liver makes the fluid that digests your food. You cannot survive without a liver. Once the virus has damaged your liver, you develop yellow skin (jaundice), fatigue and progressive weight loss.

Hepatitis is one of the most serious infections you can obtain through intercourse. It kills a moderate number of those exposed. There is no cure for this viral infection. Therefore, it is imperative that you protect yourself from exposure. Condoms provide the best protection short of abstinence.

Prevention by Vaccine

If you are at high risk of being exposed to hepatitis, you should ask your caregiver for the hepatitis vaccine. Vaccination is ideal for health-care workers, preschool teachers, prison workers, prostitutes or any woman who chooses to have multiple partners. All children should be given the hepatitis vaccine. You never know what risk-taking behavior your children will try during adolescence, so it is best to have them protected from a serious infection such as hepatitis.

The vaccine is given in three doses. After the initial dose, the second is given in one month and the third six months after the first. The Centers for Disease Control and the American Academy of Pediatrics recommend the vaccine be given to all newborns and to all children before starting school, in college or the military.

Other Forms of Hepatitis

There are other forms of hepatitis, such as hepatitis A, C and E. Hepatitis A is obtained through contaminated water or food; it causes a limited problem of fever, weakness and abdominal pain, but no serious long-term problems. Hepatitis C is obtained through blood transfusions, and can cause severe liver damage and death. Hepatitis E is rarely found in the United States, and causes the same problems seen with hepatitis A, although more intensely.

VENEREAL WARTS

The human papilloma virus, or HPV, causes venereal warts, also known as condyloma. This virus is caught through unprotected intercourse.

Symptoms

The warts grow on the labia, and they look like cauliflower. They are not painful, but when they get large they bleed when irritated. Venereal warts grow into the vagina and down around the opening of the anus. On rare occasions they grow so large that they obstruct the vaginal canal – a problem if you are about to give birth. The warts also cause pain and bleeding with intercourse.

Diagnosis and Treatment

HPV is diagnosed based on the appearance of the warts. If there is any doubt, your caregiver obtains a sample of the wart for confirmation. The most common complaint with the warts is that they are unsightly. The treatment is to remove the warts. A chemical solution is applied to the warts once a week until they disappear. Only one application is needed for most small warts. If there are multiple or large lesions, or if there is a diffuse pattern throughout the vagina, the warts are removed by laser or conventional surgery. Regardless of the method of treatment, venereal warts can reappear. While there is no treatment to permanently remove the underlying virus (HPV), it is rare for a woman to need treatment for the warts more than twice. Once you have had venereal warts, you are contagious to future partners. Men also contract and transmit condyloma, showing the same type of cauliflower lesions.

MOLLUSCUM CONTAGIOSUM

Symptoms

Molluscum contagiosum is a viral infection transmitted through unprotected intercourse. Small pimples appear all around the skin of the buttocks. These pimples are not painful, and they do not cause any serious problems. Women come in for evaluation simply because they know these pimples should not be there. No pain or vaginal discharge is associated with this infection.

Treatment

The treatment of this viral infection involves opening the pimple by squeezing its base. The base is treated with a chemical stick called silver nitrate. No other treatment is needed. The pimples typically do not return.

PUBIC CRABS

Pubic crabs are just what their name suggests – very, very small parasites that resemble crabs and accumulate on the pubic hairs around your vagina. These parasites cause a great deal of itching and irritation. The diagnosis is made by finding what look like flakes of skin at the base of the hair. Also, small specks of brown material are found on your skin and on your undergarments. Your caregiver may look at one of the hairs under the microscope. The treatment of pubic crabs is with a lotion or cream called lindane. You and your partner need to be treated at the same time. Also, your clothing and bedding must be thoroughly washed.

TRICHOMONAS

Trichomonas is an infection of the vagina that causes a discharge with a bad odor and itching. This is one of the most commonly seen sexually transmitted diseases in a physician's office. Looking at a sample of the vaginal discharge under the microscope makes the diagnosis. Trichomonas is only transmitted through sexual intercourse. Trichomonas is treated with an antibiotic called Flagyl, which may be given as one large dose or over several days in smaller doses. Flagyl causes severe nausea if you take it around the time you have had any alcohol. Therefore, make sure you tell your caregiver if you had a drink the night before if you are given this antibiotic.

Other Pelvic Infections

The vagina normally has both yeast and bacteria present. If the amount of yeast becomes too much, you have a yeast infection. If the amount of bacteria is too great, you have bacterial vaginosis. These infections cause a discharge and are not related to sexual activity. Some women also have a very heavy vaginal discharge at certain times of the month that is totally normal. Discharge usually occurs with ovulation, which is in the middle of the cycle. Unlike discharge that is symptomatic of infection, this normal discharge does not have a strong odor, and it does not cause itching or pain.

YEAST INFECTION

Symptoms

Vaginal infections caused by yeast are accompanied by a thick, white discharge. You feel strong itching around the vaginal opening, and the skin turns a burning red. Yeast infections frequently occur when you have been on antibiotics for a sore throat, sinusitis or a bladder infection, because antibiotics alter the pH balance of your vagina, making conditions more favorable for yeast to grow out of control.

Diagnosis and Treatment

A yeast infection is diagnosed after looking at a sample of the vaginal discharge under the microscope. The treatment is with a vaginal cream. Over-the-counter products include Monistat-7 and Gyne-Lotrimin, which are taken for seven days. These products will cure the majority of yeast infections. Stronger concentrations of the medications are available and are taken for only three days; these include Terazol-3 and Monistat-3. These creams are used before bedtime. The majority of the cream is placed up into the vagina with an applicator, and a small amount is spread on the skin around the vaginal opening. A new medication for the treatment of yeast infections, Diflucan, has become very popular. This is a pill that is taken only once.

For difficult-to-treat infections, tablets of boric acid are placed in the vagina. Another alternative is to paint the vagina with a solution of gentian violet. In order to increase the concentration of lactobacilli in your vagina, which prevent the proliferation of yeast, you should eat one serving of plain yogurt each day. If you have frequent recurrences, you should be tested for diabetes and AIDS, as these medical conditions make a long-term cure unlikely.

BACTERIAL VAGINOSIS

The problem with bacterial vaginosis is a heavy vaginal discharge with a bad odor. The diagnosis is made through inspection of the discharge under the microscope. The treatment is with the antibiotic Flagyl. This antibiotic may be taken as a tablet or as a vaginal cream used twice a day for seven days. Another cream called Cleocin vaginal cream is used only once a day.

COMMON SYMPTOMS, LIKELY CAUSES

When you experience symptoms of a pelvic infection, you want relief. This chart describes the most common problems that lead a doctor to suspect pelvic infection, what could be causing them, and the tests you need to find out.

Symptoms	Possible Causes	Test
Abdominal pain, nausea, fever and a heavy vaginal discharge	Gonorrhea Chlamydia	Culture of the cervix
Painful small pimples on the skin around the vaginal opening	Herpes (most likely)	Culture of the area
Vaginal discharge	Yeast infection Bacterial vaginosis Trichomonas	Inspection of a sample under a microscope
Bumps or growths of skin around the vagina	Venereal warts Molluscum contagiosum	Visual inspection
	Herpes	Culture of the area
	Syphilis	Blood test

Women's Health: Your Guide to a Healthier and Happier Life

How to Cope with the Diagnosis of Sexually Transmitted Disease
CARING FOR YOURSELF PHYSICALLY

An abnormal vaginal discharge, lumps of the vaginal skin or abdominal pain can cause great concern. You should always try to protect yourself from sexually transmitted diseases. If you think you already have an infection, seek a medical evaluation immediately. An infection that is not treated can cause permanent damage to your body. The end results can include chronic pelvic pain, infertility and death. Not all infections are transmitted by sexual contact. Only after a thorough evaluation by your physician can you know the source of an infection. However, many are related to sexual exposure. A difficult situation presents itself when one member of a monogamous couple is diagnosed with a sexually transmitted disease. Some infections can be present for years before problems develop. The presence of some of these infections does justify a candid discussion with your partner about the possibility of an affair.

If you have a sexually transmitted disease, tests should be done to make sure you do not have other infections as well. It is standard to test for gonorrhea, chlamydia, syphilis, hepatitis and the AIDS virus at the same time. You need a thorough evaluation so that all infections are treated appropriately.

DEALING WITH YOUR EMOTIONS, PLANNING FOR THE FUTURE

You also should use the time with your physician to get the support you and your partner need to get through this difficult experience. The resource list at the end of this chapter is full of additional sources of information about these diseases and sources of support. Especially if you find yourself living with an infection for which there is no cure, such as herpes or HIV, you will probably want to learn as much as you can about the latest medical research and available treatments. You also may find it helpful to talk to other people going through the same thing, either informally or in organized support groups. This experience may be more than you want to handle alone.

If you learn you have an infection, you may feel tremendous emotional pain. You may feel that you are "dirty," and this feeling can have a bad impact on your self-image. Many women have contracted pelvic infections with their first sexual experience, so having an infection does not mean that you are promiscuous. Nor does having an infection make you a bad person. But you should take this occasion to evaluate your sexual practices. If you are involved in serial monogamy, use this experience as a stimulus to develop new standards for deciding if having sex is appropriate.

Conclusion

I would like you to use this information to avoid infections by using condoms, and by limiting your exposures to multiple partners. If you have the symptoms discussed in this chapter, please go to your physician and ask for testing. When you are young, one of your major concerns should be limiting any damage to your fallopian tubes that could impair your fertility.

When it comes to your sexual life, as in all aspects of life, you have many decisions you must make, and you should have the knowledge you need to make well-informed ones.

Additional Resources
Books

- **AIDS : Etiology, Diagnosis, Treatment and Prevention,** *Vincent T., Jr. Devita,* Lippincott-Raven Publishers, 1996.

- **Sexually Transmitted Diseases Sourcebook: Basic Information About Herpes, Chlamydia, Gonorrhea, Hepatitis, Nongonoccocal Urethritis, Pelvic Inflammatory Disease,** *Linda M. Ross,* Omnigraphics, 1997.

- **Youth, AIDS, and Sexually Transmitted Diseases (Adolescence and Society),** *Susan Moore,* Routledge, 1997.

- **The Hidden Epidemic: Confronting Sexually Transmitted Diseases,** *The Institute of Medicine,* National Academy Press, 1996.

Organizations

- **American Social Health Association (ASHA)**
  P.O. Box 13827
  Research Triangle Park, NC 27709
  (202) 543-9129
  http://sunsite.unc.edu/ASHA/

- **ASHA Resource Center**
  Publications about herpes and HPV
  (800) 230-6039

- **National AIDS Hotline**
  (800) 342-AIDS (English)
  (800) 344-7432 (Spanish)
  (800) 243-7889 (TTY Service for the Deaf)

- **National Herpes Hotline**
  (919) 361-8488

- **National STD Hotline**
  (800) 227-8922

- **ASHA Healthline**
  Publications about sexual health
  (800) 972-8500

- **Association of Reproductive Health Professionals**
  2401 Pennsylvania Avenue N.W.
  Suite 350
  Washington, DC 20037-1718
  (202) 466-3825
  Fax: (202) 466-3826
  E-mail: ARHP@aol.com
  http://www.arhp.org

- **Centers for Disease Control and Prevention**
  1600 Clifton Road, N.E.
  Atlanta, GA 30333
  (404) 639-3311
  http://www.cdc.gov

- **SIECUS**
  (Sexuality Information & Education Council of the United States)
  130 West 42nd Street
  Suite 350
  New York, NY 10036-7802
  (212) 819-9770
  Fax: (212) 819-9776
  E-mail: siecus@siecus.org

Internet Sites

- **http://www.minn.net/racoon/herpes/herpes.html**
  The Herpes Home Page serves as an information and community center for people with herpes, offering research and treatment news as well as various bulletin boards and chat rooms, links and more.

- **http://www.cdcnac.org/**
  The site of the CDC National AIDS Clearinghouse shares HIV/AIDS and STD resources, information about education and prevention, published materials, research findings and other news.

- **http://www.geewiz.com/std.html**
  The U.S. Department of Health and Human Services offers facts about STDs and answers to common questions about condoms.

- **http://www.immunet.org**
  Immunet offers "easy access to quality information about HIV/ AIDS,"aimed at medical professionals as well as people with AIDS. The site presents treatment news, an online lecture series, a scientific review of alternative therapies, a resource directory and more.

- **http://edcenter.med.cornell.edu/Pathophysiology_Cases/STDs/ STD_01.html**
  Cornell University Medical College makes available this information about epidemiology and diagnosis of common STDs. This site is useful for those who want more in-depth information about the appearance of these diseases and which organisms cause them.

- **http://www.med.jhu.edu:80/jhustd/genstd.htm**
  The Johns Hopkins University STD Research Group presents this page of links to sites that offer general information about STDs.

- **http://cdc.gov/od/owh/whstd.htm**
  The office of Women's Health, a division of the Centers for Disease Control and Prevention, prevents statistics on the health impact of sexually transmitted diseases for women.

CHAPTER SEVEN

BREAST HEALTH

Staying on Top of Their Changes

F rom before the time you put on your first training bra, your breasts have no doubt figured prominently in the image you have of yourself. The female breasts are among the most noticeable organs in the human body. Made up mostly of fat with a network of milk-producing glands, the breasts are designed to nourish children. However, that true purpose is often obscured by our society's – and sometimes your own – concern with breast size, shape and appearance. Many consider the breasts to be sexual organs to be admired by men.

Misconceptions surround the problems and diseases affecting the breasts. In order to understand these problems, you first must understand the organs' development and normal function. The various problems that occur are mostly "benign," or non-cancerous, ones; however, breast cancer is one of the diseases women fear most. This chapter discusses the development of the breasts, many common non-cancerous problems that can occur in the breasts, problems that can lead to cancer, as well as breast cancer itself. We also cover how your physician evaluates a breast lump and what you should do to screen yourself for cancer.

How Your Breasts Develop
A LENGTHY PROCESS

Breast development is a continuous process from birth through adulthood. The proper development of the breast is dependent upon exposure to certain hormones. These hormones are produced at different times women grow from childhood to adulthood. The breasts are composed of several different types of tissues. There are cells that secrete milk; these are grouped together to make up the **glands**. There are cells that carry milk from the glands to the nipples; these cells make up the **ducts**. Fat cells compose most of the breast tissue; however, rarely are diseases of the breast associated with the fat cells. Most problems occur either in the ducts or glands.

WHAT HAPPENS AT PUBERTY

" I was 12 when my breasts started developing. That was the big thing to have going on in your life. It was major. If you didn't, you were like an outcast. My first bra was a hand-me-down. My best girlfriend developed a lot before I did, so I got her training bra."

In infancy, your breasts have a primary mammary cord, the main duct from which all the future ducts eventually develop. By puberty, a network of ducts and a few alveoli are present. The alveoli are the actual glands where future milk production will take place. They are composed of groups of glandular cells arranged like clusters of grapes, and the ducts are like the stems. Around age 10 or 11, girls begin to notice an increase in the size of their breasts. This change occurs because estrogen and progesterone, the two main female hormones, start to be produced. With the increase of estrogen and progesterone, the ducts and alveoli begin to multiply and develop.

By adulthood, your breasts have a complex, branched network of ducts. The cells that line the glands are not able to produce milk until pregnancy occurs. Many other hormones are needed for complete breast development and function.

THE EFFECT OF PREGNANCY

For the cells that line the glands to produce milk, **prolactin** must be present. Prolactin is produced in the pituitary gland, and the amount released is much greater after pregnancy. However, these cells must first be exposed to two other hormones – cortisol and insulin. If there are inadequate amounts of these hormones, proper development can still occur, but a larger amount of prolactin may be required. (A benign tumor of the pituitary gland, called a **prolactinoma**, causes an overabundance of prolactin to be produced. Women with this condition leak milk from their breasts without ever having been pregnant.)

The tremendous increase in the primary female hormones that occurs during pregnancy is responsible for a significant change in the breasts. Estrogen and progesterone levels rise throughout pregnancy, stimulating breast growth. Early in pregnancy, growth of the ducts and glands cause the breast to become very tender. Sometimes this tenderness is the first indication that you are pregnant.

" During pregnancy my breasts became voluminous, three times their normal size. After the birth of the baby and breast-feeding, about six months later, they really shrank and became softer. They were hanging lower."

Prolactin levels continue to rise throughout pregnancy; however, the breasts usually do not produce milk until after delivery. This is because progesterone "blocks" the action of prolactin on the glands during pregnancy. At the time of delivery, progesterone levels drop rapidly and the breasts begin producing milk. Milk is said to "come in" two to three days after delivery.

Milk is produced in the glands and stored there, as well as in the ducts. Suckling causes a hormone called **oxytocin** to be released from the pituitary gland. Oxytocin causes small muscles in the walls of the ducts to contract. These contractions force milk out of the nipple, leading to a "letdown" of the milk. The relatively high levels of prolactin at the time of delivery cause some continuous stimulation and milk production even in the absence of suckling. The breasts can become engorged with milk if the infant is not allowed to feed and drain the breast.

The medication Parlodel, which in the past was commonly given to mothers who were not breast-feeding, blocks the production of prolactin so that milk is not produced. Parlodel has been associated with a small number of maternal deaths and therefore is not usually offered to you unless you have a severe problem with engorgement. If you do not breast-feed, take three 200mg tablets of Motrin every six hours for the first three days after you deliver. To prevent engorgement, you must wear a tight-fitting bra day and night for four days, and avoid any stimulation of the breasts. If you are weaning your baby from nursing, follow the same instructions for the first four days after you discontinue nursing. Once you stop, you must not allow the baby to suckle on your breast at all. If you do allow the baby to "pacify" at the breast, you will have a tremendous problem with engorgement.

In women, as in other animals, there is the potential for more than two breasts. These are rarely seen. More common, however, are multiple nipples. These are usually along the "milk line" that runs from the axillary (armpit) area to the groin on each side. Many "moles" on the abdomen are actually these accessory nipples. These accessory nipples may enlarge and darken during pregnancy, and you may notice that a small amount of milk drains when you breast-feed. This is normal, and these changes reverse after pregnancy and breast-feeding.

Common Non-Cancerous Abnormalities of the Breast

Problems can occur in the breasts, just like in any other part of the body. We tend to divide these problems and diseases into **benign** (non-cancerous) and **cancerous** categories. There are; however, some problems that fit into an in-between **pre-cancerous** category.

PROBLEMS THAT CAUSE LUMPS

Fibrocystic changes in the breast tissue are the most common affliction of the breast. According to some estimates, fibrocystic changes affect up to 70 percent of women and lead to 30 to 50 percent of all breast biopsies. When you have this condition, hundreds of tiny cysts form in the breast, surrounded by dense, fibrous tissue. The breast becomes very tender, especially just before your menstrual period. Lump size may also increase during this time and then decrease after your period is over. Rarely, a clear to yellow discharge is noted. This condition gives the breast a "rubbery" or "bean-bag" feel. In the past this condition was called a disease; however, we now commonly refer to it as fibrocystic change. **It is not pre-cancerous;** however, small cancerous lumps can be more difficult to find when the breasts are lumpy in general.

Nobody knows why some women develop this condition. It is more common in women whose mothers are also affected, so there is probably a genetic predisposition. It also is well known that caffeine and nicotine aggravate tenderness and lump size. If you have fibrocystic changes in your breasts, avoid caffeine, chocolate, tea and nicotine. Additionally, studies suggest that taking 400 IU of vitamin E a day helps decrease the tenderness. Also, you should wear a properly fitted, supportive bra.

Simple cysts are the next most common problem of the breast. Cysts can cause a painful lump in the breast. They are more common in women with fibrocystic changes. The work-up and evaluation are simple if you have a single cyst. A cyst is a fluid-filled sac, ranging in size from ¼-inch to 2 inches. A cyst is usually easy to feel and is drained with a needle to "prove" it is a cyst. The fluid is typically a greenish-yellow color. The doctor may or may not send the fluid to the lab for analysis. If the fluid is clear, it does not have to go to the lab for analysis. If the fluid is bloody, it is sent to the lab to make sure there are no cancerous cells. These cysts are almost always benign. Unless they recur in the same place, a simple aspiration is all that is needed for treatment. When a cyst is drained and later recurs in the same location – especially if it has been drained twice before – the cyst should be surgically removed.

Fibroadenomas also cause isolated lumps in the breast and are more worrisome due to the fact they are solid (as are most breast cancers). They are found more commonly in women with fibrocystic changes. Fibroadenomas are the most common solid tumor of the breast in women under age 25. They are benign tumors and not pre-cancerous; however, if you are over age 25, they are removed to prove they are indeed benign. If you are under age 25, the area is observed with regular exams and possibly a mammogram. If you have a strong family history of breast cancer (sister or mother with breast cancer diagnosed before age 50) and have a lump at a young age, your physician may suggest you have it removed.

(For more information on what happens when you see a doctor about a breast lump, see the section of this chapter "How Breast Lumps are Evaluated.")

PROBLEMS THAT CAUSE NIPPLE DISCHARGE

Many women are taught that a bloody discharge from the nipple is always a sign of cancer; however, this is not true. Most bloody discharges are caused by small **intraductal papillomas,** which are usually benign. Papillomas are growths in the duct walls made of bundles of blood vessels. They bleed easily with even gentle rubbing of the breast. The breast ducts are arranged like spokes on a wheel converging at the nipple, and each duct has a separate opening in the nipple. By gently squeezing the nipple, you can actually identify the duct that contains the papilloma because blood comes out of only that duct. Sometimes a duct is injected with dye that shows up on an X-ray, and the outline of the papilloma can be seen. In order to remove the papilloma, the affected duct is excised. This is a simple outpatient surgical procedure that does not leave a large scar. The papilloma needs to be removed to make sure your discharge is not due to cancer. Having a papilloma removed does not alter your ability to breast-feed or significantly change the shape of your breast.

NIPPLE DISCHARGES

Many of the benign conditions we have discussed can cause nipple discharges. As part of a good monthly breast self-exam, you should perform a careful check for a nipple discharge. The presence of a nipple discharge is usually a sign of an underlying problem with the breast. The type of discharge does not always help you decide what the problem is, or even if the condition is benign or malignant. A very subtle clear discharge may be the only sign of an underlying cancer in the breast and therefore should be evaluated. Bloody discharges are most commonly found associated with benign papillomas; however, they may also be found

with an underlying breast cancer. Therefore, any new
discharge should be reported to the doctor.

In young women, intense stimulation of the breast (i.e.,
during foreplay) can actually cause a discharge to be produced.
This is a common cause of concern and testing. This sort of
discharge is usually not a symptom of any underlying breast
problem; however, you should always have a discharge evaluated.
When it comes to problems relating to your breasts, it is always
ideal to have your physician carefully examine and consider
serious possibilities before you just assume nothing is wrong.

PROBLEMS THAT CAUSE INFLAMMATION

There are two inflammatory conditions of the breast: mastitis and
mammary-duct ectasia.

Mastitis is an infection of the breast. It is most commonly found
in women who are breast-feeding. Bacteria known as "staph" cause
this infection. The bacteria usually come from the baby's mouth; therefore, the baby gives the mother the infection. The infected breast becomes warm, swollen and red. You rapidly develop a high fever, chills
and marked fatigue. You need to call your physician immediately, as
this infection develops rapidly. Rarely, an abcess forms that needs to
be drained. The infection is treated with an antibiotic and warm compresses. The baby should continue to breast-feed to help keep the breast
from becoming more swollen. The breast milk and antibiotic used to
treat mastitis are safe for your baby.

Mammary-duct ectasia also presents with a red, swollen breast,
but it is more common in women near the age of menopause. Clogged
breast ducts cause mammary-duct ectasia. This uncommon problem
occurs because normal secretions in the breast back up in the ducts and
become inflamed. This condition can cause a lump near the nipple and
is commonly quite painful due to the inflammation around the affected
duct. There can be a thick, sticky discharge that is gray-green in color.
Treatment is with warm compresses and antibiotics. Rarely, the affected
duct needs to be excised if it does not respond to antibiotics.

OTHER NON-CANCEROUS CONDITIONS

Sclerosing adenosis is a benign condition where there is excessive growth of the tissues in the glands of the breast. The changes in the breast associated with sclerosing adenosis are usually microscopic. However, when the changes occur over a large area of the breast, a lump can sometimes be felt. The areas that are growing most rapidly may develop calcium deposits within them. These calcifications are visible on a mammogram. The calcifications cause concern since similar calcifications are seen within a cancerous lesion. Therefore, it is not uncommon for a biopsy of the affected area to be done to confirm the diagnosis.

Fat necrosis causes lumps in the breast that are painless, round and firm. They are the result of degeneration or breakdown of the fatty tissue, usually following a blow to the breast that you may or may not remember. Sometimes there is a bruised look to the tissue around an area of fat necrosis. If the lumps are solid, a biopsy may be needed to confirm the diagnosis.

Pre-Cancerous Changes

There has been tremendous confusion in the past about what conditions fit into the pre-cancerous category. A good definition would be a condition that increases the risk of an invasive (malignant) cancer – not one that makes a cancer harder to find.

HYPERPLASIA

When you have a biopsy for evaluation of a lump or suspicious change in the breast, sometimes a condition is found in which there is an overgrowth of the cells that line the ducts. This overgrowth or "piling up" of the cells in the ducts is called **hyperplasia.**

The pathologist – a physician who specializes in performing and interpreting diagnostic tests – looks at the cells in this area to determine if they have any characteristics of cancer cells. A normal cell has a small amount of dark material in the middle (the nucleus). With pre-cancerous changes, the dark nucleus increase in area, and with cancer, the nucleus replaces almost the entire cell.

With normal tissue, your cells are arranged in an orderly pattern, which varies according to the type of tissue. With pre-cancerous changes, this pattern is slightly disrupted, and with cancer, there is total loss of a normal pattern. Therefore, when a breast biopsy is examined under a microscope, if the pattern of growth is relatively orderly and the cells themselves look normal, then there is not an associated increased risk of developing cancer. If, however, the overgrowth of cells obliterates the ducts, or if the cells themselves look abnormal, then there is an increased risk of developing cancer in the future. In general, the more excessive this growth is, the greater the risk of cancer development. In women with moderate to extensive hyperplasia, the risk of developing breast cancer in the future is 1.5 to 2 times the average women's risk. If "atypical" cells are seen (ones with too much of the dark nucleus), and there is hyperplasia (overgrowth of cells with a loss of the normal pattern), the risk of developing a future breast cancer is 5 percent.

CARCINOMA-IN-SITU

Ductal carcinoma-in-situ and **lobular carcinoma-in-situ** can actually be thought of as cancers that have not become invasive and are still confined. These names are bothersome because they contain the word "carcinoma," suggesting cancer. The reason they are listed under pre-cancerous conditions and not cancer is that these problems are limited to the most superficial layer. Imagine it as a skin change that has not gone under the skin. Under the top layer of your skin, there is a basement membrane that separates the top layer from the rest of the body. If cancer cells are limited to this top layer, there is minimal risk that the abnormal cells have spread. If the abnormal cells extend beyond this basement membrane, cancer cells spread freely. Therefore, if abnormal cells are limited to the top layer, even in a breast duct, they do not carry the same risk as ones that have gone beyond the basement membrane. The cells that cause these problems look like cancer cells in every way, except that they have not spread at all. Unfortunately, this process may be a diffuse one in the breast and therefore is still a concern. Typically these lesions also cause calcifications in the breast. The diagnosis is made many times on mammography due to "typical" calcification patterns the radiologists have learned to recognize. If you have this condition, you may be diagnosed after a routine mammogram detects these calcifications or through an evaluation of a bloody nipple discharge.

Women with ductal carcinoma-in-situ have a 25- to 75-percent chance of being diagnosed with a future breast cancer. Women with lobular carcinoma-in- situ have a 30-percent chance of a future breast cancer. In the past, many women with this disease had mastectomies to prevent invasive cancer. However, with careful follow-up and mammography, you may elect to follow this condition conservatively, and a mastectomy can be done only if an area of invasive disease is found. Careful discussion of the risks and benefits of various treatments is indicated if you have these lesions. The final decision of how to proceed is made case by case. Treatment of these lesions remains an area of great controversy still.

BREAST PAIN

Breast pain is a common complaint and a cause for alarm in many women. Most women with this complaint have diffuse (widespread) tenderness in both breasts. This pattern of tenderness is usually attributable to benign conditions or hormonal changes. The benign causes of pain are treated by anti-inflammatory medication like ibuprofen. A good supportive bra is helpful. In some women, treatment with low doses of a male hormone (testosterone) has been shown to be beneficial.

Of greater concern are areas of focal tenderness or pain – pain that is specific to one area. Women with fibrocystic breast changes typically experience diffuse tenderness in both breasts before their period. However, if a woman with this complaint develops an area of more intense, persistent pain, careful evaluation of that area is needed.

PAGET'S DISEASE

Paget's disease of the nipple looks like a raised red patch of skin around the nipple. It has the appearance of eczema. Despite its benign appearance, it is almost always associated with an underlying cancer. The cancer is usually a ductal cancer and may still be an in-situ lesion. If Paget's disease is noted after a breast skin biopsy, you will undergo a very thorough evaluation for underlying cancer due to the very high rate of cancer found in women who have overlying Paget's. Of all women with breast cancer, Paget's disease is found in 1 to 2 percent.

How Breast Lumps Are Evaluated
NEEDLE BIOPSY

Collecting Fluid From a Cyst

If you feel a lump in your breast, one of the easiest ways your caregiver can determine if it is solid or cystic is to place a needle into the mass and see if fluid can be removed. This process of drawing off fluid is called **aspiration**. Many doctors order a mammogram of the breast first before aspirating a breast cyst. The concern is that trauma to the breast from the aspiration may cause changes to occur on the mammogram and lead to confusion. More importantly, a mammogram allows a careful evaluation of the rest of the breasts to be performed. When you have a palpable lump, the mammogram cannot be relied on to determine if the lump is benign or malignant. If the mass is not seen on mammogram, it still must be biopsied to determine if it is cancer.

If fluid can be aspirated from the lump, then it is probably a benign, or non-cancerous, one. The fluid that is obtained from a cyst is usually discarded and not evaluated unless it is bloody. If bloody, the fluid is sent to cytology, where the cells are examined under the microscope to see if they are abnormal. A repeat exam of the breast should be performed several weeks later to make sure the cyst has not recurred. Cysts that develop from cancer cells reform quickly, because these abnormal cells produce an unusual amount of fluid. Therefore, if a cyst has clear fluid and does not reform, it is considered benign. If the fluid is bloody or the cyst reforms in the same location, additional testing with a biopsy must be done.

Collecting Cells From A Solid Mass

If no fluid is obtained during aspiration, the lesion may be solid. The doctor may still use the needle to obtain a sample of the mass. By placing the needle in the mass and pulling back on the plunger of the syringe, the doctor creates suction in the needle. As the needle is passed back and forth through the mass, cells are "shaved off" and collected in the needle. Before an aspiration or biopsy is done, your skin is numbed with a local anesthetic like lidocaine. These procedures are not very painful, but some discomfort should be expected. The cells are placed on a slide and sent for evaluation by a cytologist. The cytologist determines if suspicious cells are present and if further evaluation is needed.

Sampling a Small or Suspicious Area With the Help of X-Ray

Stereotactic needle biopsy is a relatively new procedure used in the evaluation of breast lesions. It is most useful for the biopsy of masses too small to feel and suspicious areas seen on mammograms. This procedure is done by a radiologist using specialized X-ray equipment. The breast is placed in a position so it cannot move, very similar to how a routine mammogram is done. Using X-ray guidance, a needle biopsy of the suspicious area is obtained. This technique can be used to biopsy areas of suspicious calcification if these areas are relatively localized. Unfortunately, if the area involved is diffuse, the area biopsied with this technique may be benign, but just next to it may be a cancer.

In general, if you or your doctor finds that you have a breast lump, it needs to be tested to prove it is benign. This is especially true for anybody over the age of 25. Breast cancer is almost unheard of in women younger than 25. Any localized solid mass in the breast of a woman over the age of 25 needs to be sampled in some way to rule out cancer.

SURGICAL BIOPSY
Removal of a Solid Mass

An open biopsy of a solid lump or suspicious area is still the "gold standard" to which other techniques are compared. With this technique, the area of concern is totally removed. You are taken to the operating room for an outpatient procedure. You may be put to sleep or given medication to calm your nerves through the IV, and a local anesthetic, such as lidocaine, is placed into your breast so the biopsy does not hurt. Once the mass is removed, your wound is closed with sutures just beneath the skin. This procedure leaves a small scar, but it is the ideal way to determine if a mass is cancerous or not.

While you are asleep on the operating table, your doctor may send the mass to the lab for a preliminary look at it under the microscope. This step is called a **frozen section**, and while these results are usually correct, they are considered unofficial.

Evaluation of a Larger Area of Concern

If you have diffuse, worrisome calcifications in your breast, the biopsy is performed differently. Here, a radiologist places a small needle into the middle of the area of calcifications. Once the needle is placed, a mammogram is taken to make sure the tip of the needle is in the middle of the calcifications. Your surgeon then removes the tissue around the tip of the needle. The radiologist uses the mammogram machine to determine if the area of concern has been totally removed before sending the tissue to the pathologist. This process is called a **needle localization biopsy**. It obviously takes a team of experts in various fields of medicine to perform this correctly.

What You Need to Know About Breast Cancer
HOW SERIOUS THE DISEASE IS

Breast cancer is the second most common cancer in women in the United States. It accounts for 31 percent of all cancers in women. Statistically, 1 in 8 women will get breast cancer at some point in their lives.

The risk increases significantly after age 40; the disease is very rare in women younger than age 30. The incidence of breast cancer is higher in developed countries and has slowly increased over the past several decades. Almost 70 percent of breast cancers occur in women who have no known risk factors; therefore, every woman is at risk.

Despite the increased incidence of breast cancer in this country, the death rate from breast cancer has not changed much over the past 50 years. Screening programs help increase the detection rate, and the smaller the mass when detected, the better your chance of survival. The death rate from most other female cancers has actually declined due to better screening and preventive techniques, such as Pap smears for the cervix. Breast cancer is the second leading cause of cancer death in women in this country. (Lung cancer is now the top cause of cancer death in women, due to increased smoking that began in the 1930s and '40s.)

WHAT INCREASES YOUR RISK?

Let me say again that **all women are at risk of developing breast cancer**. There are, however, women who are at greater than average risk and may require a more careful evaluation and "level of suspicion."

Family History

Your family history is important. If your mother, sister or daughter – known as a "first-degree relatives" – has had breast cancer, your risk is increased. Also, the greater the number of first-degree relatives who have had breast cancer, the greater your risk. If a "second-degree relative" (defined as a grandmother, aunt or cousin) has had breast cancer, your risk is increased minimally.

Long Exposure to Estrogen

A hormonal effect has been noticed. The greater the length of time your breast tissue is exposed to the hormone estrogen, the greater your risk of cancer. Therefore, if you start your period before age 12, you are at increased risk. If you go through menopause after age 55, you also are at greater risk. If you had your first pregnancy after age 30, you are at greater risk.

Precancerous Changes

As we discussed earlier in the chapter, atypical hyperplasia and carcinoma-in-situ increase the risk of breast cancer.

Genetic and Other Considerations

Some recent reports link excessive alcohol intake and breast cancer, but further confirmatory studies need to be performed.

The possible link between breast cancer and birth-control pill use has been extensively researched. There have been conflicting reports and studies, some showing an increased risk and others, a decreased

" I had a mammogram last week just for a baseline. I am concerned about breast cancer since my mother had it. She also had a mastectomy, but she fully recovered. It was hard on the family."

risk. In general there does not seem to be a significant increased risk associated with the use of birth-control pills.

There are families where every woman has developed breast cancer. Recently, a gene mutation that seems to be responsible for these "inherited" breast cancers was isolated on chromosome 17q21. The gene is known as BRCA1. Women with this mutation are also at increased risk of developing ovarian cancer. Of women who have this gene, 85 percent will develop breast cancer in their lifetime. It is estimated that this gene mutation accounts for 5 percent of all breast cancer cases. Twenty-five percent of women who develop breast cancer when they are younger than 35 have this mutation.

Recently, a blood test for this gene mutation became available. The problem now is deciding who should have this test and who should pay for the testing. These are still areas of controversy and debate, but eventually guidelines will be issued. In July 1996, a test for another mutated gene, BRCA2, became available. BRCA2 also is associated with an increased risk of breast cancer, but not ovarian cancer.

Of the estimated 10 percent of breast cancers that are inherited, BRCA1 accounts for 45 percent and BRCA2 accounts for 35 percent of the cases. Therefore, any screening protocols will probably require use of both of these tests. A clearer role for these tests is expected by the year 1999.

HOW YOU SHOULD SCREEN YOURSELF FOR CANCER

Screening for breast cancer involves both you and your doctor. Without both of you doing your part, screening is less than ideal. Remember, breast cancer cannot be prevented, so the only hope for cure comes with early detection.

Regular Breast Exams

You should examine your breasts monthly, looking for lumps, nipple discharge, painful areas, "dimpling" of the skin or retraction of the nipples. These exams are best performed just after a period. It is easiest to check the breasts when they are wet and soapy, so check them in the bath or shower. Afterward, inspect them in front of a mirror, looking for dimpling inward of any skin areas. Finally, gently squeeze the nipples to check for a discharge. You should report any abnormalities to a heath-care provider for further evaluation.

The importance of breast self-exam cannot be overstated. Most breast cancers are found by the woman herself. The smaller the cancer when detected, the greater the possibility for cure. Recent studies have shown that the average size lump found in women with breast cancer who did not perform breast exams is about 1.5 inches across. In women who check their breasts only occasionally, the average size lump found is 1 inch. In women who do regular breast exams, the average size lump is 0.5 inches. The main reason women do not check their own breasts, according to a recent study, is because they are afraid of finding something. **Remember: 80 percent of breast lumps are benign.**

In addition to monthly self-exams, you should have an annual exam of your breasts performed by a trained heath-care provider. This is an excellent time to report or discuss any problems with your breasts that have occurred recently, no matter how trivial they seem.

Mammograms

Mammography is an X-ray evaluation of the breasts. It is performed both to screen for cancers and to investigate lumps and other suspicious breast changes. The American Cancer Society recommends a baseline mammogram at age 35. The baseline mammogram becomes an "old" or "normal" film to compare any future films with. The American Cancer Society also recommends a mammogram every one to two years from age 40 to 50, and annual mammograms every year after age 50. These should be used as minimum guidelines. Depending on your risk factors, more frequent screening may be ordered. It is generally felt that screening mammograms in women younger than 35 are not worthwhile. Mammograms are done at these ages only if there is an abnormality on exam or unusual family history. Mammograms are useful to detect lumps as small as ¼ inch in size. These lumps are so small they usually cannot be felt.

WHAT TO EXPECT DURING A MAMMOGRAM

The best time to get a mammogram is after a period, when the breasts are the least tender and lumpy. You should wear a two-piece outfit to the mammography center, and do not use any underarm deodorant.

The procedure is quick and straightforward. Before the mammogram, you remove your shirt and bra, and either put on a hospital gown or go without a top. At most centers, a trained female technician does the actual study. The technician shows you how the machine works to help you relax. She positions one of your breasts on the flat metal plate (unfortunately, this is usually cold), arranges your arms out of the way of the X-ray machine, and then lowers a clear plastic plate down onto your breast. This plate is pressure-sensitive; it applies a moderate amount of pressure to even out your breast tissue. This provides the ideal picture for the radiologist to review and interpret.

Once your breast is under this pressure plate, the technician moves behind a protective barrier. You then hold your breath, and the X-ray is taken in one second. With the picture taken, the plastic plate is released and your breast is freed. Two X-rays are taken of each breast – one with your breast compressed

from the top and one with your breast compressed from the side.
When X-rays have been taken of both breasts, you can
get dressed and are free to go home. Your results are sent to
your primary-care physician, and either your doctor or the
mammogram center informs you of the results.

All mammography centers in the United States must meet FDA guidelines for the quality of the equipment used. There is some variation, however, in the quality of interpretation of the mammograms. In most cities, there are now radiologists who specialize in reading mammograms. It is very helpful for a radiologist to have old films to compare with when reading a mammogram. Therefore, you should avoid going to a different center each year. Prior films should be provided to a new center when you go for a mammogram.

There are two main types of mammograms; screening and diagnostic. For a screening mammogram, you make your own appointment for a regular check as long as you fit within the age guidelines noted earlier (35 years old or older). If you need a diagnostic mammogram to evaluate a lump, your physician orders it. A radiologist is present at a diagnostic mammogram in case other X-rays or ultrasounds are needed to further evaluate a suspicious area or lump. In this situation, the radiologist usually contacts your physician directly to discuss the findings.

" I examine my breasts for lumps at least once a month because of my family history. My mother had breast cancer. I found a fibroid in one breast, and I was very upset because of the family history. It was scary."

If you are asked to return for further studies after a screening mammogram, this does not mean the radiologist suspects you have cancer. Additional films are sometimes needed or ultrasounds performed to help clarify findings on an initial screening. Most of the time, these additional studies yield benign findings.

Most mammography centers do not allow you to have a mammogram if you feel a lump unless you see your doctor first. This requirement ensures you have adequate follow-up. Mammograms are not 100-percent accurate, and the concern is that if you have a negative mammogram, you may not pursue working up a palpable lump.

A breast cancer may show up on a mammogram as a solid-looking lesion. Sometimes the radiologist can tell from the mammogram that the lesion is very likely cancerous. Many times, however, a lesion is read as "suspicious," and further diagnostic tests or a biopsy is required.

Calcifications are commonly seen on mammograms. These are associated with both benign and malignant conditions. Benign calcifications tend to be larger with round edges, while calcifications associated with cancer tend to be finer and more angular. A radiologist who specializes in reading mammograms can usually tell the difference between benign and malignant calcifications. Many times, however, a biopsy of the area is needed to rule out an associated cancer.

" With one less breast, I feel like half a woman. It affects my sense of womanhood."

Sometimes a radiologist requests a follow-up mammogram be performed in six months. In these situations, the radiologist is reasonably sure the lesion is benign. The follow-up mammogram is used to make sure no changes occur during this six-month interval.

HOW BREAST-CANCER TREATMENT HAS EVOLVED

The Shift Away from Radical Mastectomy

The treatment of breast cancer has undergone a tremendous change over the past 20 years. Previously, the only treatment was a radical surgical procedure where the entire breast, the underlying chest wall muscles and the local lymph nodes were removed. This procedure often has serious side effects, such as **lymphedema**, where there is permanent swelling of the arm due to disruption of the lymph drainage. It had long been recognized that the lymph nodes needed to be removed in order to increase the cure rate, and that if just the breast was removed the cancer recurred in the local lymph nodes. Therefore, the risks and severity of this procedure seemed justified. This procedure became known as the Halsted radical mastectomy, after the doctor who originally described it. This disfiguring surgery added to a woman's horror of developing breast cancer. Later studies showed the survival rates of women who had undergone radical mastectomy were no greater than those women whose breast cancer was treated by a combination of less invasive therapies. As a result, a shift toward less disfiguring surgery and breast-conserving treatments began.

A Newer Understanding of How Cancer Spreads

Study after study has shown that women with breast cancer rarely die of a local recurrence of their disease. Most die because of recurrent cancer in other parts of the body. These recurrences elsewhere are called **metastatic disease**.

When a cancer develops, it initially spreads to the surrounding tissues. It then usually spreads to the lymph nodes in the area. The lymph nodes act like filters and collect cancer cells that are escaping out of the breast. Initially the cancer is stopped at this first line of defense; however, with time the cancer cells spread out of the lymph nodes into the rest of the body. Surgery alone can only cure those cancers in which the cancer cells have not already spread out of the lymph nodes. Once a cancer cell has escaped, it may become lodged in the bone, liver or brain and become a metastatic lesion. It was therefore known that the "cure" rate for breast cancer was directly related to the chance that cancer cells had already escaped.

Studies have shown that this risk of metastatic disease increases as the size of the original cancer increases. In these studies, if the original cancer was less than 1 centimeter in size, the risk of recurrent disease proved to be 6 percent. If the original cancer was 1 to 2 centimeters, the risk of recurrent disease was 11 percent – even if the lymph nodes were "negative" (did not contain cancer cells) at the initial surgery.

Long-term follow-up studies in women who underwent radical surgery showed a direct correlation between the number of lymph nodes involved and the survival rate. If the lymph nodes were involved at the time of the initial surgery, the risk of future metastatic disease increased significantly. The more lymph nodes that were found to have cancer in them, the greater the risk of metastatic lesions. If the lymph nodes were "negative" at the time of the original surgery, the chance of survival at 10 years (living 10 years after surgery) was 70 percent. If one to three lymph nodes showed cancer, the chance of survival at 10 years dropped to 38 percent. If more then four nodes were involved, the chance of survival at 10 years dropped to only 13 percent.

Subsequently, it was recognized that if women were dying of metastatic cancer even with small tumors and no involved nodes, cancer cells must have already escaped into the rest of their bodies. This became known as **micro-metastasis**. With the recognition that a lot of breast cancers are not truly isolated in the spot where the tumor is found came a change in strategy: doctors realized that radical surgery was not always needed and that in most cases the goal of surgery is only to control local disease. Subsequently, in order to treat these micro-metastases, other treatments were added to the initial surgery. These additional treatments are known as **adjuvant therapy**. Adjuvant therapies aimed at treating micro-metastases have changed breast-cancer treatment dramatically.

Then other, less invasive (less radical) surgical procedures were combined with these adjuvant therapies. If you develop breast cancer today, you have several different treatment options, and new treatments are being developed each year. Usually a combination approach is taken, depending on the type and size of the tumor, your age and other factors.

WHICH ADJUVANT THERAPIES ARE AVAILABLE?

Radiation

Radiation treatments are used to kill cancer cells. Radiation therapy works by disrupting the DNA in dividing cells. Cancers that are most actively dividing are usually the most sensitive to radiation treatment. Cancer cells are also more sensitive to radiation because once they are damaged they have a harder time repairing themselves than normal tissue. This fact is important, because a lot of normal tissue is exposed to radiation during treatment, and this tissue needs to survive. Radiation treatments are therefore usually spaced out over time to allow normal tissues to heal before they are exposed to more radiation. Even so, tissues that have been exposed to radiation may show changes over time, such as pigmentation changes and hardness. One other concern is the possibility that the exposure to the radiation will cause other cancers to occur that otherwise would not have. You need to be aware of these risks when deciding on a course of treatment, but sometimes there are no ideal options.

Radiation treatments are usually used now instead of removing every lymph node that might have cancer in it. Sometimes only a sample of the lymph nodes are removed, and the rest are treated with radiation. This approach reduces the chance of swelling in the arm known as lymphedema that commonly occurs if all the lymph nodes in the arm are removed.

Chemotherapy

Like radiation, chemotherapy kills cells that are rapidly dividing, like cancer cells. There is not just one chemotherapy. Rather, chemotherapy is usually a combination of various drugs that have activity against breast cancer. Most of these medicines kill cancer cells and are given by IV, thereby having an effect on cancer cells everywhere in the body. With most types of chemotherapy, you have blood drawn to be analyzed, an IV placed and then the chemotherapy solution infused. Each type of chemotherapy has its own side effects. Some cause your hair to fall out, while others may affect your heart or the production of blood cells. You may experience nausea and vomiting after receiving chemotherapy. These are serious medications that are given to you by an oncologist after you have talked about how your cancer will be treated and which side effects you can expect. An oncologist is a specialized physician who treats all types of cancer. Treatments typically last from three to six months.

The most effective chemotherapy agent available today causes loss of hair. In the past, nausea and vomiting with the chemotherapy treatments were a major deterrent to some patients; however, newer anti-nausea medicines have decreased this side effect. One other side effect from chemotherapy is that many pre-menopausal women become menopausal due to the treatment. It seems the older you are, the more likely you are to become menopausal with chemotherapy treatment.

Chemotherapy reduces your risk of dying from cancer by 17 percent. This therapy seems most effective for people who are younger than 50. Unfortunately, cancer cells tend to develop a resistance to the same chemotherapy over time, and if cancer cells are not killed by the initial treatment, recurrence with time is inevitable.

Estrogen Removal

Researchers have looked for other predictors of failure of the surgery to cure breast cancer, since 30 percent of women still died of recurrent disease even if there were no "involved" nodes at the time of surgery. It was noted early on that many breast cancers had estrogen receptors in them. This fact is no surprise since the breasts are hormonally responsive and must contain these hormone receptors in order to develop in the first place. In women with breast cancer whose tumors had estrogen receptors in them, removing all estrogen from the system decreased the risk of recurrence. This was originally done by removing the ovaries or by treating them with radiation, known as **ovarian ablation**. Ovarian ablation works best in women younger than 50, and whose tumors are estrogen-receptor positive. In these women, the reduction in the annual risk of death is 25 percent. Another treatment, tamoxifen, binds to the estrogen receptors and blocks the action of estrogen. Tamoxifen works best in women who are older than 50, reducing their annual risk of death by 20 percent.

Combination Therapies

Studies underway combine these different adjuvant therapies in an attempt to boost the cure rate further. Trials comparing tamoxifen plus chemotherapy versus ovarian ablation plus chemotherapy show these combinations increase the cure rate even greater than either therapy alone. Unfortunately, all have long-term side effects. Tamoxifen increases the risk of endometrial (uterine) cancer. Ovarian ablation can cause osteoporosis, depression and cardiovascular disease. Therapy must be individualized, and you must fully understand the risks and benefits of each treatment.

WHAT THE SURGICAL OPTIONS ARE

Modified Radical Mastectomy

A modified radical mastectomy is now the most aggressive surgery done for breast cancer. The difference between the original Halsted radical mastectomy and the modified radical mastectomy is that the muscles of the chest wall are left in place. There is still a significant risk of lymphedema in the arm, since the lymph nodes are removed just as in the original procedure. Leaving the chest-wall muscles intact makes reconstruction of the breasts easier, and less dysfunction of the arm and shoulder occurs. This procedure is usually combined with adjuvant therapies in order to decrease the risk of recurrence.

" I had surgery, a radical mastectomy of one breast, and then I had four weeks of radiation. They removed the breast, telling me I could have it reconstructed in the months that followed, but I opted to have it done four years later, because psychologically I was not ready for another surgery. That was 13 years ago. "

Simple Mastectomy

A simple mastectomy is a procedure where just the breast is removed, and the lymph nodes and chest wall muscles remain. A simple mastectomy is usually combined with other adjuvant therapy, because for most cancers the mastectomy is insufficient by itself. Since the lymph nodes are not removed, they are treated by radiation therapy to destroy tumor cells and control local recurrences in the lymph nodes. Commonly, chemotherapy with or without hormonal therapy is combined with the surgery to treat possible micro-metastasis elsewhere in the body.

Simple mastectomy has been done for years in patients with carcinoma-in-situ of the breast (non-invasive cancer) and in patients with very high risk factors and a strong family history of breast cancer. In these situations, additional adjuvant therapy may not be needed since the risk of micro-metastasis is very low. However, recent recommendations are moving away from this approach toward more conservative, non-surgical over time protocols for these specific problems.

Lumpectomy

A lumpectomy is the minimal surgical treatment for small breast cancers where the risk of local recurrence in the breast itself is small. With this procedure, only the cancer and a small amount of the surrounding breast tissue are removed. The lymph nodes may be removed, or they may be treated with radiation therapy. The majority of the breast is left alone, and there is usually no noticeable disfiguration, other than a small scar. This treatment is almost always combined with chemotherapy, with or without hormonal therapies. For smaller cancers, lumpectomy preserves the breast and, when combined with appropriate adjuvant therapy, has an outcome as good as – if not better than – the outcome with more radical surgeries.

> *"I would tell other women to be courageous, to be willing to undergo surgery, not to give up hope and to fight against this disease. I recommend reconstructive surgery."*

HOW THE BREAST CAN BE RECONSTRUCTED AFTER BREAST-CANCER SURGERY

Unlike years ago, today women who undergo breast-cancer surgery have many options available to help restore their appearance. Reconstructive procedures are some of the most important treatments to discuss with a woman who has breast cancer. Because of the amount of attention and importance our society places on breasts, women who lose their breasts due to cancer commonly become depressed and withdrawn. These reconstructive procedures help many women regain a positive self-image quicker and allow them to lead a more normal life without the constant reminder they are breast-cancer survivors.

Many times the reconstructive surgery is done at the same time as the cancer surgery. Skilled plastic surgeons usually do the reconstructive work, working together with the general surgeons who do the cancer surgery. (In some parts of the country, gynecologic surgeons do the original cancer surgery.)

Breast Implants

One of the simplest reconstructions is the placement of implants under the skin. In the past, these plastic-type bags were filled with either silicon or water; recently, silicon implants were withdrawn from the market in this country. An implant creates some problem in detecting a recurrent cancer under the implant by a physical exam alone. However, your follow-up after treatment for breast cancer includes frequent mammograms as well as a physical exam.

In many situations after mastectomy, there is too large a defect for implants to be effective right away. In these situations, the skin is closed after surgery but tissue expanders are placed under the skin. These can be enlarged over time by injecting through the skin. The surrounding skin and tissue slowly stretch, allowing the surgeon to either place implants later or do other reconstructive procedures.

Flap Procedures

Now there are several "flap" procedures performed. The most common of these is known as a TRAM flap. With this procedure, after the breast is removed, excess tissue of the lower abdomen (muscle, fat and skin) is moved to create a "new" breast and fill the defect formed by the mastectomy. This flap of tissue is carefully formed to recreate as closely as possible a normally shaped and sized breast. Later, a second operation is done to create a new nipple. Sometimes this is combined with either a reduction or implant of the other "normal" breast to allow you to feel good about the outcome.

Conclusion

Throughout this chapter, your breasts are discussed as if they were separate from your body, and nothing could be further from the truth. Your breasts are an integral part of your body as it relates to your self-image as well as to your ability to nourish your children. They are central to your sense of being a woman and feeling sensual. The fact that so many different problems occur to the breasts – most benign but some very serious – makes dedicating an entire chapter to this subject appropriate. Breast cancer is the number-two cause of cancer deaths among women, so it is impossible to overstress the importance of regular exams, mammograms and medical attention to anything that seems out of the ordinary to you.

If you are over age 25 and have a breast lump that has not been sampled in some way, please get a second opinion to make sure your health-care provider has not overlooked a problem. If two physicians agree you do not need a biopsy, then you can feel more reassured. This advice may sound unusual coming from a physician, but every good physician should welcome your need to get a second opinion.

Additional Resources
Books

*   **The Nursing Mother's Companion,** *Kathleen Huggins,* Harvard Common Press, 1995.

*   **Breast Cancer,** *Elaine Landau,* F. Watts, 1995.

*   **Breast Self-Exam,** *Albert R. Milan,* Workman, 1980.

*   **The Complete Book of Breast Care**, *Niels Laurersen,* Fawcett Columbine, 1996.

*   **A Practical Guide to Human Cancer Genetics,** *S.V. Hodgson and E.R.. Maher,* Cambridge University Press, 1993.

Organizations

*   **National Cancer Institute's Cancer Information Service** (800) 4-CANCER
    This organization gives the names of certified mammography providers in your area, and you can ask them for support-group suggestions.

*   **American Cancer Society** National Headquarters 1599 Clifton Road, N.E. Atlanta, Georgia 30329 (404) 320-3333
    The Society can recommend and give you the numbers of local support groups.

- **National Lymphedema Network**
  Suite 3, 2215 Post Street
  San Francisco, California 94115
  (800) 541-3259
  This organization helps women with lymphedema learn about up-to-date treatment options.

- **National Coalition for Cancer Survivorship**
  1010 Wayne Avenue, Suite 505
  Silver Spring, Maryland 20910
  VOICE: (301) 650-8868 FAX: (301) 565-9670
  This organization helps cancer survivors and their families start local support groups or contact existing ones, sponsors a clearinghouse of national resources for support and information on life after a cancer diagnosis, provides advice to reduce cancer-based discrimination, and serves as a unified voice of cancer survivors.

- **Y-ME's**
  (800) 221-2141
  This organization has a national support hotline where you can speak with a breast-cancer survivor.

Internet Sites

- **http://nysernet.org/bcic/**
  Breast Cancer Information. This site gives medical information, lists of health-care providers, 1-800 hotlines, support group, and political updates.

- **http://nysernet.org/bcic/nci/bcpubs/after-bc-90-2400/ resources.html**
  After Breast Cancer: A Guide to Follow-up Care. This site, provided by the U.S. Department of Health and Human Services, is full of resources and publications available from the National Cancer Institute.

- **http://www.cancernews.com/breast.htm**
  This site provides links to information ranging from breast self-exam to breast-cancer treatment and cancer prevention, as well as a link about tamoxifen.

CANCER SCREENING & PREVENTION

Learning to Save Your Own Life

Cancer is one of the scariest things that we all fear may happen to us or our loved ones. You may know someone who has had to face the challenges that the diagnosis of cancer brings, both physically and emotionally. In order to minimize your risk of having advanced cancer, you must take a proactive approach to your health. Please read this chapter to learn how to reduce your risk of cancer and how to detect a cancer at a very early stage. The earlier a cancer is detected, the greater your chance of cure. Do not let the fear of cancer prevent you from establishing a cancer-prevention and early-detection plan for yourself and every woman in your life.

According to the National Cancer Institute, more than half a million Americans died of cancer in 1997, approximately half of them women. In addition, nearly 600,000 women were newly diagnosed with cancer the same year. Considering these statistics, more than 3,000 women either died of or were diagnosed with cancer *every day* in 1997. With numbers like these, you probably know someone whose life has been touched by cancer.

The good news is that overall death rates due to cancer are very slowly declining, in large part because of screening tests that detect cancers earlier, when they are more easily treated and cured. Unfortunately, most Americans do not put into practice what we know to be good prevention against cancer.

In this chapter, we:

❧ Discuss risk factors for different cancers – those personal characteristics that predispose you toward a particular disease

❧ Describe warning symptoms of the most common malignancies in women

❧ Review screening tests – usually inexpensive, non-invasive tests that can be performed in the office to assist in early detection of cancer and

❧ Share tips for cancer prevention

Included are the latest information on genetic screening tests for breast and ovarian cancer, and a discussion of the relationship between human papilloma virus (HPV) and cervical cancer.

Before beginning, you should have a basic understanding of what cancer is and know a few definitions to make reading the sections on family history and cancer risk more accessible.

Your cells divide and multiply in order to maintain healthy tissue. For example, dead skin cells slough off from your skin's surface and are replaced by cells underneath. Almost all cells have cycles of rest and growth, and a cell's **DNA** (or genetic material) controls this cycle. **Cancer** arises from a single cell that loses control of its own growth — analogous to a switch stuck in the "on" position. Cancer does not develop overnight, because it generally takes many years to develop the abnormalities in the DNA, which eventually alter the growth "switch." In other words, it is a multi-step process. When we talk about **inherited cancers**, we refer to DNA changes (called **mutations**) in the "switches" that can be passed from parent to child and predispose us to cancer. Cancer may develop from additional mutations that come from years of exposure to chemicals, poor diet, tobacco smoke, etc. Most cancers are not inherited and result from being exposed too long to irritants or

> *"Cancer is in our family – a lot of lung cancer, a lot of colon cancer. Lung cancer was from the smoking. They all passed away. I don't smoke."*

for unknown reasons.

Finally, when we talk about **first-degree relatives**, we mean your parents, siblings and children; **second-degree** refers to grand-parents, aunts, uncles and cousins.

Lung Cancer
WHO GETS IT?

Lung cancer is the leading cause of cancer death in women. This year, 66,000 women will die from lung cancer. Despite the connection between tobacco use and cancer, more than 22 million American

" When people in my generation started smoking 30 years ago, nobody said it was bad for your health. We just thought it was cool. But it's hard for me to understand why anybody would start today."

women smoke cigarettes, putting themselves at 12 times the risk of dying of lung cancer as women who have never smoked. Women who smoke cigarettes, pipes or cigars, or who use chewable to-bacco are also more likely to develop cancers of the mouth and throat, kidney and bladder, pancreas and cervix.

Ninety-five percent of all lung cancers are made up of four ma-jor cell types: squamous cell, small cell, large cell and adenocarci-noma (glandular) cell. More than 90 percent of people with lung cancer of all cell types are cigarette smokers; the rare non-smoker who develops lung cancer usually has adenocarcinoma. **There are no tests to reliably detect lung cancer at an early stage.** Lung can-cer spreads quickly, when the initial tumors are very small. Lung cancer is not considered an inherited cancer; however, if several smokers in your family have lung cancer, or you have multiple relatives with other types of cancer, and you also smoke, your risk of developing lung cancer is greater than the average smoker's.

HOW TO DETECT IT

If you are a smoker and notice any of these symptoms, see your doctor immediately. The doctor may order a chest X-ray or request a sample of your sputum to look for abnormal lung cells. If either one of these tests shows abnormal results, your doctor obtains a biopsy of the tissue by either placing a lighted tube through your airway and into your lungs or by passing a needle through your chest wall into the tissue. If the biopsy shows you have cancer, you and your doctor will discuss treatment options such as surgery to remove as much of the cancer as possible, chemotherapy and radiation therapy.

THE WARNING SYMPTOMS OF LUNG CANCER

🦋 *Persistent cough*

🦋 *Sputum streaked with blood*

🦋 *Multiple attacks of pneumonia or bronchitis*

🦋 *Wheezing*

🦋 *Chest pain, especially with deep breathing*

🦋 *Shortness of breath*

🦋 *Unexplained fever or weight loss*

🦋 *Hoarseness*

HOW TO PREVENT IT

Since there are no good tests available to detect lung cancer at the stage when it is curable, and the overwhelming majority of lung cancers occur in smokers, the best way to reduce your risk of developing lung cancer is to never smoke or to quit if you do. Ten years after you quit smoking, your lung-cancer risk is reduced to that of a non-smoker. Use this information to help motivate you to quit.

Studies show that most smokers want to quit and have tried to stop unsuccessfully in the past. If this is true for you, take heart: the same research suggests that the more you try, the more likely you are to be successful. So be persistent and try, try again!

MORE REASONS TO QUIT SMOKING

Money

The financial rewards of smoking cessation are considerable. A pack-a-day smoker spends approximately $1.50 per day to smoke if she buys cigarettes by the carton. If you place this money weekly in a

---

savings account or money-market account at a measly 3-percent interest, you would have almost $600 at the end of one year. Think about what this money could mean in 10 or 20 years if placed in a retirement or mutual fund… a new car, a family trip or an educational degree.

Healthier Children

Your family and friends also benefit if you give up cigarettes. Exhaled or "second-hand" smoke is unhealthy because it contains the same 2,500 chemicals found in inhaled smoke, including carbon monoxide, arsenic and nicotine. Children in homes where at least one parent smokes have more colds and ear infections, and are more likely to become smokers them-

> " I have a friend whose baby was premature, and she brought him home hooked up to monitors that went off if he had trouble breathing. I found it so sad and ironic to see her put down a cigarette to rush to his side when that thing began beeping."

selves. Since adolescence is the critical period during which most women begin to smoke, you can have a major impact on your children's choices by setting a good example.

Other Health Benefits

If you stop smoking, you also enjoy improved fertility as well as a reduction in your risk of coronary artery disease (heart attack), premature menopause, and miscarriage. If you smoke while pregnant, you increase your risk of having a low-birthweight baby, early rupture of the amniotic sac or premature separation of the placenta. Some of these complications could be fatal for your baby. You can significantly reduce your risk of these events by quitting smoking.

HOW TO QUIT

Plan Your Strategy

Should you go "cold turkey" or taper gradually? Use the patch? The best way to quit is going to be different for everyone. Planning a strategy, though, should be a key component for every woman who tries. Use all of the resources available to you – your physician, family and friends, educational materials and support groups. At the end of this chapter are names and phone numbers of organizations with smoking cessation kits, videos and information on support groups in your area.

Pick a Date

Smoking cessation counselors recommend that you pick a quit date about four weeks in the future. Talk to your doctor to see if you are a good candidate for nicotine patches. If you have a cigarette within 30 minutes of rising in the morning, or you smoke a pack or more a day, you are addicted to nicotine and would benefit from using the patch. An antidepressant, Zyban, has recently been approved by the FDA for use as a smoking-cessation aid. It reduces cigarette cravings and alleviates anxiety symptoms commonly experienced during nicotine withdrawal. You may want to ask your doctor for more information.

Avoid Situations Where You Smoke

Think carefully about the times you smoke and what triggers your desire for a cigarette. Is it stress? Being with with a particular group of friends? A particular time of day? If you can identify your smoking triggers, you can plan ahead to avoid them. Plan to stay busy and exercise a little every day. Drink plenty of fluids. Develop a new hobby. Notify family and friends about your desire to quit, and join a support group through the American Lung Association or the American Cancer Society.

Prepare For The Side Effects

What can you expect to experience when you give up cigarettes? Nicotine withdrawal is responsible for most of the unpleasant symptoms you might have. These symptoms can include feeling blue, irritable, anxious, restless and hungry; and gaining weight. Many women who quit do report eating more: food may taste better, or eating may relieve tension. Be prepared — exercise, stay busy, keep low-calorie snacks around or try chewing gum.

While going through this time, please remember there is no advice in this entire book more important to your enjoyment of a healthy and happy life than this issue of quitting smoking. Good luck!

Women's Health: Your Guide to a Healthier and Happier Life

Breast Cancer
HOW OFTEN IT OCCURS

Cancer of the breast afflicts 1 woman in 8, and it is the second most common cause of cancer death in women, after lung cancer. In 1997, approximately 180,200 new cases of breast cancer were diagnosed – a number that reflects an increase in the incidence of breast cancer. The death rate has remained constant, which suggests more women are being cured.

WHAT INCREASES YOUR RISK

Some of the risk factors for breast cancer relate to levels of estrogen you are exposed to throughout life. Estrogen stimulates growth in certain types of tissue, such as glands in the breast and uterus. The following list summarizes the risk factors for breast cancer.

Age

The risk of developing breast cancer increases steadily as you grow older. Breast cancer is uncommon in women in their 20s. The risk increases to 1 in 65 for women in their 40s, 1 in 29 in their 60s, and is 1 in 8 in their 80s.

Reproductive History

The longer you have menstrual cycles, the higher your risk of developing breast cancer. If you menstruated for 40 years – you began having periods earlier than the average age of 12 or 13, and you went through menopause after 50 – then your risk of breast cancer is greater than that of a woman who menstruated for only 20 years because she had to have her uterus and ovaries removed in her 30s. Childbearing reduces your cancer risk, and the earlier your age at pregnancy, the greater the reduction in risk. Breast-feeding, pregnancy termination and oral contraceptives do not increase your risk of getting breast cancer.

Diet

Consumption of a high-fat diet and more than one alcoholic drink per day has been linked to increased breast-cancer risk. Obesity also has been linked to breast cancer, possibly because fatty tissue

" I had just turned 30 when I was diagnosed. I knew I was at risk beforehand, because my mom had cancer when she was 31. And then about a year ago, two of her sisters had breast cancer as well. I found my own with self-exam. When I was interested in getting a mammogram at 30, they told me I was too young. And when I switched gynecologists, I told them, 'I feel two lumps and they hurt, and since my mom had cancer and it's in my family, I want to do something about it.' And they said, 'No problem; we'll go ahead and get you in.' I had a mammogram and also an ultrasound, and they actually found a third lump in the same breast."

produces a form of estrogen that is metabolically active.

Previous Breast Cancer

If you have previously been diagnosed with breast cancer, you are at very high risk for being diagnosed with breast cancer in the other breast. Breast cancer of the lobular type is more likely to occur in both breasts than ductal breast cancer. Fibrocystic change is a benign breast condition that is not associated with an increase risk of breast cancer unless a past biopsy showed atypical or precancerous cells. More information on non-cancerous and precancerous breast conditions is presented in Chapter 7, "Breast Health."

Family History

If your first-degree relative had breast cancer after menopause, your own risk is not significantly increased. However, when the relative's breast cancer occurred before menopause, your risk increases 30 percent if the cancer was in one breast, and 40 to 50 percent if it occurred in both breasts.

There are five known changes in your chromosomes that predispose you to breast cancer. Mutations in genes known as BRCA1 and BRCA2 are the most common inheritable defects associated with breast cancer. When they are in their normal form, these genes help prevent cancer. If you inherit a mutated form of these genes, they lose their protective effect, and you have as high as a 90-percent lifetime chance of developing breast cancer. Approximately 1 in 50 women of Ashkenazi descent carry one of the two defective genes.

How do you know if you carry these defective genes? A number of commercial labs perform highly technical analyses of your chromosomes from a blood sample, looking for mutations in your BRCA genes. However, at present the usefulness of this test is severely limited because the results are difficult to interpret. Your chance of having an abnormal BRCA gene is increased in the following situations:

- *Having ovarian cancer in the family*
- *Having a family member with both breast and ovarian cancer*
- *Being diagnosed with breast cancer at an early age*
- *Being of Ashkenazi Jewish ancestry*

If you fit the above description, you may be a candidate for this test. Talk to your doctor, who can help you schedule an appointment with a cancer-genetics counselor (see the mailing and Internet addresses for the National Society of Genetics Counselors at the end of this chapter). Together, the three of you can decide if you should have the test and interpret the results when they return.

WHAT THE SYMPTOMS ARE

Most breast masses do not cause pain or a discharge, which is why performing breast exams is so important. In addition to breast lumps, be aware of the following warning signs of breast cancer:

- *Nipple discharge, bleeding or pain*
- *A change in size or contour of one of your breasts*
- *Nipple distortion, retraction or scaliness*

HOW TO DETECT IT

The topic of breast cancer-screening is thoroughly covered in Chapter Seven, "Breast Health." Breast-cancer screening consists of the breast self-exam, the professional exam and mammography.

Surviving Breast Cancer

*I am 48, and I was diagnosed with breast cancer six years ago. I
didn't know I was at risk. I didn't have regular physical exams. I
would normally go to the doctor when I was sick. It might be two
years in between exams. I had had one mammogram before,
because I had found a lump. The first lump was nothing – it was
a cyst, and they aspirated that. Then, a year later, I didn't feel
any lump; it was just time for my second mammogram.*

*I'm a runner, so I am more in tune with my body and its reac-
tions. I started feeling strange. Normally, I could run 15 miles;
now, after a few miles I had to stop. I felt a burning sensation in
my breast. All these things made me think. So I made another
appointment for a mammogram. After that, I went to the surgeon immediately. I had a lumpectomy and radiation and chemotherapy at the same time.*

*I felt terrified at the time of diagnosis. The surgeon told me in the
recovery room that she looked over the pathologist's shoulder
because she felt the lump was malignant. So she told us before we
even left the hospital, and then I didn't have to wait. That was
very good. And I guess after the shock wore off, it seemed like I
was able to pull myself together even before my husband did. As I
look back on it now, I think I separated myself from what was
going on. It was like it was happening to someone else.*

*The lumpectomy was in August, and I had my last chemotherapy
treatment on December 31st, about five months later. My family
was very supportive. My husband, my son and daughter, they
were wonderful. I have very close friends. My parents, of course,
my in-laws – all of them were supportive.*

*Basically, I just wanted to be around people. All of the sudden –
even though I kind of separated myself with what was going on
and it really wasn't me that was sick in my mind – I realized how
very important all these people were to me. And, you know, they*

called and sent cards. They visited. People took me to the grocery store. They took me to have my hair done. I was always surrounded. Plus I was working, and everyone at work was the same way. They made me take a nap every afternoon. They did my work for me a lot.

I keep going back to what my husband said one time: "We were supposed to grow old together, and that's my plan, just for us to grow old together. And nothing can happen to you." And he didn't care that I didn't have any hair, that I had no energy. He just wanted me to get well.

One of the great, great things in the middle of all the chemo-therapy, was that a friend and I ran a race. And it was just a 3-mile race. After a mile and a half, she would just hold me, and we were crying, and there must have been 15 to 20 friends waiting for us at the end. You know, you just forget how important family and friends are. And how grateful you are for the sunset and the rain and the wind. I guess it just makes you more aware of everything around you.

For the first five years, I was terrified the cancer would return. But now, it's not that big a deal. I go to the oncologist once a year now, and I had a mammogram this year. I worry about my daughter, of course. I need to make sure she knows those risk factors.

Breast self-exams are monthly exams you perform on your own breasts, chest wall and armpits beginning at 18 years of age. The goal of these exams is to familiarize you with what your normal breast tissue feels like so that if anything changes, you know you need to be evaluated as early as possible. You should perform these exams several days after your period ends, when your breasts are least swollen and tender.

Also beginning at age 18, you should have annual professional breast exams by a doctor or other health-care professional.

Routine screening mammography begins between 35 and 40 years of age with a baseline film, increases to every other year between 40 and 49 years of age and takes place annually after age 50. If you have risk factors for breast cancer, discuss with your doctor whether more frequent screening is warranted.

Colorectal Cancer

HOW COMMON IS IT?

Cancer of the colon and rectum is the third highest cause of cancer death in women. You have a 1-in-17 chance of ever developing this type of malignancy. The majority of cases occur sporadically, meaning they are not inherited. Excellent screening tests are available to detect colon cancer in its early stages, and healthy eating habits (to be discussed later) are a known preventive measure.

HOW TO DETECT IT

The presenting symptoms of carcinoma of the colon and rectum are rectal bleeding (either visible blood in your stool or noted on rectal exam at the doctor's office), abdominal pain, change in bowel habits, nausea, vomiting, abdominal swelling or bloating, weight loss, fatigue and anemia. If you have any of these symptoms, consult with your physician immediately for a full physical exam and possibly a **sigmoidoscopy** or **colonoscopy**. These are tests where a flexible tube is inserted into your rectum in order to look for precancerous or cancerous growths in your colon. With sigmoidoscopy, the tube looks through your rectum and up into the lower one-third of your large bowel. With colonoscopy, the tube extends further, looking at your entire large bowel.

The goal of these studies is to find a problem at an early stage, allowing either a cure of the cancer or the removal of any areas that are about to become a cancer. By having your rectal exams annually each year after age 40 and a screening sigmoidoscopy every three to five years after age 50, you reduce your risk of dying from colon cancer by 70 percent.

WHAT TO EXPECT DURING COLONOSCOPY OR SIGMOIDOSCOPY

With either test, you are first given medication to make you relax, to prevent your bowel from going into spasm and to help you not remember having the test. Plan to have someone drive you home after this test. You are positioned on your side, with your knees pulled up toward your chest. Your anal opening and the scope are well-lubricated. The physician inserts a finger into your rectum and gently slides in the tube. The tube is advanced from your rectum into your large bowel. While advancing the tube, the doctor inflates the bowel with air. It is this air in your bowel that makes this test uncomfortable, as it gives you cramps like gas pain. The doctor inspects the lining of your intestinal tract as the tube is inserted and also while it is removed. If any abnormalities are noted, a biopsy is taken to see if you have an early cancer or any precancerous changes.

WHAT INCREASES YOUR RISK?

Your risk for colon cancer increases if you have:

- ♣ *Inflammatory bowel disease such as ulcerative colitis or Crohn's disease*
- ♣ *A history of radiation treatments to your pelvis (for treatment of other cancers, not just having an X-ray of your abdomen)*
- ♣ *A family history of colorectal cancer*
- ♣ *A personal history of breast, ovarian, endometrial or colon cancer*
- ♣ *A personal history of colon polyps*

If any of the above conditions apply to you, you should discuss colorectal cancer screening with your physician (see the American Cancer Society guidelines on page 220) in order to tailor testing to your particular needs.

AMERICAN CANCER SOCIETY GUIDELINES

The American Cancer Society Recommends These Screening Guidelines for Colorectal Cancer:

🐾 If you are age 50 or older and have no family history of colorectal cancer, you should have a yearly digital rectal exam, yearly test for blood in your stool (a fecal occult blood test) and sigmoidoscopy. If the sigmoidoscopy is normal, it should be repeated every three to five years; otherwise it should be repeated in one year to make sure there are no new polyps.

🐾 If you have a family history of colorectal cancer (one or more first-degree relatives), the above testing should be started at age 40.

The majority of colorectal carcinomas develop from an initially benign growth called an **adenomatous polyp**. Nineteen percent of the general population develops these polyps.

Less than 10 percent of colorectal cancers are inherited as problems with your chromosomes such as the BRCA gene changes. There are two inherited syndromes your physician looks for in your history: familial adenomatous polyposis (FAP) and hereditary nonpolyposis colorectal carcinoma (HNPCC). The HNPCC is characterized by a history of colon cancer in three first-degree relatives in two generations. At least one of the cancers occurs in someone less than 50 years old. HNPCC has two variants — Lynch Syndrome I, where cancers are confined to the colon, and Lynch Syndrome II, where, in addition to colon cancer, relatives also have cancers of the endometrium, breast, pancreas and gallbladder.

If you have a family history of these types of cancers, your risk for having colorectal cancer (as well as these other cancers) is increased. The American Cancer Society recommends you follow these screening guidelines:

& *If you have a known family history of FAP, each member of the family should have annual rectal exams and sigmoidoscopy or colonoscopy **starting at age 10**. If no polyps are found, these tests are repeated every three to five years. If polyps are seen, colonoscopy is performed annually.*

& *If your family history is consistent with HNPCC, screening is the same as above but should start in the late teen years.*

HOW IT IS TREATED

The treatment of colon cancer is surgical removal of the involved section of your intestine. Depending on the location, size of the cancer and whether cancer cells have spread to the liver, you may need additional treatment with chemotherapy. The details of treatment vary for each person, and your surgeon will describe your options if you develop colon cancer.

Uterine Cancer
HOW COMMON IS IT?

There were 34,900 cases of uterine cancer in the United States in 1997, making it the most common malignancy of the female reproductivity tract. Seventy-five percent of uterine cancers occur in postmenopausal women. Uterine cancers are divided into two broad categories — those

" I had an anal hemorrhage. I could not have a colonoscopy because I had diverticulitis, but I had a barium enema and that showed a mass. I was not too surprised because of the cancer in my family and my age. I was 76 when the cancer was discovered. I had 18 inches of my intestines taken out. Then I had a year of chemotherapy. I finished the treatment in 1990. I was in treatment every week for a year. I had sores in my mouth, I had nausea and fatigue. But I could rest. I did what I had to do."

involving the muscle of the uterus, called **sarcomas,** and those related to the endometrium (lining of the uterus), called **adenocarcinomas.** Sarcomas are uncommon (representing 3 percent of uterine cancers) and have no certain predisposing factors; therefore, the remainder of this discussion will focus on endometrial cancer.

WHAT INCREASES YOUR RISK?

Roughly half of all endometrial cancers occur in women with risk factors. Endometrial cancer is similar to breast cancer in regard to risk factors, because estrogen made by the ovaries or taken orally stimulates the lining of the uterus, causing it to grow. Progesterone prevents growth of the endometrium; it is made by the ovaries if you menstruate regularly or is taken orally with hormone replacement therapy.

Any factor that increases exposure to estrogen or decreases exposure to progesterone increases the risk of endometrial cancer. These risk factors include beginning menstruation at an early age, going through menopause late, taking estrogen supplementation without progesterone, having ovarian tumors (they make estrogen) and having irregular menstrual cycles (increased estrogen and low progesterone levels characterize irregular cycles). If you have never been pregnant, the uninterrupted stimulation of estrogen from repetitive menstrual cycles also increases your risk of uterine cancer. Use of tamoxifen, a breast-cancer treatment drug, likewise increases the risk of endometrial cancer. This drug stimulates the lining of the uterus in the same fashion as estrogen.

Obesity increases estrogen exposure because fatty tissue contains an enzyme that manufactures a form of estrogen called **estrone.** Estrone also stimulates the endometrium to grow. The level of risk is related to the degree of obesity; risk increases ten-fold for women who are more than 50 pounds overweight. Consumption of a high-fat diet also is linked to endometrial cancer.

Finally, as discussed previously with breast and colon cancer, individuals with family members who have had colon, breast or uterine cancers may have a gene that predisposes them to uterine cancer as part of the Lynch II syndrome.

WHO SHOULD BE SCREENED?

The American Cancer Society does not recommend testing all women for endometrial cancer because testing is neither cost-effective nor warranted. There are, however, certain groups for whom screening is justified. You should be screened for endometrial cancer if you:

- ♣ *Are postmenopausal and take estrogen without progesterone*
- ♣ *Experience postmenopausal bleeding*
- ♣ *Are obese*
- ♣ *Experienced menopause after 52*
- ♣ *Have family members with colon, breast, ovarian or uterine cancer*
- ♣ *Are over age 40 and have bleeding between periods*
- ♣ *Are over 40 and have increasingly heavy periods*
- ♣ *Have endometrial cells on a Pap smear*

All women with bleeding after menopause should be screened for endometrial cancer. The likelihood that postmenopausal bleeding is caused by endometrial cancer is dependent on your age: 9 percent if you are in your 50s, 16 percent in your 60s, 28 percent in your 70s, and 60 percent in your 80s.

HOW SCREENING IS PERFORMED
Endometrial Biopsy

Most of the time, evaluation for endometrial cancer is performed in the office with an endometrial biopsy. A thin, flexible plastic device is inserted through your cervix into the uterus to obtain endometrial tissue. You are placed in the same position as for a Pap smear. You can expect to feel mild to moderate cramping when the soft plastic tube is placed through the cervix and again when the biopsy is taken. The tissue is examined microscopically by a pathologist. Occasionally, the cervix is too tight to allow passage of this device comfortably, and you need to undergo surgical dilation of the cervix and endometrial sampling by curettage, or "D & C." This procedure is usually done under general anesthesia, or with a spinal as an outpatient.

Depending on your age, the symptoms of your bleeding and your general health, your doctor may elect to perform hysteroscopy or transvaginal ultrasound to evaluate bleeding in addition to or instead of an endometrial biopsy.

Hysteroscopy

Hysteroscopy is a visual exam of the inside of the uterus using a lighted scope. It is useful in identifying polyps (fragile, benign gland growths that can cause irregular bleeding), fibroids and cancer. With this procedure, commonly done in the office setting, you are placed in the same position as for a Pap smear. Your cervix is made numb with lidocaine and slightly dilated. A metal scope is inserted through your cervix and into the uterus. The scope has a light, and sterile saline or CO_2 gas is infused to dilate the uterine cavity. This procedure allows excellent visualization of the uterine lining.

Transvaginal Ultrasound

A transvaginal ultrasound is used to measure the thickness of the uterine lining. An endometrial thickness less than 5 millimeters has a very low chance of being cancer. While the presence of a thin endometrial lining is reassuring, few physicians feel this finding alone is enough evidence that you do not have a polyp or cancer. The reliability of this test is being evaluated, and until we feel confident we are not missing women with cancer, I suggest this test not be used without additional tests such as the endometrial biopsy.

Sonohysterography

A new method to evaluate the lining of the uterus is sonohysterography. With this procedure, a small plastic catheter is inserted through your cervix and into the uterus. Sterile saline is inserted, dilating the uterine cavity and allowing an excellent view of the lining of the uterus with the ultrasound. Polyps or other growths that are difficult to see with routine ultrasound stand out clearly when the uterine cavity is filled like a water balloon. The advantage of this procedure over hysteroscopy is that your cervix does not have to be dilated as much since a small catheter is used, resulting in less discomfort.

I still feel an endometrial biopsy is needed to rule out cancer. Many physicians prefer the hysteroscopy because it allows them to actually see inside the uterus.

HOW IT IS TREATED

If you are diagnosed with endometrial cancer, your doctor will recommend surgery to remove your uterus, fallopian tubes and ovaries in order to determine the extent of spread or stage of the cancer. You may also have lymph nodes removed from within your pelvis at the time of surgery for the same purpose. After surgery, depending on the stage and other prognostic factors, your doctor may advise you to have radiation therapy to improve your chances of being cured.

Ovarian Cancer

HOW COMMON IS IT?

The death of comedienne Gilda Radner from ovarian cancer focused a good deal of attention on this form of cancer in the 1980s. You may already know that ovarian cancer is less common than endometrial cancer, but that it is responsible for more deaths per year: 14,200 women were expected to die of ovarian cancer in 1997, and 26,800 were expected to be diagnosed. The high death rate is due to the fact that ovarian cancer is without symptoms in its early stages; more than two-thirds of cases present with advanced disease. In addition, there are no good screening tests to detect ovarian cancer in women without symptoms.

WHAT THE SYMPTOMS ARE

The symptoms of ovarian cancer develop late and are often vague and difficult to relate specifically to the ovaries. You might experience menstrual irregularities, changes in bladder or bowel habits, abdominal swelling, pelvic pain or pressure, or painful intercourse.

WHAT INCREASES YOUR RISK?

Your lifetime risk of ovarian cancer is 1 percent. That risk increases very slightly if you have never had children, have frequently used talcum powder on the genital area, consume a high-fat diet, have used fertility drugs for a very long time, are descended of Ashkenazi Jewish ancestry, or are very tall.

Approximately 5 percent of ovarian cancers are inherited; therefore, having family members with ovarian cancer is also a risk factor for developing the disease yourself. There are three hereditary patterns of ovarian cancer: a site-specific familial ovarian cancer, a breast and ovarian cancer syndrome, and the Lynch II syndrome (discussed previously in this chapter in the section on endometrial cancer). Some of the inherited ovarian cancers are due to the BRCA1 and BRCA2 mutations mentioned previously, for which a blood test is now available. The same precautions regarding genetics testing for breast cancer discussed earlier apply to ovarian cancer as well. You should be tested only after discussion with your physician and a session with a genetics counselor who specializes in cancer genetics (see the National Cancer Institute web site for information or write to the National Society of Genetic Counselors; these addresses are listed in the Resources at the end of this chapter). The test results could have a profound affect on you emotionally, financially and socially. You could lose your health insurance or your job, have unnecessary surgery, suffer depression, or be afraid to start a family for fear of passing on the defective gene.

HOW IT IS TREATED

The treatment of ovarian cancer involves the surgical removal of the uterus, tubes, ovaries and a layer of fat in your abdomen called the omentum. After surgery you are given chemotherapy. Radiation therapy is rarely used to treat ovarian cancer.

WHEN OVARIAN CANCER RUNS IN YOUR FAMILY

If you have a strong family history of ovarian cancer,
The American College of Obstetricians and Gynecologists
recommends the following:

☙ *If you want to have children, you should have screening*
with a vaginal ultrasound every six months [age not
specified]. If you are putting off childbearing, you may
want to use birth-control pills for contraception since
they have been shown to be protective in low-risk women.
You should consider having your ovaries removed when
your family is complete.

☙ *If you are in a family with a known familial ovarian or*
hereditary breast and ovarian cancer syndrome and you
do not want children, you should consider having your
ovaries removed. Unfortunately, having this surgery does
not guarantee you cancer protection, but it greatly
reduces the risk.

Measuring blood levels of Ca-125, a protein frequently produced on the surface of ovarian cancers, has not shown to
be a good screening test because many benign conditions,
such as fibroids and endometriosis, cause elevated levels.

Cervical Cancer
HOW COMMON IS IT?

The gradual decline in cervical cancer over the years is a tribute to
the success of the Pap smear as a screening test. Since its introduction
into medical practice in the 1940s, rates of invasive cervical cancer have
decreased by 50 percent, while diagnosis and treatment of precancerous cervical changes – known as dysplasia or cervical intraepithelial
neoplasia (CIN) – have increased.

HOW CERVICAL CANCER DEVELOPS

The most common cervical cancers arise from squamous cells, the same type your skin is made of. Just as are other cancers, cervical cancer is the result of a multi-step process. It begins with the introduction of human papilloma virus (HPV) into the cells of your cervix through exposure during sexual intercourse. HPV is the same virus that causes venereal warts, but it is very rare for women to get warts after exposure to this virus. Nearly 50 percent of women carry the HPV virus in their cervical tissue, but less than 5 percent ever develop dysplasia or venereal warts.

WHAT INCREASES YOUR RISK?

Most women who have had intercourse have been exposed to this virus, but many of the risk factors for cervical cancer have to do with the likelihood that you acquired this virus during a susceptible time (puberty and pregnancy). You are considered to be at higher risk of developing cervical cancer if you:

- ❦ *Have had two or more sexual partners*
- ❦ *Have had a sexually transmitted disease like gonorrhea or chlamydia*
- ❦ *Had first intercourse before age 18*
- ❦ *Have had cervical dysplasia in the past*
- ❦ *Smoke cigarettes*
- ❦ *Had your first pregnancy as a teenager or had multiple pregnancies*
- ❦ *Have a history of genital warts*

Not all human papilloma viruses are created equal. Approximately 80 subtypes have been identified. Different subtypes of HPV are linked to different cancer risks. Low cancer risk is associated with types 6, 11, 42, 43, and 44, and high risk with types 16, 18, 45 and 56. Although subtyping of HPV infections is available to your doctor, it is not routine practice to have this test performed. The results do not change the way you are taken care of, and there is no change in how often you should have a Pap smear. Studies are ongoing that may eventually enable your doctor to use HPV serotyping to individualize your treatment and follow-up should you have cervical dysplasia. A new Pap-smear collection and processing system, known as ThinPrep, is being evaluated in hopes of reducing the number of missed cases of dysplasia.

WHAT THE SYMPTOMS ARE

Precancerous cervical lesions are generally without symptoms, but may be associated with spotting or abnormal discharge. Late warning signs of cervical cancer are:

- ❧ *Bleeding after intercourse*
- ❧ *Bleeding between periods*
- ❧ *Abnormal vaginal discharge*
- ❧ *Pelvic pain*
- ❧ *Swelling in one or both of your legs*

As with most cancers, early diagnosis of cervical dysplasia and careful follow-up will virtually eliminate the possibility of developing cervical cancer.

HOW SCREENING IS PERFORMED

If you are 18 years of age or older, or are younger but sexually active, you should have yearly Pap smears. The Pap smear is a screening test for cervical cancer that samples cells from the outside (or ectocervix) and the inside (or endocervix) in order to find precancerous changes.

Like most screening tests, the Pap smear is not perfect. It can be read as normal when there is actually dysplasia present (a false negative test), and abnormal when there is no dysplasia (a false positive test). You reduce your chance of missing an abnormality by having a Pap smear every year. If you have had several normal annual Pap smears or have had a hysterectomy for reasons not related to cervical disease, you may be a candidate for less frequent testing — ask your doctor.

WORDS TO KNOW WHEN GETTING A PAP SMEAR

Do not be baffled by the words your doctor uses when discussing your Pap-smear results. **Dysplasia** is a pre-cancerous change of the top layer of the cervix, and it can range from mild to moderate to severe. Between a normal result and mild dysplasia is **atypia**, which is not treated as a precancerous condition. Inflammation from a yeast or bacterial infection can make a Pap smear return with atypia. On the other end of the spectrum, one step past severe dysplasia, is cervical cancer.

WHEN THE RESULTS ARE ABNORMAL

Precancerous Conditions

If you have atypia or mild dysplasia, your physician may follow the situation with Pap smears every three months. If dysplasia or persistent atypia results again, you are further evaluated with colposcopy. **Colposcopy** is an office procedure where a microscope is used to examine the cervix and look for abnormal areas. If abnormalities are noted, biopsies are taken, because a pathologist can make a more accurate diagnosis with a biopsy specimen than with a Pap smear.

The treatment for any abnormalities that are confirmed by biopsy depends on the following issues:

🐾 *The severity of the lesion (mild dysplasia versus severe dysplasia versus cancer)*

🐾 *The location of the lesion (ectocervix versus endocervix versus the entire cervix or more)*

🐾 *Your plans for future childbearing*

Low-grade or mildly abnormal lesions can be monitored over time with repeat Pap smears and colposcopy, and may regress on their own. Freezing the top layer of the cervix, an office procedure known as **cryotherapy**, can also destroy them. If your cervix has severe dysplasia or abnormalities within the canal, the affected area is excised in the office using **LEEP** (loop electrocautery excision procedure, where an electric knife is used to shave off the top layer of the cervix) or destroyed via **laser ablation**. In certain situations, you may be best served by having the abnormal cells removed by **cone biopsy**, a same-day outpatient surgery in which a cone-shaped portion of the cervix is excised. If you are done with childbearing, or do not want children, **hysterectomy** (surgical removal of the uterus and cervix) might be your best treatment.

CANCER

If you are diagnosed with cancer, your doctor needs to know how much it has spread. This is known as the stage of the cancer. With cervical cancer, the stage is assessed by physical exam, including a thorough pelvic exam. If physical exam reveals that the cancer is confined to your cervix, you will have a cone biopsy to determine the microscopic depth and width of the cancer. This information helps guide further surgical treatment. If the cancer has spread just beyond the cervix, your options are radiation therapy and surgery, which have identical rates of cure. Any further spread cannot be cured with surgery, and radiation therapy is your best hope for a cure.

Cancer Prevention

The American Cancer Society estimates that one-third of the 500,000 cancer deaths each year have a dietary contribution. This is an empowering statistic, because diet is something we have control over; however, Americans choose to eat high-fat, low-fiber diets with inadequate intake of fruits and vegetables. The goal of this segment is to give you the information you need to eat healthier. By making small, gradual changes in your diet, you can learn new habits that significantly reduce your chance of developing cancer.

Healthy eating habits have been specifically linked to a decreased risk for cancer of the colon (high-fiber, low-fat), breast (minimal alcohol consumption, low-fat) and uterus (low-fat).

The American Cancer Society's guidelines on diet, nutrition and cancer prevention are summarized below. You may find you have the greatest success in revamping your diet if you make small changes gradually. It takes time to adjust to the differences, especially if you are a sedentary person who enjoys meat and is accustomed to regular alcohol consumption. Be creative and persistent in your goal to eat a "cancer-preventive" diet. For example, perhaps focusing solely on regular exercise for the first month or two will reduce cravings for high-fat snack foods. A 60-year-old sedentary, obese man in Sacramento, California, completely changed his life by making a serious vow to exercise every day. Although he did not alter his diet for the first three months and consumed his usual high-fat, junk-food-laden diet, he still lost 37 pounds in three months. This weight loss boosted his morale and encouraged him to eat better. After one year, he had lost 71 pounds and had completed a marathon!

Choose Most of the Foods You Eat from Plant Sources

- Eat five or more servings of fruits or vegetables each day.
- Eat other foods from plant sources – such as
breads, cereals, grain products, rice, pasta or beans –
several times each day.

Normal metabolism in cells produces oxygen-induced DNA damage associated with the development of cancer. Antioxidant nutrients are thought to protect against cancer and include vitamin C, vitamin E, selenium, and carotenoids such as beta-carotene. Clinical studies have shown that people who eat more fruits and vegetables, which contain relatively high doses of these nutrients, have a lower risk for cancer. Antioxidant supplements have not demonstrated a significant reduction in cancer risk.

If you think about it, adhering to this guideline is not difficult if you spread the recommended servings over the course of a day: a banana with whole-grain cereal for breakfast, some raisins for mid-morning snack, a can of minestrone soup and salad for lunch, an apple in the afternoon, and rice and beans with cornbread for dinner.

Limit Your Intake of High-Fat Foods, Particularly from Animal Sources

- Choose foods low in fat.
- Limit consumption of meats, especially high-fat meats
such as beef, pork and lamb.

Foods that get less than 25 percent of their calories from fat are considered low-fat. The FDA's new food-labeling requirements make calculating the percentage of fat in foods easy. If the label lists the number of fat calories in a food serving, take this number and divide it by the total calories per serving.

For example:
140 fat calories ÷ 230 total calories = 61% of total
calories per serving from fat.

If only the "total fat" in grams is listed, multiply this number by 9 (the number of calories per gram of fat) to calculate the number of fat calories per serving, then perform calculations as above.

For example:
Total fat grams = 1 gram
1 gram x 9 cal/gram = 9 calories per serving from fat.

If the total number of calories per serving is, for example, 100 calories, then
9 fat calories ÷ 100 total calories = 9% of total
calories per serving from fat — a much better choice!

You may want to shop with a calculator or consider buying a pocket-sized calorie and fat counter to help you plan your meals. If you are unsure how fat-laden a food is, keep in mind that generally speaking, the more closely a food resembles its original, unprocessed form, the less fat it has. For example, a plain baked potato is barely altered and low in fat, but a potato chip is fat calorie-laden.

Be Physically Active;
Achieve and Maintain a Healthy Weight

You should be moderately active for 30 minutes every day of the week. Ideally, this 30 minutes of activity should be for a continuous stretch of time, at your target heart rate. Your target heart rate is calculated as follows:

220 – (your age) = maximum heart rate (MHR)
Target heart rate (THR) = (.75 - .85) x MHR

For example:

If you are forty years old, your **MHR** is 220 – 40 = 180. Your THR is 180 x (.75 - .85) = **135 – 153 beats per minute**. Thus, when you exercise, your heart rate should stay between 135 and 153 beats per minute in order to gain the maximum calorie-burning and cardiovascular benefits of exercise.

If you are overweight, 40 years old or over, a smoker or extremely sedentary, get clearance from your physician before you begin an exercise program.

Choose a form of exercise you enjoy that fits easily into your schedule. Vigorous walking and jogging require no special equipment and can be done almost anywhere, including malls if the weather is bad and airports if you are a frequent traveler. Exercise in the morning if at all possible — you are less likely to skip it due to changes in daily work or family responsibilities. If you would find it more enjoyable, enlist a friend to join you. If you have difficulty making time because of parenting responsibilities, ask a neighbor if she would be interested in taking turns babysitting to give you both time to exercise.

Limit Consumption of Alcoholic Beverages,
If You Drink at All

Studies have noted a link between alcohol consumption and increased breast cancer risk. The mechanism for this effect is unknown.

Women with an unusually high risk for breast cancer (see the risk factors in the section on breast cancer) may want to consider total abstinence from alcohol. If you are 60 years of age or older and have minimal risk for developing breast cancer, the cardiovascular benefits from a glass of red wine a day may outweigh the risk of cancer.

Excess alcohol consumption increases the risk of mouth and esophageal (food tube) cancers as well.

Other Recommendations

- Quit smoking to reduce your risk of lung and cervical cancer.
- Set up an appointment with your doctor to review your timetable for cancer screening — mammograms, Pap smears and sigmoidoscopy. Have a thorough knowledge of your family's cancer history before you go, including specific diagnoses and age at diagnosis.

Conclusion

Please do not ignore the topic of cancer screening and prevention. Ignorance is not bliss, and burying your head in the sand could result in your having to deal with an advanced cancer. There are few areas of medicine where you can have a greater impact on your health. Please read this chapter several times and speak with your caregiver to develop a personal plan of cancer prevention and screening. By following such a plan, you can reduce your risk of dying from cancer by over 50 percent.

Additional Resources
Books

- **Living With Lung Cancer: A Guide for Patients and Their Families,** *Barbara G. Cox, David T. Carr, M.D., and Eloise Harmon, M.D.,* Triad Publishing, 1997.

- **American Lung Association Seven Steps to a Smoke-Free Life,** *Edwin B. Fisher and Toni L. Goldfarb,* John Wiley & Sons, 1998.

- **The Breast Sourcebook: Everything You Need to Know About Cancer Detection, Treatment and Prevention,** *M. Sara Rosenthal and Karen Keiser,* Lowell House, 1997.

- **Causes and Control of Colorectal Cancer: A Model for Cancer Prevention (Developments in Oncology, No. 78),** *Gabriel A. Kune,* Kluwer Academic Publishing, 1996.

- **Ovarian and Uterine Cancer: Reducing Your Risk (If It Runs in Your Family),** *Sherilynn J. Hummel and Marie Lindquist,* Bantam Doubleday Dell, 1992.

- **New Developments in Cervical Cancer Screening and Prevention,** *Eduardoluiz Fabiano Franco and Joseph Monsonego (Editors),* Blackwell Science, 1997.

Organizations

- **American Cancer Society**
  1599 Clifton Road, NE
  Atlanta, GA 30329
  (800) ACS-2345

- **National Society of Genetic Counselors**
  Attn: Ms. Bea Leopold
  233 Canterbury Drive
  Wallingford, PA 19086-6617

- **American Lung Association**
  1740 Broadway
  New York, NY 10019
  (800) 586-4872

- **Health Promotion Resource Center**
  Stanford Center for Research in Disease Prevention
  1000 Welch Road
  Palo Alto, CA 94304-1885
  (415) 723-00003

- **National Cancer Institute**
  Office of Cancer Communications
  31 Center Drive, MSC 2580
  Building 31, Room 10A-29
  Bethesda, MD 20892-2580
  (800) 4-CANCER

Internet Sites

- **http://www.cancer.org**
  The American Cancer Society site has information about each of the cancers discussed in this chapter as well as links to additional Internet sites.

- **http://cancernet.nci.nih.gov/patient.html**
  This National Cancer Institute site offers "a wide range of accurate, credible cancer information" about treatment, detection, genetics and prevention, as well as a homepage for bids, facts for ethnic and racial groups, and more.

- **http://www.biostat.wisc.edu/bca/bca.html**
  Breast Cancer Answers, a serivce of Wisconsin Comprehensive Cancer Center, gives up-to-date information about breast-cancer screening recommendations and much more.

- **http://www.mskcc.org/document/CN970401.htm**
  This page offers the most current guidelines for colon-cancer screening from Memorial Sloan-Kettering Cancer Center.

- **http://oncolink.com/**
  University of Pennsylvania Cancer Center's Oncolink shares facts on cancers and their treatment, clinical trials, cancer screening, and stories from cancer patients and survivors.

- **http://www.med.upenn.edu/gdrs/tests/brca/consent-brca1mut.html**
  Reading this consent form for BRCA1 mutation screening from the University of Pennsylvania Health System's Genetics Diagnostic Library & Referral Service helps you to understand the complexity of the genetic testing issue.

CHAPTER NINE

MENOPAUSE

Preparing for "The Change"

The hot flashes. The sleepless nights. You can no doubt identify these symptoms from jokes on television comedies or those "horror stories" from an older aunt or grandmother.

Do most women look forward to menopause? Probably not. But menopause — sometimes called "the change of life" — is a natural part of every woman's life cycle, not something to be dreaded or ignored.

A good time to read this chapter is before you experience any of the symptoms of menopause. If you educate yourself about this process, you will be able to experience the changes of menopause with less apprehension. Reading about these changes, as you are doing now, is a good start. Communicating with friends and family members also will help. Share with them what you are learning and experiencing. If you and your partner are familiar with the changes you are undergoing, your partner can be more supportive and will be less likely to misunderstand your emotions. Your partner should allow you the emotional flexibility to adapt to your body's changes. A good knowledge base will help both of you avoid a great deal of anger, frustration and fear. And remember to bring any questions you have to your doctor or health-care provider.

" Because of what my mother went through and how she experienced menopause, I was not looking forward to it. Because even though they had replacement therapy at that time, it was not really improved, and she had mood swings and hot flashes. So the first time I had a hot flash, I took an appointment to get some sort of therapy, because I wasn't going to go through it the way she did. But… my Mom was not a very positive woman. I'm more like my Dad, much more positive. And I think that plays a role."

Change is part of life, and like many other changes, menopause may have its difficult moments. A woman who is approaching menopause is likely to have weathered such stressful times as puberty, marriage, parenthood and separation from adult children. You may have found that preparing for such stresses helped you handle them better. Likewise, this chapter serves in part to offer you guidance and help you prepare for another of life's changes.

The first portion of this chapter explains a normal menstrual cycle and the role of the ovaries in menstruation and menopause. The chapter also addresses the changes that occur with menopause, both the ones you can feel and the ones you do not feel, and puts into perspective the benefits and risks of hormone replacement therapy. The chapter also offers strategies for coping with the changes of this phase of life, and includes a list of resources where you might turn for more information and support.

Why Does Menopause Happen?

The best way to understand menopause is to first understand a normal menstrual cycle. Your menstrual cycles, or periods, are controlled by the ovaries, which are under the control of the brain. Your brain produces FSH, or follicle stimulating hormone, which goes through the bloodstream to the ovaries. FSH stimulates the ovaries to produce estrogen and progesterone, which make the uterus produce a menstrual cycle. The estrogen and progesterone make the uterine lining thicker in preparation for pregnancy, when a growing baby implants in the lining. If you do not get pregnant that cycle, the lining comes out as menstrual flow.

In menopause, the ovaries stop responding to FSH. The brain increases the amount of FSH in an attempt to keep the ovaries active. Your doctor tests for an elevation of FSH to determine if you are entering menopause. When the ovaries stop responding to FSH, there is no longer any production of estrogen, which means your periods will stop. The cessation of periods is the most noticeable sign that menopause is occurring.

The average age at menopause is 51. It may occur as early as 30. If you enter menopause before age 30, your doctor will order a blood test to make sure your chromosomes are normal. If the test reveals any Y chromosomes (normally found only in men), you are at high risk of having a tumor of the ovary. If you have this Y chromosome, you should have both ovaries removed now to avoid the risk of cancer.

Menopause also occurs whenever the ovaries are removed surgically. Surgery results in an abrupt loss of estrogen, frequently causing more dramatic symptoms. With the surgical removal of the ovaries, you also lose the small amount of testosterone normally made in the ovaries. Even after natural menopause near age 50, the ovaries continue to produce testosterone. The loss of testosterone can lower some women's libido, or sexual drive. If you have had your ovaries removed and notice a decline in your libido, ask your caregiver about medicine that combines estrogen and testosterone, Estratest.

To summarize, menopause is a stage in your life, usually near age 50, when your ovaries no longer function; the term also covers the surgical removal of the ovaries. This change results in the loss of estrogen, and the end of monthly menstrual cycles.

Below we will review the impact of losing estrogen on osteoporosis, heart disease and menopausal symptoms.

" I didn't feel I was very well versed on the subject of menopause; I didn't have to be, because I didn't think I was going through pre-menopausal stages yet. So my menopause was brought on overnight. As I look back, I bet I was having symptoms and could have benefited from mild doses of Premarin. What I remember most vividly after I had my hysterectomy were the night sweats and hot flashes. And that was before they gave me hormone replacement – after I left the hospital and before I went back for my checkup. I'd wake up in the middle of the night soaked, absolutely sweaty, and I thought I had fever from the surgery. It never occurred to me that I was having night sweats, because I had some complications after the surgery. So I just figured this was more of that. That went on until I went in for my first checkup."

Menopause: Preparing for "The Change"

Osteoporosis: A Problem You Can Prevent

WHAT CAUSES BRITTLE BONES?

Osteoporosis is the loss of bone strength. Most women have strong bones as they enter menopause. Bone strength is greatest in your 20s and 30s, and it declines slightly by age 50. In the first five years following menopause, bone strength declines rapidly because of the loss of estrogen. Thereafter the bones continue to get weaker, but at a slower rate.

Before menopause, your bones usually are strong enough to withstand a small fall or accident. However, after menopause and years of weakening from the lack of estrogen, your bones are more likely to break during the same sort of fall, and you could end up with a broken hip. The risk of dying from the complications of a broken hip in an elderly woman is very high. By avoiding osteoporosis, we can avoid 40,000 to 50,000 hip fractures each year in the United States.

In addition to the hips, the wrists and the spine are common areas for fractures. Fractures in the spine cause chronic severe back pain and the poor posture that many elderly women assume. The impact on society is great from all these fractures, both in terms of financial costs and reduced quality of life. In order to avoid having daily pain as part of your elderly years, you need to take steps to prevent osteoporosis when you enter menopause (and, ideally, throughout your life). At menopause, you can help ward off the loss of bone with hormone replacement therapy, extra calcium, vitamin D and regular exercise.

HOW TO KEEP YOUR BONES STRONG

Take Hormone Replacement Therapy

Hormone replacement therapy is replacing the estrogen your body made before you went through menopause with estrogen in the form of a pill, patch, cream or injection. Some people worry about taking anything "artificial" and avoid hormone replacement. We will discuss the different methods and the risks of taking estrogen later in this chapter. For now, you should know that the dose of estrogen in hormone replacement therapy is much lower than the dose in birth-control pills. The estrogen in birth-control pills is ethinyl estradiol, which is four times more potent than the conjugated estrogen of hormone replacement therapy. Women have been well-educated about the risks associated with taking birth-control pills after age 35, and you may mistakenly think the same risks are associated with taking estrogen for hormone replacement therapy. Remember, the amount of medicine is not the same; the amount of estrogen in hormone replacement therapy is very low.

Without hormone replacement, you experience a rapid loss of bone strength, putting yourself at a far greater risk for osteoporosis. Even if you exercise and take calcium and vitamin D, without the estrogen, you lose bone strength. Estrogen has to be present to keep the bones strong.

It is difficult to persuade someone to take medicine in order to prevent a problem from occurring in the future. Osteoporosis is a condition that develops without your feeling any pain. Once bone strength is lost, there is no regaining it. Therefore, once osteoporosis causes pain, it is too late to start hormones. Large studies show us that taking estrogen has a great effect on preventing osteoporosis. From the study by Ettinger published in the *Journal of Obstetrics and Gynecology* (issue 72, 1988), we know that up to 50 percent of bone strength is lost during the first 10 to 15 years after menopause. You must understand this fact in order to help you know why you need to take medicine when you do not feel sick or in pain.

" I have come to the conclusion for me that definitely I will continue to take my Premarin until the day I die, unless something comes up in the future that we don't know about now. For one thing, the studies have shown that calcium isn't absorbed properly or as well without the presence of that hormone in your body. I've seen what osteoporosis can do to you, and it's sure not something I want to deal with if you can take a pill and avoid it. Secondly, the studies have shown that if you pop that little pill, you've got an edge against heart attacks. And every time I think about that, I have to smile. Give me a pill! I don't want to have a heart attack. Wouldn't it be nice if we could give our men a pill, other than a baby aspirin?"

Exercise

Now that you know the essential role estrogen plays in preventing osteoporosis, we can now discuss other ways to keep your bones strong. Exercise is known to help maintain bone strength. Ideally, you would exercise three or more times per week. You need to find an exercise that you can enjoy, afford and do conveniently. It should involve weight-bearing, such as lifting weights, dancing or taking an aerobics class. Walking by itself is not ideal for the promotion of bone density, but it is much better than no exercise at all. As with all exercises, you need to progress slowly to avoid injury.

Get Plenty of Extra Calcium

In addition to estrogen and exercise, taking extra calcium helps the bones remain strong. You need a total of 1500 mg of calcium each day. Most people can get about 1000 mg a day from a healthy diet; after menopause, you should try to get an extra 500 mg of calcium each day. You can get this extra calcium in two to three glasses of milk each day. If you do not like milk, you can take the antacids that contain calcium, such as Tums, as a daily calcium supplement.

Take Vitamin D Supplements

In addition to estrogen, vitamin D supplements are important, especially if you live in an area where winters are long, and the sun is rarely seen. If you live in a long-term health center, supplements with vitamin D are critical. Vitamin D is made in the skin when exposed to sun. This vitamin helps estrogen maintain bone strength.

In summary, to protect yourself from osteoporosis after menopause, I suggest taking estrogen, getting weight-bearing exercise at least three times a week, and taking supplements of 500 mg of calcium and 400 to 800 IU of vitamin D each day.

Heart Disease: Not Just for Men

THE CRAMP THAT CAN KILL

The heart muscle pumps blood throughout your body. Blood vessels deliver energy to this muscle, like the muscles in your legs. If the blood vessels that feed your heart are blocked, you get a muscle cramp, usually felt as chest pain – which is a heart attack. If the blood vessel does not open, the muscle stops working, and you may die.

Before the age of 50, your risk of heart attack is much lower than a man's. After menopause, your risk is equal to that of a man. The number-one cause of death for women over age 50 is now heart attacks – a statistic we can attribute to the increase in women smokers that began during the World War II era.

HOW TO LOWER YOUR RISK
Keep that Cholesterol Under Control
You can lower your risk of having a heart attack in several ways. Taking estrogen in hormone replacement therapy is one of the most significant ways to protect your heart. The estrogen works in two main ways: it keeps the blood vessels open, which allows the heart muscle to get all the blood it needs, and it improves the blood lipids. Lipids are the blood component that accumulates in the hearts' blood vessels, not allowing the blood to pass through to the heart muscle. By improving the lipids, there is less chance of blocking these important vessels. To keep your cholesterol and lipid levels in a healthy range, you should avoid obesity, get regular exercise and eat well.

Throw Away the Cigarettes
Another way to avoid a heart attack is to stop smoking. Smoking increases the risk of heart attacks and lung cancer. By quitting smoking, you can markedly lower your chance of dying from one of these two problems.

ESTROGEN FOR MEN?

When the scientific community learned that estrogen prevents many women from having heart attacks, researchers designed studies to see if the same effect would occur with men. In men who were given estrogen after age 50, however, there was no protection from heart attacks. While estrogen appears to protect a women's heart, it does not have the same benefit for men.

Get Up and Move

The third way to lower your risk of heart attacks is to get regular exercise, at least three times per week, preferably walking one or two miles every day. This exercise keeps the heart muscle in good shape and the vessels clean and open. A regular exercise program is also good for lowering your stress level. You can make it a sociable activity and have fun while staying in shape.

FOODS TO AVOID
FOR A HEALTHY HEART

The key is to avoid foods high in saturated fats, such as:

🐾 *Whole milk* 🐾 *Chocolate*
🐾 *Butter* 🐾 *Shellfish*
🐾 *Cheese* 🐾 *Fatty meats*
🐾 *Corn oil*

To summarize: in order to remain healthy and free of heart disease, you need to take estrogen in hormone replacement therapy, avoid smoking, get regular exercise and eat low-fat foods.

The Symptoms of Menopause

The traditional complaints associated with menopause include hot flashes, mood swings, crying spells and vaginal dryness. It is also not unusual to develop urinary incontinence and a decreased enjoyment of sexual intercourse. Until recently, these complaints were the only issues discussed when talking about menopause. Now, we realize most women go through menopause with very mild symptoms. The issues of osteoporosis and heart disease have become the main focus when preparing you for this period of life. However, let us discuss ways you can cope with these less serious, but still bothersome, conditions.

HOT FLASHES

The most frequent complaint among women in menopause is hot flashes – a sudden flushing of the skin, usually on the face. In an instant, the body feels very hot, and the room temperature seems high. These hot flashes frequently occur during the night. After several nights of losing sleep due to hot flashes, you tend to become very tired and irritable. If you are constantly denied regular sleep, it is understandable that you would become irritable, grouchy, moody and depressed.

This experience is not unlike the first few months of life with a new baby. The lack of regular sleep is a major part of the stress of a newborn. Women who adapted to the stress of caring for a newborn tend to do well with the stress of menopausal changes. If you have learned to cope with the stresses of life up until menopause, you will probably continue to handle difficult situations well through this new phase of life. However, if you have never developed good coping skills, you may not do as well with the stress and changes of menopause.

" Migraines, tight headaches, hot flashes, night sweats... My whole body would be covered with perspiration and hot, hot, hot. I just knew what was happening, so I didn't let it last very long."

Fortunately, hot flashes respond to hormone replacement therapy. If you only need estrogen (i.e., Premarin), your hot flashes may continue; if they do, let your caregiver know. The addition of progesterone (i.e., Provera) may alleviate hot flashes. If you are one of the few women who continue to have problems, special medications, such as Buspar and clonidine, may help. If you experience difficulty in controlling hot flashes, know that hot flashes tend to stop by themselves after less than five years.

MOOD SWINGS

Another feared complaint associated with menopause is mood swings. While hot flashes are related to hormonal changes, mood swings and crying spells are not hormonally controlled. As mentioned earlier, the general bad mood some women exhibit in menopause can

" I didn't really know what to expect with menopause. I had just heard of those hot flashes... And I knew someone who had just gone through it, and I thought she was like Dr. Jekyll and Mr. Hyde! Crying and then angry and then fine for a few minutes and there we go again... And I thought, 'Oh, God! Please, never! Don't let it happen to me!'"

be related to the lack of good rest. Chronic fatigue sets in, and many other complaints begin to emerge. This time of life can be full of challenges other than menopause, such as the death of a spouse, divorce or an "empty nest." As you cope with these situations, you may feel depressed or sad – a normal response in a demanding time.

With hormone replacement therapy, you are more likely to get rest. Sleep helps you avoid the tremendous fatigue, forgetfulness and crying spells sometimes attributed to menopause. You should plan to get some rest during the day, and adjust the amount of work you expect from yourself during the first years of menopause.

VAGINAL DRYNESS

The last symptom associated with menopause that we will discuss is vaginal dryness. The skin of the vagina is sensitive to estrogen. If the estrogen level is not maintained, vaginal skin becomes thin. The skin loses its ability to lubricate and stretch, resulting in less enjoyment of intercourse. The use of estrogen in hormone replacement therapy helps maintain a youthful vaginal lining – allowing a couple to continue the same sexual habits they have enjoyed throughout their life together.

DEBUNKING THOSE MENOPAUSE MYTHS

A few myths about menopause need to be addressed. Menopause is not associated with a high rate of true clinical depression. While many women have periods of feeling blue, true depression is rare. As we discussed earlier, the women who are depressed during menopause are more likely to have had problems with depression when they were younger. It again relates to the coping skills they bring to this special and stressful time of their lives.

MENOPAUSE AND DEPRESSION
In a study by J.B. McKinley published in the **Journal**
of Health and Social Behavior *(volume 28, 1987),*
depression in menopausal women was associated with
social stressors and was not a result of menopause itself.

The other myth associated with menopause is that you lose your interest in intercourse. Your desire to remain intimate remains strong; however, your vaginal walls become thin with the loss of estrogen, causing pain with intercourse. Hormone replacement therapy prevents this thinning and pain. The estrogen works regardless of how it is taken, but a vaginal estrogen cream is the ideal treatment for this situation. Also, your vaginal walls remain healthier if you have frequent intercourse. If you are taking HRT, after menopause and have less intercourse than you did before menopause, the cause could be stress in the relationship or another health problem that is making intercourse difficult. For example, a man could be taking medications that make having an erection difficult. If you take HRT, and if you and your partner are both in good health and have a loving, nurturing relationship, you can expect to continue enjoying the sexual relationship you have built together.

" *I wouldn't wish to go back to having periods. I mean, I'm so thankful to be where I am right now! I love my age. My sex life is better than it has ever been in my whole life. Ever. It's just a great feeling. I like where I am right now. I just try to tell everybody how wonderful I think it is. And I'm being sincere when I say it. Your hair? Yes, it turns gray. Wrinkles? Yes, they come – but who cares?"*

A Closer Look at Hormone Replacement

So far this chapter has explained the changes that occur with menopause. Now it is time to discuss how hormone replacement can help you avoid some of the serious problems. After describing hormone replacement therapy, we will review the benefits, risks and various methods of taking the medicine.

WHAT IS HRT?

Hormone replacement therapy involves taking estrogen, with or without progesterone. If you have a uterus, estrogen without progesterone increases your risk of developing uterine cancer. If progesterone is taken with estrogen, your risk of uterine cancer is minimal. If you do not have a uterus (because of hysterectomy), you do not have to take progesterone. If you have a history of endometriosis, however, some physicians keep you on progesterone even if you have had a hysterectomy. The fear is that the sites of endometriosis in your abdomen could respond to estrogen and develop cancer.

WHICH REGIMEN IS BEST?

There are many ways to take hormone replacement therapy. The main difference is the absence or presence of a monthly period. The traditional method is to take estrogen (i.e., Premarin or Estratab) on days 1 through 25 of the month, and progesterone (i.e., Provera) on days 15 through 25. There are two main problems with this system. First, you continue to have monthly bleeding episodes, and most women at this point in life would like to stop having periods. The other disadvantage is that you go one week each month without taking hormones. During this time you may experience menopausal symptoms, such as hot flashes.

The most current HRT regimen is to take both estrogen and progesterone every day of the month. Estrogen may be prescribed in several forms. The most common is Premarin 0.625 mg or 1.25 mg. If your ovaries have been removed, or if your sex drive has decreased, some caregivers are adding the male hormone testosterone. This estrogen-testosterone combination is given as Estratest. Some women prefer avoiding pills, especially if they do not need progesterone. For these women, there is an estrogen patch, Estraderm. This adhesive patch, in the usual dosage of 0.05 mg, is applied to the skin anywhere except the breast, and is changed twice per week. A new patch called Climara is changed once per week. Estrogen also can be given in a monthly injection called Delestrogen. If you still have problems with vaginal discomfort or urinary incontinence, estrogen is given as a vaginal cream (Premarin vaginal cream) you apply three times a week.

With this continuous estrogen therapy, progesterone is also given every day. The advantage of this method is you have no menstrual periods. (It may take up to six months before all bleeding stops.) Progesterone is given as Provera 2.5 mg or 5 mg. A new pill containing both estrogen and progesterone is available, called Prempro.

> " I wear a seven-day-long patch (which really only lasts about five days). As long as I have it on, I don't feel any discomfort."

WEIGHING THE BENEFITS AND RISKS

The benefits of taking hormones are the reduction of bone loss, the reduced risk of a heart attack and the decrease in menopausal symptoms. There are risks associated with HRT. These include the risk of uterine and breast cancers.

Estrogen taken alone increases the risk of cancer of the uterus five times the normal rate of 1 per 1,000 women per year. When progesterone is taken with estrogen, this risk is minimized. Therefore, if you have not had a hysterectomy, you should be on both estrogen and progesterone to avoid increasing your risk of cancer of the uterus.

The effect of estrogen on the development of breast cancer is not clear. The addition of progesterone does not affect your chance of getting breast cancer. Most studies have shown no increased risk of breast cancer; some studies have shown a decreased risk, while others have shown an increased risk. The Nurses' Health Study, a study of 20,000 women done from 1976 to 1988, showed no increased risk of breast cancer in women who had previously been on estrogen. Among women who were on estrogen at the time of the study, there was a 30-percent greater risk of breast cancer. The researchers found that women with breast cancer who were on estrogen were 20-percent less likely to die from the cancer. These findings suggest that women on estrogen are going to the doctor for their yearly exams and finding cancer more frequently and at earlier stages, leading to fewer deaths. A study by the Centers for Disease Control called the "Cancer and Sex Hormone Study" found no increased risk of breast cancer with the use of estrogen. When you ask physicians who study this issue closely, most feel that taking estrogen slightly increases the risk of breast cancer.

In order to understand all of these issues regarding risks and benefits of HRT, consider a study by Ettinger published in the *Journal of Obstetrics and Gynecology* (volume 87, 1996). The researchers compared overall mortality in women taking estrogen with women not taking estrogen. If you follow 1,000 women in each category, 20 in the group without estrogen died each year, while in the group taking estrogen, only 11 died each year. I feel the bottom line is that if you want to have a greater chance of being alive and feeling well at age 70, you need hormone replacement therapy. Because of the small increased risk of breast cancer associated with HRT, I strongly support your doing breast self-exams each month, having a yearly breast exam by a physician and getting a yearly mammogram.

The future promises many advances in hormone replacement therapy. There are plans for an injection that can be taken routinely throughout the year to give all the hormones you need. But these advances are of little use if women are not willing to take hormonal therapy. When you have all the information, you should see that the overall effect of HRT is very beneficial. With this knowledge, you are equipped to evaluate what you read in the women's journals. If you have any concerns about a particular aspect of hormone replacement therapy, it is important to discuss them with your caregiver.

Cancer Screening: What to Watch For

In addition to hormone replacement therapy, menopause is a time to begin cancer screening. Your chance of having cancer before age 50 is low. However, the risks start to increase after menopause. Menopause itself is not the reason for an increased risk of cancer; nonetheless, this is a time when you need to know what could happen. (Chapter 8, "Cancer Screening & Prevention," is an additional source of information on this topic.)

CANCER AND YOUR AGE

According to the American Cancer Society, someone's probability of developing cancer up to age 39 is 1 in 52. The risk is 1 in 11 from age 40 to 59, and from age 60 to 79, the risk is 1 in 4.

The three most common cancers are lung, breast and colon cancer. In the 1980s, breast cancer was the leading cause of cancer deaths among women. The rate of breast cancer has not declined; instead, the incidence of lung cancer has risen greatly since 1970. As a woman, you also should be aware of female organ cancers – cancer of the uterus, ovary and cervix. We will review which cancers are screened for, and how the screening is done.

1997 CANCER DEATHS FOR WOMEN

♣	Lung cancer	66,000
♣	Breast cancer	43,000
♣	Colon cancer	24,000
♣	Pancreas cancer	14,600
♣	Lymphoma	12,060
♣	Ovary	14,200
♣	Uterus	6,000
♣	Cervix	4,800

LUNG CANCER: MOSTLY FOR SMOKERS

Lung cancer is the number-one cause of cancer deaths among women. Currently, lung cancer claims 64,300 women per year in the United States, while breast cancer is responsible for the deaths of 44,300 women each year. One reason is the tremendous increase of the number of women smoking since World War II. Lung cancer is very rare among non-smokers. Even if you have smoked for many years, upon stopping your chance of getting lung cancer rapidly declines.

There are no screening tests available for lung cancer. Therefore, I strongly suggest that you stop smoking now. After five years as a non-smoker, your risk of getting lung cancer will be near the level of a person who has never smoked. Speak to your caregiver about getting a nicotine patch to make the change to being a non-smoker more tolerable. However, the patch is no good until you have decided to become a non-smoker. Without the strong desire to stop smoking, the patch alone will not make you change.

BREAST CANCER: THINK EARLY DETECTION

Your risk of breast cancer increases as you age. A family history of breast cancer, especially in a sister or mother, also increases the risk. The ideal screening program for breast cancer includes monthly breast self-exams, annual exams by your caregiver and routine mammograms. The first, or baseline, mammogram is done between ages 35 and 40. You should get a mammogram every other year between 40 and 50, and yearly after age 50.

How to Perform a Breast Self-Exam

A breast self-exam is not difficult to perform. Press down on your breast with your fingertips, moving your hand in small circles. It is important to cover the entire breast, even the part that goes into your armpit. The two most common approaches are to cover the entire area of the breast by going around it, like a clock, or to examine your breasts in rows, up and down, until you have felt the entire surface. Feel for a mass like a marble under the skin. Do not think you need to find a mass the size of a grain of sand. Women who do regular self-exams do not make a big deal out of the process. You can quickly perform the exam while bathing.

COLON CANCER: SCREENING IS IMPORTANT

Colon cancer is the least well-known of the three common cancers. It is a cancer of the digestive tract (intestines). Colon cancer results in 27,500 deaths per year. The screening process involves testing your stool (bowel movement) for blood, and having a sigmoidoscopy done to look for areas that may become cancer. After age 40, you should have a rectal exam during your annual visits. During this exam, the caregiver will feel for any abnormal areas, and test the stool for blood. Also, you should test your stool at home on three occasions with a test kit, following instructions given to you at your annual visit. After age 50, a flexible sigmoidoscopy is done every three to five years. This test involves passing a flexible tube into the rectum, searching for any areas that may become cancer. If anything is noted, it usually can be removed through a very simple procedure. By following this protocol, you can reduce your chance of having a deadly colon cancer by 70 percent.

CERVICAL CANCER: THE REASON YOU HAVE PAP SMEARS

Cervical cancer is cancer of the cervix – the lowest part of the uterus, the part at the upper vagina. The screening test for cervical cancer is a Pap smear. A Pap smear is done each year at your annual exam. This test involves passing a small instrument over the cervix to sample the top layer of skin. The cells are inspected for changes that could become cancer. If any are noted, a more thorough exam of the cervix, called colposcopy, is done with a microscope. The goal is to find an abnormal area and treat it with a simple procedure before it becomes cancer.

UTERINE CANCER: IT BEGINS WITH BLEEDING

Uterine cancer involves the uterus, or womb. This cancer is more common among obese women, and women with a history of very irregular periods. The most common complaint in a person with uterine cancer is abnormal bleeding after menopause. If you have abnormal bleeding, a biopsy or sampling of the uterus will be done to make sure there is no cancer. There are no screening tests available to find this problem before it becomes cancer. Therefore, if you are not having any bleeding problems, you will not be tested for uterine cancer. The Pap smear does not test for problems in the uterus.

Cancer deaths from cervical and uterine cancer are at 6,000. The death rate from these cancers has declined dramatically – 67 percent – since the 1950s, around the time the Pap smear was introduced.

OVARIAN CANCER: HARDER TO DETECT

Ovarian cancer occurs mainly in women in their 60s. The current death rate per year from ovarian cancer is 14,800. At first, there are no symptoms. As the cancer cells spread through the abdomen, they tend to surround the digestive system (intestines). The cancer blocks the digestive tract, causing a swollen abdomen, and at the same time loss of appetite and usually nausea and vomiting. Unfortunately, there are no good methods to find ovarian cancer before it spreads to the intestines. Studies are being done to see if routine ultrasounds detect early problems. Also, the blood test Ca-125 is being investigated as a screening method. Currently, these tests have not been shown to be of any benefit. As they are expensive and can lead to inappropriate surgeries, they should not be routinely offered. If you have a strong family history of ovarian cancer, however, you should discuss these tests with your caregiver. If two close family members (your mother or sisters) have ovarian cancer, you might consider having your ovaries removed as a preventive measure when you are finished having children. Again, the Pap smear does not test for any problems with the ovaries.

Reducing Your Risk of Cancer

Reading so much about cancer may overwhelm you. While you need to know about the seriousness of this topic, you should not feel helpless. The suggestions below, developed by the American Cancer Society, can help keep you from ever getting cancer.

- Stop Smoking.
- Nutrition and Diet
  - *Maintain a desirable weight.*
  - *Eat a varied diet.*
  - *Include a variety of vegetables and fruits in your daily diet.*
  - *Eat more high-fiber foods, such as whole-grain cereals, breads and pastas; and vegetables and fruits.*
  - *Cut down on your total fat intake.*
  - *Limit your consumption of alcohol, if you drink at all.*
  - *Limit your consumption of salt-cured, smoked and nitrite-cured foods.*

- Minimize your exposure to the sun.
- Stop chewing tobacco or dipping snuff.
- If you are on estrogen and have a uterus, make sure you also take progesterone.
- Avoid such occupational hazards as radiation, asbestos, nickel, chromate and vinyl chloride.
- Have a mammogram at age 35 to 40, then one every two years from 40 to 50, and one every year after age 50.
- Have an annual exam with a Pap smear.
- Get your stool checked for blood yearly after age 40, and have a flexible sigmoidoscopy every three to five years after age 50.

Feeling Well After Menopause: The Big Picture

Reading this chapter probably does not make you look forward to the changes associated with menopause. However, now you are armed with the knowledge you need for this new stage of life. When you understand what is occurring during menopause, you are better able to judge the need for hormone replacement therapy. The roles of estrogen in reducing bone loss and lowering the risk of a heart attack are well documented in medical literature. The risks and benefits need to be put in perspective. The articles in most women's magazines tend to focus on the potential negatives instead of giving a clear view of all the considerations. While the risk of breast cancer may be slightly increased by taking hormonal therapy, it has been proved that women on hormones live longer and healthier lives than women not on hormones.

Menopause is also the time in life to stop taking good health for granted. If you continue to do that, you can expect to lose that good health earlier than necessary. You are more likely to enjoy good health if you use hormone replacement therapy, eat well, get regular exercise, stop smoking and get routine exams. The exams will include screening for breast, colon and cervical cancer.

Finally, communication is key. If you communicate with your partner, your caregiver and your friends, you can get through menopause with more understanding and less stress.

Additional Resources

Books

- **The Pause: Positive Approaches to Menopause,** *Lonnie Barbach, Ph.D.,* Penguin Books, 1993.
- **The Estrogen Decision Self-Help Book,** *Susan Lark, M.D.,* Westchester Publishing, 1994.
- **Natural Progesterone: The Multiple Roles of a Remarkable Hormone,** *John R. Lee, M.D.,* BLL Publishing, 1994.
- **Women's Bodies, Women's Wisdom,** *Christiane Northrup, M.D.,* Bantam Doubleday Dell, 1994.
- **Perimenopause: Preparing for the Change.** *Nancy Lee Teaff, M.D., and Kim Wright Wiley,* Prima Publishing, 1995.

Organizations

- **Jacobs Institute of Women's Health**
  409 12th Street, S.W.
  Washington, DC 20024-2188
  (202) 863-4990
  http://www.jiwh.org/

- **The North American Menopause Society**
  P.O. Box 94527
  Cleveland, OH 44101
  (216) 844-8748
  E-mail: nams@apk.net
  http://www.menopause.org/

Internet Sites

- **http://www.pslgroup.com/MENOPAUSE.HTM**
  Doctor's Guide to Menopause Information and Resources offers medical news and alerts, discussion groups and newsgroups, links to related sites and more. This site is an excellent resource for getting information about menopause and the related issues.

CHAPTER TEN

INCONTINENCE

Breaking the Silence

a woman and a group of friends made plans to eat at a restaurant near their hotel. Dread enveloped her as they walked the few blocks to the shopping complex. Her bladder felt so full. She feared she would not get to a bathroom soon enough. She stepped onto the escalator, and there was nothing she could do. "I went all over the escalator," she recalls. "It's a good thing I had on a denim dress, so I could try to hide it." As soon as she walked into the restaurant, she hurried for the restroom and rinsed out her underwear. Nobody said a word about the dark, wet splotches on her dress. She still wonders who knew what happened.

Many, many women feel this shame, suffering in silence with a condition they are embarrassed to talk about. Urinary incontinence is a major health problem in the United States and around the world. It affects 15 percent of women younger than 60, 25 percent of women older than 60, and up to 50 percent of all nursing-home patients. Many women avoid social and sometimes sexual activities because of incontinence, which can lead to depression and a loss of self-worth. Because of what they hear from family and friends, and what they see on TV, they use pads and adult diapers prematurely. Even when seeing their family doctor for an annual check-up, they rarely bring up their incontinence. Only about 50 percent of incontinence sufferers seek medical attention.

> " I haven't brought this up with a doctor in years. It hasn't been a big enough concern. When you go to the doctor, you try to think of the big questions, and the little ones slip through the cracks."

Unfortunately, the cost of *not* treating the problem can be staggering. Government statistics show that the cost of untreated incontinence is around $11.2 billion annually for outpatients and around $5.2 billion for nursing-home patients. I have found that about half the sanitary napkins and pads purchased are used for the control of urinary leakage instead of menstrual flow. And then there are the products made specifically for adult control of incontinence. Recent estimates show that an average user will spend around $1,000 to $1,500 per year on these adult diapers.

"It makes me feel stupid! You can't get to the bathroom, and urine leaks down your leg, and you think, 'Isn't this a fine kettle of fish!' And there's nothing you can do to stop it. Luckily, it doesn't happen that often and not all the time — and that's another thing that's confusing!"

Incontinence is **not** an inevitable part of aging. Successful treatments are available. You should not let incontinence lower your quality of life. Although the subject may be embarrassing to discuss, you must be willing to talk to your caregiver. Incontinence is a common, serious and treatable problem, and the cost of not getting treatment is very high, not only financially, but also emotionally.

The purpose of this chapter is to help you understand incontinence. There is a review of the process of urination, an explanation of the causes and evaluation of incontinence, and a discussion of treatment options.

How Urination Should Work

In order to understand the kinds of problems that can lead to incontinence, it is important to understand how the bladder works. We all tend to take our bladders for granted until they cause problems, but this is actually how it is supposed to be. You are busy enough without having to constantly worry about how your bladder is working.

Urine is made in the kidneys, transported down the ureters and stored in the bladder until you find a socially acceptable place to empty. Think of the bladder as a plastic bag that you can fill easily until the bag is full, then suddenly the pressure shoots up and it becomes hard to fill. At capacity, when the bladder walls are starting to become stretched, the bladder signals your brain that it is getting full. When you get the original "urge to go," you can usually suppress that urge for a while in order to reach the bathroom. You then consciously allow the bladder muscle to contract and empty. The contraction of the bladder is what allows you to urinate. In order to stay dry, the bladder must not contract unless you are on the toilet.

Also important to this process is the external sphincter muscle, which functions to hold the urine in the bladder until you are ready to void. To again use the analogy of the plastic bag: If you took a plastic bag full of water and turned it upside down, the water would pour out of the bag. So in order to keep water in the bag, you hold the neck of the bag shut with your hand. To let water out, you relax your grip, and the water begins to flow. Like your hand around that plastic bag of water, the external sphincter controls the flow of urine.

The tube that drains the bladder is called the urethra. It is much more than a tube leading from the bladder to the outside; it also acts to help keep you from leaking. The urethra is composed of two layers — an outer one of muscle fiber and an inner one called the mucosa — that contribute to the counter-pressure, or resistance, that urine coming down from the bladder must overcome in order to escape. The urethra and its support tissues, along with the external sphincter, are responsible for keeping urine in the bladder. Damage to the urethra, its support and the external sphincter are the main reasons that women leak.

What is Incontinence?

Incontinence is the *involuntary* loss of urine. This is the simple definition. For our purposes it is important to add to this. I doubt there is a person alive who has not occasionally leaked a little urine when rushing out of the bathroom, or laughing hysterically with a full bladder, or trying to hold urine way beyond normal. So how should we define incontinence more specifically? Incontinence can be defined as the involuntary loss of urine of sufficient volume and frequency such that it interferes in some way with your normal function. It may prevent you from doing activities that you normally would do. It may make you do things that are uncomfortable for you, such as wearing pads. It may alter the way other people perceive you or interact with you. In light of our discussion of normal function, another definition would be the uncontrollable loss of urine when bladder pressure is too strong for the urethra to resist.

The Main Types of Incontinence

There are several different types of incontinence, each having a different cause and treatment. For each of the different types, we will discuss the common symptoms, the cause or causes, the appropriate diagnostic tests and the various available treatments. The main types of incontinence are:

> *"I think twice before I do anything. I don't participate much in sports anymore, and I sure don't want to wear a bathing suit."*

♣ *Transient incontinence*
♣ *Stress incontinence*
♣ *Overflow incontinence*
♣ *Mixed incontinence*
♣ *Urge incontinence*

There are other rare causes, such as fistulas (holes) caused by prior surgery or radiation treatments, that we will not cover in this discussion. We will cover each of the other types in some detail beginning with transient incontinence.

What is Transient Incontinence?

As the name implies, transient incontinence comes and goes, or is of short duration. This is usually not due to a problem with the bladder or urethra itself. However, there may be changes in the function of the bladder or urethra caused by other medical or psychological problems. The incontinence these women have may be caused by infections, medications, weakening of the tissues after menopause, or confusion and immobility. Transient incontinence is one of the major causes of incontinence in the elderly. It is, therefore, important to discuss your general health, living arrangements, medications and psychological problems during any evaluation. Also, it is important to think of any changes in daily routines that may have occurred at the time of onset of leakage problems. A bladder infection is one of the most common conditions that leads to a brief episode of incontinence. Infection causes the bladder to have very strong, uncontrollable contractions, resulting in incontinence. Bladder infections are many times overlooked and easily treated with antibiotics.

Many medications have an effect on the bladder and urethra. These may be medicines prescribed by your physician but may also be medications that you buy over the counter. Diuretics can cause excessive urine production and worsen incontinence in people who otherwise would only have minimal problems. Many medications used to treat allergies, depression, spastic bowel problems and dizziness contain anticholinergics, compounds that can prevent the bladder from contracting, and thus cause you to retain urine. The bladder becomes too full, and urine starts to leak. Some cold medications contain agents that increase the pressure, or tone, in the urethra and lead to urinary retention and overflow of urine. Blood pressure medication can lead to leakage by decreasing the tone in the urethra. Alcohol can increase urine production and result in incontinence due to the confusion and impaired mobility. As you can see, it is important to review with your doctor all the medications you are taking, as they may be a factor in causing or contributing to incontinence.

Drugs That Can Cause Transient Incontinence

- **Diuretics** — Aldactone, Dyazide, HCTZ, Lasix, Maxide
- **Antidepressants** — Adapin, Asendin, Effexor, Elavil, Ludiomil, Norpramin, Pamelor, Sinequan, Surmontil, Tofranil
- **Spastic bowel medicines** — Bentyl, Levsin, Librax
- **Dizziness medicine** — Antivert
- **Antihistamines** — Actidil, Actifed, Allegra, Atarax, Benadryl, Chlor-Trimeton, Claritin, Clistin, Dimetane, Dimetapp, Hismanal, Periactin, Phenergan, Rondec, Seldane, Tavist, Zyrtec
- **Blood-pressure medicines** — Cardura, Hytrin, Minipress

Physical limitations, such as severe arthritis, can make getting to the bathroom a very strenuous activity. The time and effort required to get to the toilet may result in leakage of urine. A bedside commode can help people get relief in time and prevent incontinence.

One of the most common and easily treated causes of transient incontinence is the change in the tissues that occurs after menopause. The tissues that make up the urethra and bladder neck, as well as the tissues in the vagina, are all responsive to estrogen. After menopause, with the decline in estrogen levels, there is a simultaneous atrophy of the vaginal, urethral and bladder-neck tissues as well as weakening of the surrounding muscles and support tissues. Very commonly, urinary incontinence begins or worsens at this time.

Estrogen replacement, given as a pill or as a vaginal cream, reverses these atrophic changes and increases the resistance in the urethra that counteracts the pressure in the bladder. Treatment with estrogen may prevent or decrease episodes of incontinence. Typically one half an applicator (2 grams) of estrogen cream is placed in the vagina at bedtime three times a week. If you have a uterus, your doctor should also prescribe progesterone to prevent abnormal tissue build-up in the uterus that could lead to cancers.

Transient incontinence, therefore, may have many different causes, but the treatment is usually straightforward and aimed at trying to return the bladder and urethra back to their baseline function. For the other major types of incontinence, more testing is usually indicated. We will first discuss these tests and then proceed to a discussion of stress, urge and overflow incontinence.

How is Incontinence Evaluated?

Most women first discuss incontinence with a family doctor or other primary-care provider, who treats transient causes of incontinence. However, frequently there are other reasons why you are incontinent, and you can expect to be referred to a specialist for more testing. Many obstetricians and gynecologists have special training to evaluate and treat urinary incontinence.

At this point, I will explain the simple and also the more advanced tests you may encounter while being evaluated and treated. Read this section two or three times to have a good understanding of why these tests are being performed. This way, you will be more relaxed and less anxious about the entire process.

SIMPLE TESTS FOR URINARY INCONTINENCE

Your doctor will first obtain a history and do a complete physical exam. Be ready to discuss any prior surgery, back injury, stroke, chronic medical problems or cancers you have experienced. Also, be able to tell the doctor when the leakage began, what makes it worse, how much leakage occurs each time and any other symptoms that occur at the time of leakage. Do you have pain or burning with urination? Do you urinate more frequently than other people do? Do you feel a strong urge or pressure sensation when your bladder is full? After a thorough history and physical, a few basic tests are needed.

A **urine sample** is checked to make sure there is no infection or blood present. If there is blood in the urine without any infection, other tests are done to rule out bladder cancer. A urologist performs the evaluation for cancer.

A **Urolog,** or voiding diary, is a very effective way to determine the extent of your incontinence. You are asked to keep a diary of the fluids you drink, when you void, how much you void and any leakage episodes. You also document any other symptoms, such as urgency, pain, burning, etc. An example of a simple voiding diary is included on page 266.

A **post-void residual (PVR)**, obtained by draining the bladder with a catheter immediately after voiding, is useful if you feel you are not emptying your bladder well, or have difficulty starting to void.

A **pad test** determines how much urine you are leaking. With this test, a pad or diaper is weighed and then you wear it for an hour, at which time the pad is weighed again. Any increase in weight over 2 grams is significant. This test is also useful to see how therapy is progressing. If therapy is helping, the weight of the pads will decrease, indicating less leakage.

Simple cystometry, done in the doctor's office, detects abnormal contractions in the bladder as it fills. The bladder should fill without an increase in pressure and without any contractions until it is full. During this test, a small catheter is placed in your bladder, and the

VOIDING DIARY

Date_____

FLUID INTAKE		VOIDED VOLUME	
TIME	VOLUME/FLUID TYPE	TIME	AMOUNT VOIDED/PROBLEMS

A voiding diary is an effective way to determine the extent of your incontinence.

other end is connected to a funnel-like syringe. Water is poured into the syringe and flows into the bladder. If there are no bladder contractions, water will continue to flow into the bladder. If your bladder contracts, it will force water back out through the catheter and into the syringe. The doctor or nurse can see a rise in the water level in the syringe and determine at what volume this occurred. Usually, you will feel an urge to urinate at the time of any abnormal bladder contraction.

WHEN MORE ADVANCED TESTS ARE NEEDED

In some women, the simple, basic tests do not provide enough information to make an accurate diagnosis and plan appropriate therapy. This may be true for anyone with a complex medical history with lots of medical problems, or if you have had previous treatments or surgery for incontinence that did not work. In these cases, more complex testing is indicated.

With special equipment and an appropriate understanding of your problem, even the most complex problems can be solved. Some of the typical tests done with this equipment are:

- ❧ *Uroflow testing*
- ❧ *Multi-channel cystometry*
- ❧ *Voiding pressure-flow studies*
- ❧ *Urethral pressure profiles*

Each of these tests provides different and valuable information about a how your bladder is working.

A **uroflow test** is usually done first. You are asked to urinate into a special toilet that measures the speed and volume of urine produced. Afterward, a small catheter is placed in your bladder to drain the remaining urine, and this post-void residual (PVR) is recorded. This information may help the doctor understand how you void. Most people void in a continuous fashion once they start, until the bladder is empty. Some women have to strain and push on the bladder in order to empty. They void in an intermittent fashion, and have a weak stream. If the amount of urine remaining in the bladder after you urinate is very high, you may have overflow incontinence. Overflow incontinence is discussed later in this chapter.

Multi-channel cystometry involves placing one small catheter in your bladder to measure pressure, and a second catheter in your vagina or rectum. You stand or sit as sterile water is slowly pumped into your bladder. As your bladder fills, you are asked to do things that typically would make you leak urine, which might be walking, standing, jumping, coughing and laughing. The catheters are connected to a computer that records and plots the measured pressures. At the same time, small electrodes measure how well the external sphincter muscle

> "There's nothing worse than wet underwear. It's like wearing a wet bathing suit. It's so uncomfortable."

is contracting. The results help your doctor determine the cause of your incontinence. If your bladder contracts inappropriately, the problem is called urge incontinence. If the urethra is poorly supported, the problem is called stress incontinence. Both of these types of incontinence are explained in detail later in this chapter.

Voiding pressure-flow studies are usually done next. With your bladder full and the catheters and electrodes in place from the previous study, you are again asked to void on a special toilet. This time, not only are the speed and volume of urine recorded, but also bladder pressure and the activity of the external sphincter muscle activity. With this test, your doctor determines the strength of the bladder muscle and also checks to see if the urethral sphincter muscle is relaxing the way it should.

Urethral pressure profiles can be done in the same session. The catheter in your bladder from the previous study is slowly pulled down into your urethra, and pressure in the urethra is recorded. This pressure is an important part of the system to keep urine in the bladder. Women who have a damaged urethra — from previous surgery, injury to nerves in the pelvis, or multiple dilatations — can have very low pressure in the urethra, with a resulting loss of urine during any activity, especially standing.

How Incontinence is Treated Without Surgery

Let me repeat: There is help for incontinence. Please do not avoid evaluation by telling yourself that your incontinence is not that bad, or live in embarrassment and misery instead of discussing the problem with your doctor. For each major type of incontinence (stress, urge and overflow), there are several therapeutic approaches, and there are many options other than surgery. In many cases, surgery is not beneficial, and can be detrimental. Only a few types of incontinence are best treated surgically, but even in these cases there are other options that can be tried.

In the later sections on stress, urge and overflow incontinence, we will discuss specific drug therapies, surgical options and supportive devices. However, some behavioral and exercise treatments are helpful for all types of incontinence. These treatments may not always lead to a cure, but they may decrease the amount and frequency of leakage significantly. First we will discuss:

❧ *Bladder training*
❧ *Timed voiding*
❧ *Prompted voiding*
❧ *Kegel, or pelvic-floor muscle, exercises*
❧ *Biofeedback training*
❧ *Vaginal cone retention*
❧ *Electrical stimulation therapy*

During **bladder training,** you learn to delay voiding for progressively longer intervals. This technique is used if your bladder has inappropriate contractions with the presence of very little urine. Normally the bladder does not contract unless it is completely filled. Initially, urinate every 15 to 20 minutes during the day. The interval is increased every few days. Ignore the desire to urinate, and void only at the allowed time. You learn relaxation techniques to help you. If you leak while waiting for the allowed time, that is OK; you still continue with the schedule. The goal is to build up to an interval of two to three hours. This technique produces few cures, but most women have a 50-percent reduction in the amount of urine loss.

With **timed voiding,** you are asked to void at certain predetermined times. These times are selected based on your activity level and fluid intake to coincide with increased urine production. You learn to void only at these times. This technique is used in many nursing homes, and there is generally a decrease in the number of patients who are incontinent in a given day.

Prompted voiding is also used in nursing homes and by people who depend on others for their care. The idea is to teach you to be more aware of your bladder signals. You are constantly asked if you have leaked, and the interval between episodes is documented. You are then "prompted," or asked to void, before this interval is reached.

Kegels, or exercises of the pelvic-floor muscles, help strengthen the support of the bladder and urethra. These exercises help increase the resistance to urine outflow and keep the urethra closed, and they work with almost all types of incontinence. To do the exercise, contract or draw up the vaginal and anal muscles and hold for a count of 10. You can repeat this process multiple times a day.

" You can do the exercise anywhere at any time, and unless you're making a funny face, nobody knows you're doing it."

It is important to do these exercises correctly to have a beneficial effect. The hardest part is identifying the muscles that need to be worked. One way is to place a finger in the vagina and try to squeeze the finger. Another way is to try to stop urinating in the middle of the stream. If you do these exercises incorrectly, you may not notice an improvement and actually can make the problem worse. You will not notice an effect from these exercises for several months, because the muscles are very small. As with any other exercise, you may need to continue to do them forever to have a beneficial effect. Otherwise, the muscles will shrink, and the problem will get worse again. However, these exercises are free, painless and easy to perform with minimal effort. All women would benefit from doing these exercises as a preventive measure.

Occasionally, a woman is unable to identify the appropriate muscle groups. One problem many women have is that they contract the abdominals, or stomach muscles, in their attempt to contract the vaginal muscles. Contracting the abdominal muscles places additional downward force on the bladder, and that can make the bladder fall down worse. We can use **biofeedback training** to help you isolate the right muscles. Biofeedback training involves monitoring the activity of the abdominal and vaginal muscles. A monitor is connected to a TV screen, and you can see the activity of the different muscles. You learn to contract the appropriate vaginal muscles without contracting the abdominal muscles. In this way, you can learn to do Kegel exercises correctly and do them at home.

Vaginal cones are also used to strengthen the pelvic-floor muscles. These small, egg-shaped plastic devices come in a set of different weights. You place a weighted cone in your vagina and squeeze your vaginal muscles to hold the cone in place. The lightest cone is used first, and progressively heavier cones are then used as the muscles get stronger.

Electrical stimulators are becoming available to help strengthen the vaginal muscles. These devices cause the muscles to contract and relax every 5 to 10 seconds for about 10 minutes. You repeat the treatment a couple of times a day. These stimulators are useful if you are unable to do Kegels — that is, if you cannot consciously contract your vaginal muscles. The muscles may be so small that you cannot get them to contract by yourself. The electrical stimulators work directly on the muscles and get them to contract. In time, as the muscles get stronger, you may be able to take over again and stop needing the help. Studies have shown some benefit in all types of incontinence; however, they are most effective for urge incontinence.

There are also some new devices coming on to the market that are designed specifically for the control of incontinence. These devices do not cure the underlying condition; however, they may be alternatives to using pads. These new devices are:

   ❧ *Reliance Insert*
   ❧ *Introl device*
   ❧ *Impress Softpatch*

The **Reliance Insert** is recommended mainly for women with stress incontinence. This small, flexible device looks like a little catheter, with a balloon on one end and a string on the other. You insert the device in your urethra and inflate the balloon with air from a small syringe. The device acts like a cork, sealing the urethra so urine cannot leak. When you want to void, you pull the string and the balloon deflates. You then discard the insert, using a new one the next time you need one. This insert is helpful if you leak only with certain activities, such as dancing or playing tennis. You are then free from wearing pads and worrying about odor problems. However, it cannot be worn all the time, and it increases the risk of bladder infections. Also you have to

> "Whenever I am participating in any sexual activity, I have an extra towel there, just in case."

learn how to place and remove the insert.

The **Introl** device is about the same size as a diaphragm, and you insert it into the vagina the same way. It looks like a ring with two extensions, which gently lift up on either side of the urethra and prevent leakage of urine in women with stress incontinence. The device can be worn all day and only needs to be removed at night for cleaning. The biggest problem is getting the device fitted correctly. Also, if you have a large cystocele (bladder prolapse), you may have a hard time keeping the device in the vagina with any activity.

A device called the **Impress Softpatch** may soon be widely available. This soft foam patch has adhesive on one side. You place the patch over the opening to the urethra, sealing it from leakage. You remove the patch when you need to void and put a new one in place afterward. These patches are currently available from a company named Uromed, although the Impress Softpatch is not scheduled for release until sometime this year.

Next, we will discuss the major types of incontinence: stress, urge, overflow and mixed. For each type we will discuss the typical symptoms, causes, special tests and treatments.

What is Stress Incontinence?
WHAT THE SYMPTOMS ARE

Stress incontinence is one of the most common types of incontinence in women. The name has nothing to do with emotional stress, but rather physical stress on the bladder that causes leakage. If you have stress incontinence, you:

- ✿ *May leak urine with coughing, sneezing, laughing, running or jumping*

- ✿ *Usually can sleep through the night but may leak when getting up*

❧   *Leak less with an empty bladder*

❧   *May avoid exercise, intercourse or other activities
because of leaking*

Women with stress incontinence tend to leak a small amount. If you have this problem, you probably lose a "squirt" or "spurt" of urine with activities, not a large volume of urine. If you are like most women with stress incontinence, you control leakage by wearing a pad or pantyliner rather than bulkier products, like diapers, that are made to catch larger volumes of urine. When stress incontinence is the only cause of your leakage, you have no problems with pelvic pain, and you can empty your bladder completely.

WHAT CAUSES STRESS INCONTINENCE

Stress incontinence has two causes. It is important to make an accurate diagnosis, because the treatment is different for each. The most common cause is damage to the ligaments that support the bladder and bladder neck. The medical term for this condition is hypermobility of the bladder neck; it also is referred to as the bladder "falling down." The other cause is damage to the urethra (called intrinsic urethral sphincter deficiency or "low-pressure urethra").

When you have a "fallen" bladder, the tissues and ligaments that support the bladder and the neck of the bladder have been damaged. This damage commonly occurs during childbirth but can also result from repeated heavy lifting or from a chronic cough. Once these supportive tissues and ligaments are damaged, any

---

Tips for Preventing Stress Incontinence

❧   *Do Kegel exercises regularly.*

❧   *Quit smoking (or do not start), and alleviate
a likely source of chronic cough.*

❧   *Avoid straining when you urinate or have
a bowel movement.*

❧   *Maintain an appropriate weight.*

---

straining causes the bladder to fall downward. The muscles that retain the urine do not function as well, and leakage occurs. In severe cases, the bladder protrudes out of the vagina. You may notice a painful mass (a cystocele) coming out of the vagina when standing. In many cases, there is damage to the support of the uterus and rectum as well, causing a "dropped" uterus (prolapse) or bulge from the rectum (rectocele).

If your stress incontinence is due to loss of support to the bladder neck, you have leakage of urine with coughing, sneezing and laughing. One of the most beneficial findings is being able to see this leakage during the exam. Other tests confirm the diagnosis.

A **cotton-swab test** is almost always performed. The doctor places a cotton swab in your urethra and notes the angle that the swab makes in relation to the floor. You then are asked to cough, sneeze or bear down, and any change in the angle is documented. Any change greater than 30 degrees is abnormal.

Urethroscopy is commonly used to look inside the urethra, and to see if the urethra is functioning correctly. In the doctor's office, a small "scope" is placed in the urethra. This relatively painless test allows the doctor to see if the urethra is damaged or scarred in any way.

Simple or multi-channel urodynamic studies are often performed to confirm a diagnosis of genuine stress incontinence. They also can rule out other causes of incontinence such as abnormal bladder contractions or spasms.

Urethral pressure profiles (UPP) are sometimes obtained by directly measuring the pressure at multiple points along the length of the urethra. If, when you cough, the pressure in the urethra is less than the pressure in the bladder, you will leak urine. This by definition is stress incontinence.

The other cause of stress incontinence is damage to the urethra itself. If you have a low-pressure urethra, you may lose a large amount of urine, especially when standing with a full bladder, because there is no resistance to urine flow. This form of incontinence is most common in women who have had several failed surgical incontinence procedures. Upon examination with a small scope, the urethra appears scarred and open. Women with this condition usually are leaking constantly, pouring out urine like water out of a pail with a hole in it. Fortunately, this kind of stress incontinence is very rare.

WHICH MEDICINES IMPROVE STRESS INCONTINENCE

The previously described behavioral treatments and exercises can cure about 15 percent of patients. Another 60 percent will see improvement if they stick to their treatment. In addition, various medications can increase pressure in the urethra, and thus prevent loss of urine.

Estrogen is very useful for post-menopausal women who have thinning of the tissues around the bladder. Beneficial effects can usually be noted within a few weeks of taking estrogen. With a healthier urethra, there is more resistance to the loss of urine. Estrogen is most helpful in the treatment of stress incontinence.

Phenylpropanolamine, a drug commonly found in many cold preparations (such as Entex-LA), causes contractions of the muscles around the urethra. The squeezing of the urethra helps hold back urine. Most people tolerate this drug well after a few days. The most common complaints are restlessness and insomnia. The typical dose is one pill twice a day.

The antidepressant **imipramine** is especially useful for people who have both stress incontinence and urgency. It also, indirectly, causes the muscles around the urethra to contract. Typical dose is 10 to 25 mg, two to three times a day. This drug may cause drowsiness initially.

HOW THE URETHRA CAN BE RE-SUPPORTED SURGICALLY

If behavioral treatments and medications fail to keep you dry, surgery is the next step. Many different procedures can correct more severe forms of stress incontinence. The goal of each is to re-support the urethra to prevent it from falling down with stress. The operation is chosen based on your symptoms, medical condition, risk factors for failure (such as obesity, chronic cough and heavy lifting), and the skill and training of the surgeon. It is very important to correct all support problems at the time of surgery. If the uterus or rectum has lost its support, that problem is also corrected.

Abdominal Approaches

These approaches (Burch, MMK and paravaginal repair) have the best chances for success. However, they are also the hardest to perform and take longer to recover from. With these procedures, a bikini-cut incision is made in the lower abdomen, and the urethra is reattached to the back of the pubic bone with permanent sutures. Only rarely does this sort of repair give way, but failures can still occur if the sutures pull away from the urethra.

After this procedure, you may be unable to urinate immediately. In that case, a catheter is placed in your bladder until you can urinate on your own. Some surgeons are teaching women how to catheterize themselves for this period after surgery. Most women are able to urinate on their own within a few days; however, some need up to a week. Rarely, a woman may take longer. Recently, more of these operations are being done through tiny incisions in the abdomen and using a "scope" called a laparoscope. This smaller incision can speed up recovery.

Vaginal Approaches

This kind of surgery is done through the vagina by passing an instrument on each side of the urethra, avoiding any large incision on the abdomen. The three most common procedures done in this fashion are the Pereyra, the Stamey and the Raz. In each, the tissue around the urethra is tied to a leather-like layer surrounding the muscles of the abdomen. The urethra is therefore better supported. These procedures have a cure rate of greater than 90 percent. However, with time, there is a risk the incontinence will return. Recent reports show five-year cure rates of 30 to 60 percent. In some hands, however, there are excellent long-term cure rates. As these procedures are done within the vagina, the repair of other vaginal problems such as rectocele or cystocele is easily accomplished.

It is important to remember that any surgical procedure has risks, and complications can occur. These include bleeding, infection and damage to the surrounding tissues (e.g., blood vessels, nerves, bladder and rectum). The complication rate with surgery is around 20 percent, with most complications being very minimal and no long-term adverse effects expected.

HOW A DAMAGED URETHRA CAN BE TREATED

As we discussed earlier, the treatment for stress incontinence due to a damaged urethra is different than for stress incontinence due to a urethra that has fallen down from loss of support. While the behavioral, exercise and drug therapies are the same, the surgical options are different. With the previous surgeries, the goal was to re-suspend the urethra and prevent it from moving downward with coughing, laughing, etc. If you have a damaged urethra, these surgical procedures do not work well because the urethra is already well-supported. The problem with a damaged urethra is that the pressure in the urethra is too low to keep urine up in the bladder. Subsequently, if drug and exercise therapies are not successful, surgical procedures that *increase* the pressure in the urethra are used.

" Here I am 28 years old, and I don't want to wear the Depends or the maxipads. I want to learn to try and hold it."

Surgical Procedures

In the past, a sling procedure was commonly used to treat this condition. In this procedure, a strip of leather-like tissue is obtained from a leg muscle or the abdominal wall. This strip is looped around the urethra and tied to the abdominal wall. The loop pulls up the urethra and squeezes in on it, increasing the pressure inside — much like a string tied around the neck of a blown-up balloon. The five-year cure rate is about 89 percent. Unfortunately, sometimes after this procedure, women are unable to void at all and need to drain their bladders with a catheter several times a day. This may sound awful, but if you are hopelessly leaking all the time, this would seem like a good trade-off.

Collagen Injection

Recently, a new technique has been devised to treat stress incontinence due to a damaged urethra. This is a much simpler and quick procedure called **peri-urethral collagen injection.** Collagen is a naturally occurring fiber in living tissues. A small amount of a paste-like material made up of collagen is injected on each side of the urethra, near where it enters into the bladder. This material squeezes in on the urethra and closes it, much as your hands would if you pushed in on each side of a garden hose. This procedure has a cure rate of around 70 percent initially. Unfortunately, some people are allergic to collagen, and it cannot be used for them. Also, the collagen itself tends to break down and the effect wears off with time. Retreatment may therefore be needed in the future, but the complication rate with this procedure is minimal and recovery is very quick. The average number of sessions required to stop the leakage completely is around three.

Supportive Devices

Finally, some supportive devices can be used for stress incontinence. Everyone is familiar with ads on TV for "adult diapers." Various pads made for menstrual flow control also can absorb urine leakage. There is nothing wrong with this approach as long as you know this is not the only option.

" It even happened at work one day. I couldn't get to the bathroom quick enough. I couldn't get away from my desk, and I wet myself. It's a terrible feeling."

Many women leak only when playing sports or during certain scheduled activities, like aerobics classes. Many of these women have found that placing a tampon or two in the vagina or inserting a diaphragm before these activities prevents them from leaking. The diaphragm and tampons help support the top wall of the vagina and prevent the urethra from falling down with stress. Due to the risk of infection, these approaches should not be used constantly, but for intermittent use they can be very helpful.

Some women who have damage to the support of the vagina should not have surgery because of poor health. In this situation, a pessary can help correct relaxation problems, and at the same time support the urethra and decrease incontinence episodes. These devices have been around for years and years, and some women use them successfully. Pessaries are usually plastic rings of various shapes and sizes that are fitted to the woman by a doctor. They are designed for continuous wear but need to be periodically removed and cleaned.

What is Urge Incontinence?
WHAT THE SYMPTOMS ARE

" It all started with my back problem. After my back surgery, I figured the incontinence would gradually go away and things would get back to normal. Well, things didn't get back to normal."

Urge incontinence is another major type of incontinence. With this type, you may have the sensation that you are about to lose urine and try to get to the bathroom quickly before you leak. You probably void frequently to keep your bladder empty. With urge incontinence, you leak a larger volume of urine than someone with stress incontinence does; a pantyliner is not enough protection. You may avoid social gatherings because of the embarrassment of wetting yourself and, over time, could become depressed. One medication used to treat urge incontinence (imipramine) is an anti-depressant; its beneficial effects on urge incontinence may have been discovered after the medicine was given to depressed people with this problem. Certain foods can irritate this condition, especially caffeine. Unlike with stress incontinence, with urge incontinence you may lose urine at night. Not uncommonly, women with urge incontinence have a childhood history of late bed-wetting.

WHAT CAUSES URGE INCONTINENCE

Urge incontinence is due to abnormal contractions, or spasms, that occur in the bladder as it fills. Normally your bladder fills completely before any contractions occur. When a contraction occurs, you feel a sensation of urgency — the feeling that you are about to leak. If you have urge incontinence, you can try to suppress the contraction or "hold your urine" until the contraction quits, but often you will leak during the contraction. There is no problem with the urethra or its support of the urethra. The problem is with the control of the bladder muscle. A bladder infection or any

> " My husband understands and my mother understands, but other people don't — when I say I've got to go, I've got to go; get me to the bathroom now, or there's going to be an accident. Biofeedback has helped with that."

process that can damage or stimulate the nerves that control the bladder can cause urge incontinence. A bladder infection can do this. This condition is commonly seen in people with:

- 🦋 Back problems (spinal tumors, disk rupture)
- 🦋 Strokes
- 🦋 Birth defects
- 🦋 Multiple sclerosis
- 🦋 Infections
- 🦋 Bladder tumors

If you suddenly develop urge incontinence without a recent back injury or pelvic surgery, you must undergo a neurological evaluation to look for problems with the nervous system (spine, brain, etc.). If blood is found in the urine and there is no infection, you should see a urologist to rule out bladder cancer.

WHICH TESTS DETECT URGE INCONTINENCE

Since the underlying problem is bladder contractions causing leakage, testing is performed in order to prove that this is your problem. A urine sample is checked for infection or blood. If you are elderly, your urine also is checked for cancerous lesions in the bladder. Many times the doctor looks in your bladder and urethra with a small scope to check for changes in the bladder or urethra that may be triggering abnormal bladder contractions.

The physical exam needs to include a careful evaluation of the nerves of the back and pelvis to rule out lesions in these areas. Several pelvic nerve reflexes can be checked to make sure that the nerves to and from the spinal cord are intact and functioning.

HOW URGE INCONTINENCE IS TREATED

Treatment of urge incontinence is usually non-surgical, because the problem is not anatomical as it is in stress incontinence, but rather is due to a problem with how the bladder muscle works. Behavioral techniques, exercises, biofeedback and electrical stimulation (discussed earlier) work very well. These treatments are usually combined with some type of drug therapy initially. Typically, Kegel exercises combined with bladder training and a medication to help decrease the bladder spasms are employed. After a time, medications are discontinued if possible.

Medications to treat urge incontinence relax the bladder muscle and prevent spasms and contractions. These medications have expected side effects. Most cause problems with dry mouth, dizziness, blurred vision, constipation and dry skin. The side effects are related to how much medicine is required to control the bladder. If you have glaucoma, you should not use these medications, because they may make the glaucoma acutely worse. Side effects are so common, however, that if you report none you are probably not taking the medication as prescribed.

Oxybutynin (brand name Ditropan) is the most common medicine used. The dose is 5mg taken two to four times a day. Some of the drugs used to treat irritable bowel syndrome (or spastic colon), such as **Bentyl** and **Levsin,** are good alternatives.

Imipramine is especially useful for those with both stress and urge incontinence. It is also useful if you leak urine at night. It has few side effects other than sleepiness, but is not as strong in preventing bladder contractions. It is useful if you cannot tolerate the other medications.

Cure rates with a combination of the above treatments are around 40 percent, with up to 80 percent of people having marked improvement in symptoms.

What is Overflow Incontinence?
WHAT THE SYMPTOMS ARE
Overflow incontinence is the last major type of incontinence. It is also relatively uncommon in women who come to a doctor's office. It is more commonly seen in nursing-home patients. If you have overflow incontinence, your bladder contracts poorly or not at all. The

bladder fills to capacity, then any additional urine runs out of the bladder, like a pail overfilled with water. In women, obstruction of the urethra is rarely the cause of overflow incontinence; in men, this is common due to enlargement of the prostate.

With overflow incontinence, your bladder never feels empty — it is constantly full. Since your bladder does not contract, you may push on your lower abdomen and lean forward to help compress the bladder and thereby urinate. Overflow incontinence produces classic complaints of:

🐾 *Constant dribbling*
🐾 *Not feeling empty after urination*
🐾 *Taking a long time to start voiding*
🐾 *Producing a weak stream of urine*
🐾 *Needing to push on the abdomen to void*
🐾 *Dribbling urine when standing*

WHAT CAUSES OVERFLOW INCONTINENCE

Overflow incontinence is caused either by a bladder muscle that does not contract or by a blockage. As mentioned earlier, obstruction is rare in women. A bladder that does not contract can be due to weakness or damage to the muscle fibers of the bladder. It may also be due to damage to the nerves that help the bladder contract — commonly seen with medical conditions like diabetes that affect the function of nerves.

WHICH TESTS DETECT OVERFLOW INCONTINENCE

The biggest clue to overflow incontinence is the large amount of urine left in the bladder after voiding. This remainder can easily be measured by draining the bladder with a catheter after voiding (a post-void residual, or PVR, described above). Uroflow studies, also described above, will usually show that you take a long time to empty your bladder. You void in an intermittent fashion, pushing down on your abdomen, getting out a small amount of urine each time.

Obviously, because of the high likelihood of a nerve problem, testing is indicated. Also, you are screened for medications that might interfere with the bladder's ability to contract. *Quite a few prescription and over-the-counter medicines can cause the bladder not to contract well.* Medications that might be causing overflow incontinence can usually be changed.

HOW OVERFLOW INCONTINENCE IS TREATED

In general, if you have overflow incontinence due to obstruction or treatable medical conditions, you should have these treated to see if your bladder function improves. Also, you can learn techniques to help you empty your bladder during voiding. One of these techniques is the **crede** maneuver, where you place both hands over the bladder area and lean forward on the toilet. By doing this, you tend to compress and empty the bladder.

Treatment of overflow incontinence is aimed at keeping the bladder empty and preventing loss of urine. After proper instructions, you can easily drain your bladder. This is called self-catheterization. Using self-catheterization, you can drain your bladder regularly to prevent it from becoming overly distended. Women use short catheters to drain the bladder, and with proper technique, infections are infrequent.

What If I Have "Mixed" Incontinence?

Unfortunately, you may fall into the category of women who do not have just one type of incontinence, but some element of each. Many women have symptoms of both stress and urge incontinence. If that is the case for you, you need to determine which one is causing the biggest problem. It is inappropriate to have surgery for stress incontinence if 90 percent of your episodes of incontinence are due to urgency, or bladder contractions. You need very careful evaluation and testing. Your doctor should also set realistic goals with you and discuss fully the anticipated outcomes of your treatment. If 80 percent of your problem is stress incontinence and the rest is due to urge incontinence, you should be told that if you have surgery to fix the stress incontinence, that most likely the urge incontinence will not go away. The urge component may still need to be treated after the surgery, perhaps with medication.

Conclusion

If you leak urine, you should discuss this problem with your physician. Please do not allow yourself to suffer physically or emotionally from this problem; seek help. After a thorough exam and a few tests, your caregiver can explain why you leak and review with you what treatments are appropriate. At that point, your input — how strongly you feel about medication versus conservative treatment versus surgery — helps guide the course of action. The goal of this chapter is to educate you about each of these options. The bottom line is that incontinence is a very treatable condition. Incontinence should not prevent you or your loved ones from enjoying life to its fullest.

Additional Resources
Books

- **Bladder Control for Women,** National Kidney and Urologic Diseases Information Clearinghouse, 1997.

- **Overcoming Bladder Disorders: Compassionate, Authoritative Medical and Self-Help Solutions for Incontinence, Cystitis, Interstitial Cystitis, Prostate Problems and Bladder Cancer,** *Rebecca Chalker and Kristene E. Whitmore,* HarperCollins, 1991.

- **Urinary Incontinence in Adults: Clinical Practice Guidelines,** Agency for Health Care Policy and Research, revised 1996.
  This booklet, published by a division of the Department of Health and Human Services, is aimed mainly at health providers; however, it is an excellent source of basic information for the public. A patient's version is also available. Ask for AHCPR Publication No. 96-0682 from:
  AHCPR Publications Clearinghouse
  P.O. Box 8547
  Silver Springs, MD 20907

Organizations

- **American Uro-Gynecologic Society**
  401 N. Michigan Ave.
  Chicago, IL 60611-4267
  (312) 644-6610

- **Continence Restored, Inc.**
  407 Strawberry Hill Ave.
  Stamford, CT 06902
  (914) 285-1470 (day) or (203) 348-0601 (evening)

- **National Association for Continence**
  (formerly Help for Incontinent People)
  P.O. Box 8310, Spartanburg, SC 29305-8310
  (864) 579-7900 or (800) 252-3337 (800-BLADDER)
  E-mail: lverdell@globalvision.net
  http://www.nafc.org

- **The Simon Foundation for Continence**
  P.O. Box 835
  Wilmette, Illinois 60091
  (800) 237-4666 (800-23SIMON) (24 hours / 7 days)

- **Uromed Corporation**
  64 A St.
  Needham, MA 02194
  (615) 433-0033
  http://www.uromed.com

Internet Sites

- **http://www.incontinet.com**
  InContiNet, which is self-proclaimed "the Web's leading resource on incontinence and pelvic muscle disorders," reaches out to the incontinence sufferer as well as the medical professional. Offerings include a discussion group, a mailing list and critical reviews of incontinence literature.

- **http://www.nafc.org**
  The National Association for Continence (see Organizations, above) offers the latest edition of its quarterly newsletter online — as well as a wealth of other information.

- **http://vhp.nus.sg/~sfcs/continet/**
  Global perspective is available from the International Continence Society. This home page features a message board and mailing list as well as articles of interest.

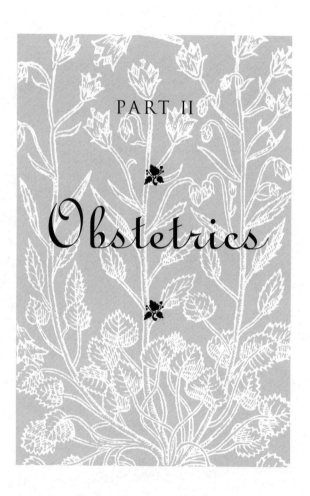

PART II

Obstetrics

With Birth

As is In Life,

Your Greatest Challenges

Often Produce

Your Greatest

Gifts.

CHAPTER ELEVEN

PRE-PREGNANCY CONSULT

Preparing Yourself for Pregnancy

hen you plan to begin your family, having a normal, healthy baby is your primary concern. Although there are no guarantees, we can address some issues that can help bring about the best outcome from your pregnancy. Among the general public, there is a 3-percent risk of having a baby with a malformation. The goals of this chapter are to help you keep this risk as low as possible, and to help couples facing high-risk pregnancies to approach them with more confidence and comfort.

The best time to have a visit with your caregiver is three months *before* you start trying to become pregnant. An exam before conception allows a thorough evaluation of any special problems. With pre-pregnancy counseling, we can have you in the best possible shape, both physically and mentally.

Use this chapter to help you understand some of the many factors that can impact a pregnancy. The chapter is not all-inclusive, and it does not replace the advice of your physician. Instead, it will allow you to understand what he or she advises, and why certain tests and procedures are done during pregnancy.

The Main Topics Include:
- *Review of family history*
- *Racial and ethnic considerations*
- *Evaluation of medical problems*
- *Complete physical exam*
- *Lab evaluation*
- *Healthy habits*
- *The role of prenatal vitamins*
- *Ways to increase your chances of becoming pregnant*

Reviewing Your Family History

In reviewing your family history, the goal is to find any conditions that could be passed on to your children. It is important to provide a thorough and accurate medical history of both your and your husband's parents, brothers and sisters, aunts and uncles, cousins and grandparents.

If any of these relatives has had a baby with a birth defect (including a loss during the second half of pregnancy), obtain medical records relating to that baby's condition. This information helps your physician decide if your risk of having a similar problem is increased.

A family history of multiple miscarriages may be important. (Multiple miscarriages means that a woman has had three or more miscarriages.) This history becomes very important if that relative has never had a live baby. In this situation, there may be a defect in the family genes, or chromosomes, that could be passed on to your future offspring. Therefore, a consultation with a specialist in this area, called a geneticist, would be appropriate.

Racial and Ethnic Considerations

WHITE POPULATION

Cystic fibrosis is a condition found in the genes of 1 in 25 whites. If both parents have the gene for cystic fibrosis, their baby has a 1-in-4 chance of inheriting this condition. With time, thick mucus accumulates in many important organs of a person with CF. The parts of the body that help digest food – such as the pancreas, biliary tract and intestines – become blocked. When this blockage occurs, food is not absorbed and cannot be made available to the body. The body responds as if the person were not eating, and general weakness develops. In the lungs, the small openings are blocked, which in turn makes breathing more difficult. Because of their weakness and blocked lungs, people with cystic fibrosis have problems with frequent pneumonia.

A baby born with cystic fibrosis appears normal. Problems develop over the years; average life span is 20 to 30 years. Occasionally, a baby has problems from birth, with poor feeding and weight gain. Of babies not diagnosed at birth, most are identified by their first birthday due to chronic cough, a swollen stomach and poor weight gain.

A test for cystic fibrosis has only recently been found. At present, the testing of all whites is not suggested. It is ideal to test couples if someone in their family has cystic fibrosis. If you do have someone in your family with cystic fibrosis, talk with your physician. You also should see a geneticist, who specializes in finding these conditions for couples.

AFRICAN-AMERICAN POPULATION

In the African-American population, **sickle-cell disease** is the most common condition that can be passed from parents to children. Sickle-cell disease is a problem with the red blood cells. The cells change shape when there is not enough oxygen in the bloodstream. A normal red blood cell is round and slightly depressed in the center. With sickle-cell disease, the cells bend in the middle, resembling a sickle. A blood cell with this shape does not travel through the blood vessels very well, and the vessels become blocked. If this blockage is in the stomach, the person has severe stomach pain. If blockage occurs in the joints, the person has intense joint pain. Over time these blocked vessels cause permanent damage to the internal organs. People with sickle-cell disease often cannot get enough air during heavy exercise or an infection. Therefore, they must avoid both situations, and get treatment quickly if they ever develop an infection. People with sickle-cell disease may live into their 40s.

All African-American couples should be tested for this serious condition before attempting to conceive. One in 10 has the ability to pass this disease on to a child. If both parents carry the gene, the chance their baby will have sickle-cell disease is 25 percent – 1 in 4. If just one parent has this gene, the baby has no chance of contracting the disease.

If you are already pregnant and you learn that you and your partner both carry the gene for sickle-cell disease, you can have your baby tested. Testing is done early in pregnancy by either amniocentesis or chorionic villus sampling. (Both of these procedures are explained in the section "Advanced Maternal Age" in this chapter.) If your baby is found to have sickle-cell disease, you will face a difficult decision. You can choose to terminate the pregnancy (have an abortion), or you can begin preparing for the birth of a baby with a special problem.

JEWISH POPULATION

Tay-Sachs disease is a fatal condition involving the brain. Among Jewish people of Eastern European descent (Ashkenazi Jews), 1 in 30 has the ability to pass this gene to a baby. If both the man and woman have this gene, there is a 25-percent chance the baby will have Tay-Sachs disease. A couple should be tested for this fatal problem before trying to conceive. If you are already pregnant, the baby can be tested for this condition by amniocentesis or chorionic villus sampling.

Babies with Tay-Sachs disease usually die by age 4. Excess fat accumulates around the brain cells, causing paralysis, blindness and eventually death. At this time, there is no cure or treatment. Therefore, if your baby is found to have Tay-Sachs disease, you must decide whether to terminate the pregnancy, or accept the birth of a baby with a special problem.

ASIAN, MIDDLE EASTERN, NORTH AFRICAN, INDIAN & MEDITERRANEAN POPULATIONS

Thalassemia, a condition involving components of the blood cells, can vary in severity. There are mild forms, where the person has no problems, and there are also other forms so profound that the baby dies before birth. A blood cell is made from four building blocks. If just one block is missing, the condition is not very severe. If the main blocks are missing, however, the blood cells will not work, becoming the cause of the baby's death.

People of Asian, Middle Eastern, North African, Indian and Mediterranean descent are most likely to carry the gene for thalassemia. If you fall into one of these groups, you can be a carrier of the disease without knowing it – that is, you might have no symptoms yet still give this disease to a baby, who could die very young. Through blood tests, we can determine if you carry the gene for thalassemia. If you are already pregnant and find out that you and your partner both have the ability to pass on this disease, you can have your baby tested. If the baby has thalassemia, you will have to make a decision about the birth of the baby.

Common Problems in Pregnancy

This section reviews how certain common problems can affect a pregnancy, and it also explains how to prepare yourself for becoming pregnant. There are many other problems that affect pregnancy, and you should discuss any medical or social problem you have with your doctor.

DRUG USE

It is of major importance to openly discuss drug use, including alcohol and tobacco, with your doctor. These problems have a very negative impact on a developing baby. To stop using drugs is difficult at any time in your life; however, the anticipation of pregnancy is an excellent inspiration. Do not try to fool yourself into believing you will stop during pregnancy. Trying to stop a drug habit while pregnant is very hard, due to the demands that pregnancy puts on your system. Do not think you have developed a sudden ability to be strong. Realize your problem, and stop the drugs before becoming pregnant.

ADVANCED MATERNAL AGE

Every young woman should know how the age of a mother affects her baby. The term **advanced maternal age** applies to a woman who will be 35 or older when she delivers her baby. Thirty-five is very young to be considered advanced. However, this age group can have special problems, including greater incidence of infertility, miscarriage, chromosome abnormalities, and difficulty at the end of pregnancy. In general, the older the woman is, the more likely – and more severe – her problems with pregnancy will be. Use this information when you try to choose the best time to begin a family. (See Chapter 18, "Pregnancy After 35," for more details.)

Infertility and Miscarriage

Women over age 35 can have problems with infertility; the older you are, the more difficult it can be to become pregnant. If you are in your 20s, your chance of experiencing infertility is 7 percent. If you are in your early 30s, that risk increases to 15 percent; in your late 30s, it is 20 percent; and in your 40s, the chance that you will experience infertility is 30 percent. Once pregnant, you have a higher rate of miscarriage with advancing age. Before age 35, your risk of miscarriage is 10 percent. From 35 to 40, the risk is 20 percent, and after age 40, your risk of miscarriage is higher than 30 percent. (Chapter 19, "Infertility," provides a broader discussion of these issues, as well as resources for support and education.)

INFERTILITY

A couple is considered infertile if unable to conceive
after one year of unprotected intercourse.

Chromosomal Abnormalities

The greatest risk for women over age 35 is having a baby with a chromosome problem. There are many types of chromosome problems, with Down's syndrome being the best known. Normally, a person has two exact copies of chromosomes 1 through 22, plus XX for a girl and XY chromosomes for a boy. A baby with Down's syndrome has an extra copy of chromosome 21 (thus the other name for this disorder, Trisomy 21). Certain characteristics are common in people with Down's syndrome: their mouths are slightly open, and their tongues protrude somewhat; their eyes are slanted; and they frequently have heart problems and some degree of mental retardation. Some people with Down's syndrome are only mildly retarded and live with minimal problems into adulthood. Others have severe retardation and require complete, long-term care. The average life span of a person with Down's syndrome is 40 to 50 years.

Living With The Diagnosis of Down's Syndrome

I was a little upset when I first found out; you know, I always wanted a girl after two boys, and something was wrong with her. But we were glad that she didn't have a lot of medical problems unlike some children have; some have heart problems and other problems, but she didn't have any of those.

I had four ultrasounds, and they never picked up on it. I had no idea. I had a perfect pregnancy 'til the end; she came a little early. They told me right after I delivered. After half an hour, they came and said she had Down's syndrome – they suspected it because her eyes are a little bit more slanted. I just had high blood pressure at the end of my pregnancy, but that's pretty normal with the third pregnancy. You know, I'm 33, and they say that if you're over 35 there's a high risk because your eggs are getting older, but there are a lot of younger people who have children with Down's syndrome. It depends on every individual person.

We wouldn't change anything. Even if we had known before, we still would have kept her! We moved here when she was 7 months old, and now she's 2½. We belong to an active Down's syndrome association. We have meetings on different topics going from babies to teenagers. It gives you some support, and it might give you some ideas that you haven't tried before. You know anytime you have a problem, you're not the only ones to confront that problem.

Her brothers love her to death; she's a spoiled little girl! She loves books. We are just very fortunate; she's a high-functioning child. You never know; every child is different. You never know what kind of child you're going to have until they're born and start growing up. She's going to live a good life for herself. She's a giggly, typical little girl.

Pre-pregnancy Consult: Preparing Yourself for Pregnancy

If you are of advanced maternal age, it is suggested that you have genetic studies done early in your pregnancy to determine if your baby has Down's syndrome or any other chromosomal problem. There are risks involved with the studies, but if you are older than 35, the risk of having a baby with Down's syndrome is greater than the risk of the tests. (For comparison, your risk of having a baby with a chromosome problem at age 20 is 1 in 500; at 35, the risk is 1 in 200; and at 40, the risk is 1 in 60.)

The current studies available are chorionic villus sampling (CVS) and amniocentesis (for more detailed information about these tests, see Chapter 18, "Pregnancy After 35"). CVS is done between the 10th and 12th weeks of pregnancy. The test involves passing a catheter through the upper vagina (cervix) or through the lower abdomen into the uterus. When the catheter is passed through the cervix, you are in the same position as during a Pap smear. Your cervix is cleaned with a sterile solution to minimize the risk of infection. The catheter then collects cells from the placenta. During the procedure, ultrasound is used to make sure the baby is not touched. The results are available in seven to ten days.

Amniocentesis is done during weeks 15 through 20. A catheter is passed through your lower abdomen and fluid is collected. Again, the baby is not touched. There are cells from the baby that float in the fluid, and these are the cells that are tested. The results are back in ten to fourteen days.

Both CVS and amniocentesis tell you not only whether your baby has normal chromosomes, but also whether the baby is a boy or a girl. The tests do not detect birth defects, such as an abnormal heart. The risk of miscarriage after an amniocentesis is 1 in 200; after a CVS, the risk is 1 in 100.

The advantage of CVS is that it is done earlier in your pregnancy – an important issue when deciding what to do with the results. If the baby has a chromosomal problem, like Down's syndrome, you may choose to terminate the pregnancy. If you have an abortion, it is safer and easier to perform at an earlier stage of pregnancy. Another option is to use the information to prepare yourself and your family for the birth of a baby with special problems. With either decision, you will have lifelong consequences to address. It is very important that you freely discuss all your concerns with your doctor.

The advantage of amniocentesis is that another test is done on the fluid other than the one for Down's syndrome. The other test is for alpha-fetoprotein (AFP). The AFP test detects birth defects associated with the digestive system, spine and brain. If the AFP value is high, your doctor further evaluates the baby with a special ultrasound.

End-of-Pregnancy Issues

If you are older than 35, you are also more likely to have problems near the end of your pregnancy. Therefore, your doctor monitors your baby very closely during this time with a non-stress test (NST). This test involves monitoring the baby's heartbeat during regular visits. If the baby appears to be stressed, noted by decelerations in the heart rate, your physician may want to induce labor or do more advanced tests.

Pregnancy for women over age 35 is not to be feared, but there are issues that must be addressed. With good care, you should be able to have a wonderful pregnancy and a healthy baby even if you are of "advanced maternal age." This overview is meant to help you approach the many decisions that face you better-informed and more confident.

DIABETES

Diabetes is a condition where the body does not process sugars very well. Whenever we eat food, particularly sweets, the body absorbs the sugar into the blood. The body's cells use sugar for energy to do work, such as walking for a muscle cell or thinking for a brain cell. In order to get the sugar from the blood into the cells, your body releases insulin. Without enough insulin, the sugar is too high in the blood and too low in the cells. With diabetes, the body is not producing as much insulin as it requires. Someone with diabetes can give herself a shot of insulin with meals to provide the extra that is needed.

If you are diabetic, you need to inform your physician if you are planning to start a family. Your risk of having a baby with a malformation is higher than for someone who is not diabetic. The problems seen in babies born to diabetic mothers include a hole in the middle of the heart, anencephaly (defect of the top of the skull), spina bifida (incomplete closure of the spine), absent kidney and shortening of the lower extremities. The risk of malformations gets worse the more out-of-control your diabetes is at the time you conceive. Therefore, you should get your diabetes under control as best you can *before* you start trying to get pregnant. The most important aspect is your control at conception, not whether your form of diabetes is juvenile-or adult-onset. If you find yourself pregnant at a time of very poor control of your diabetes, you may wish to discuss the option of abortion with your physician. This decision is very personal and not to be chosen without fully understanding all the options.

YOUNG WOMEN
WITH DIABETES, TAKE NOTE

This information about diabetes and pregnancy is of particular use to you if you are dating and not using adequate contraception. Young women in your situation are usually under fair control, but that is not good enough when it comes to pregnancy. If you accidentally become pregnant, you put a child at greater risk of being born with a malformation. By getting excellent control of your diabetes before conceiving a baby, your risk of having a baby with birth defects is only slightly higher than the general population's.

While you are at increased risk of having a baby with a malforma-tion if you have diabetes, you are not at increased risk of having a baby with chromosomal problems. This is an important difference, as the tests to look for these problems are not the same. If you are dia-betic, a special ultrasound evaluation of your baby is done to detect malformations. In order to rule out chromosome problems, as in ad-vance maternal age, an amniocentesis or CVS is performed.

To understand how pregnancy affects diabetes, you need to know that a pregnancy consumes insulin. Early in pregnancy, the effect is minor, because the pregnancy is small. By the end of pregnancy, a great deal of insulin is being taken up by the placenta. The placenta (also called the afterbirth) is the organ in the uterus (or womb) that feeds blood to the baby from the mother's circulation. The umbilical cord connects the baby to the placenta. As pregnancy advances, the placenta becomes larger. It is this larger placenta that consumes insulin. Therefore, if you are diabetic, you should expect to increase your dose of insulin during pregnancy. This increased dosage does not mean the diabetes is getting worse, or that you are not doing a good job at taking care of yourself. Instead, it is a natural, expected part of the process and should not cause alarm.

There are other issues involved with pregnancy and diabetes; this basic explanation covers only the main ideas. The purpose of this section is to show why a visit to your doctor prior to pregnancy is crucial if you have diabetes.

ASTHMA

Asthma is a breathing problem in which the lungs do not allowing air to pass through easily. If you have asthma, you have to work harder to breathe, especially when exposed to something that irritates your lungs. You can control your asthma with medications, such as an inhaler or pills that help keep the lungs open.

If you have asthma and become pregnant, you have a 60-percent chance that your asthma will stay the same during pregnancy, a 20-percent chance that it will get better and a 20-percent chance it will get worse. Your asthma does not increase the risk of malformation for your baby, but asthma is associated with an increased risk that your baby will not gain the appropriate amount of weight. The most common mistake that pregnant women with asthma make is to stop taking their medication. If you stay on your medication and control the asthma, you should be able to enjoy being pregnant.

If you have severe asthma that has required admission to a hospital during the past five years, you should discuss the safety of your becoming pregnant with your physician. If you have had to be on a ventilator due to asthma, it may be wise to consider adoption of a baby. At some point the risks of pregnancy are too high to both you and a baby. If it appears that your asthma is so severe that pregnancy could result in your death, then you should be using a very reliable method of birth control.

SEIZURE DISORDERS

Seizures result from abnormal brain signals. They may cause you to simply stare out into space (petit mal seizure) or cause your body to jerk violently all over (grand mal seizure). There are many different causes for seizures – ranging from brain trauma to tumors to infections of the brain – and many seizures have unknown causes. Seizures are treated with medication to control these abnormal brain signals. If you have not had a seizure over the past three to five years, you may be able to discontinue all medication, and then try to become pregnant. You should not stop this medication without the knowledge of your physician.

If you have a seizure disorder, the main risk in pregnancy is an increased rate of birth defects. That risk is elevated whether or not you are on medication. The normal population's risk of birth defects is 2.5 percent, but if you have a seizure disorder for which you do not take medication, the risk is 4.2 percent. And with medication, the risk is 6 percent. If you depend on medication to be without seizures, you should stay on medication during the pregnancy. While you may be afraid to take medication during pregnancy, you need to realize that having a seizure while pregnant can cause problems much worse than the medication could. During a seizure, the amount of oxygen available to the baby decreases. Also, if you have a seizure while driving, you could hurt yourself (pregnant or not) and anyone you collide with; and of course, you have an extra "passenger" to consider while pregnant.

It is common to need an increased dose of medicine to control seizures during pregnancy. As pregnancy advances, the body has more blood. The medication dilutes in a larger volume of blood, resulting in a lower concentration of medicine and allowing seizures to return. By increasing the dose, your doctor maintains the concentration of the drug in your body at the level it was prior to pregnancy.

DEPRESSION AND ANXIETY

Depression is a very common condition involving feelings of worthlessness. When depressed you can vary from being blue, or in a down mood, to being dysfunctional. You tend to not enjoy things in life, and have nothing to look forward to in the future. If you are depressed, you should acknowledge that you have a serious condition and seek help from your doctor. This condition is as real and potentially life-threatening as a brain tumor. No person with a brain tumor would go without medical care; nor should a person with depression.

Depression may get worse during pregnancy, but most women with depression remain stable during pregnancy and have healthy babies. It is the first month after delivery that is the most problematic. During this month, even with a healthy baby, you get very little sleep. You have new demands placed on you that can make you very stressed and more depressed. It is important to arrange as much support as possible to be available during this very difficult time. Also, if you have depression, you should schedule regular visits with your counselor during the pregnancy. During the first months after the baby is born, these visits are even more important.

When you want to become pregnant, it is best to discontinue taking medication for depression as long as your counselor advises you that you can do so safely. However, if you need to be on medication during pregnancy, accept that fact and continue to take it. While there is some risk involved with taking most prescription drugs, these risks are usually small. If you are able to do without the medicine during the first 12 weeks of pregnancy, you greatly lower the risk involved with taking the drugs. However, not taking the medicine when you need it could prove much more dangerous than the medicine itself could ever be to the baby. Serious depression can lead to poor eating habits, abuse of drugs, or even attempted suicide – obviously dangerous to the baby's development.

Anxiety is a condition of feeling very stressed. It is very normal to feel anxious and stressed at times during pregnancy as you contemplate the changes and responsibilities a new baby will bring. (And you may feel that parenthood and anxiety go hand in hand.)

But a true anxiety disorder is a crippling thing. When you have an anxiety disorder, you are not able to relax and sleep well, and your ability to think and reason worsen over time. No good drugs for this condition can be used safely in pregnancy. The best approach to managing an anxiety disorder during pregnancy is to work with your counselor to find ways to control the problem without medication. If you cannot do so, it may not be wise to get pregnant. The other option is to get pregnant and accept the risks involved with the available medicines. The problem is that if you have an anxiety disorder, you are probably not able to cope with this option. You may be very stressed with the thought you may have harmed your baby. This stress can continue even as the baby grows up and is developing normally.

WAYS TO LOWER ANXIETY DURING PREGNANCY

🐾 *Read a lot to know about normal changes.*
🐾 *Take daily walks for a mile.*
🐾 *Take relaxing baths each evening. (Warm, not hot.)*
🐾 *Surround yourself with happy people. Do not commiserate with someone who had a bad outcome.*
🐾 *Avoid all caffeine, alcohol and other drugs.*
🐾 *Stay active in your community – helping, but not taking on a leadership role.*

HYPERTENSION

High blood pressure is becoming more common in pregnancy because more women over age 35 are getting pregnant. The main risks of high blood pressure are poor growth of the baby and worsening of blood pressure at the end of pregnancy. Your blood pressure will be closely monitored during pregnancy. If you have a history of hypertension, you may be placed on a baby aspirin a day to lower the chance that your blood pressure will get much higher at the end of pregnancy.

A history of hypertension increases your risk for having **toxemia,** also called pre-eclampsia. Toxemia is a serious problem with high blood pressure that occurs at the end of pregnancy. With toxemia, blood pressure increases dramatically, and you may have swelling of your hands and face, pain under your right ribs, dark spots floating in your vision, a progressively worsening headache and, in the worst situation, a seizure. Toxemia is treated by delivery of the baby and also with the medication magnesium sulfate to prevent you from having seizures. If the baby is not fully developed, delivery could result in problems due to prematurity, but to not deliver the baby could be life-threatening to both you and the baby due to damage to your kidneys, liver and brain.

If you have high blood pressure, you also may have problems with maintaining adequate blood flow for the needs of your developing baby. Your physician will monitor the baby through ultrasounds, assuring normal growth. During the last months of pregnancy the baby is tested with a non-stress test. This simple test involves listening to the baby's heartbeat during weekly visits. If a problem is noted, more advanced tests are used to see if the baby should be delivered.

A very serious problem related to hypertension is **abruption,** where the placenta separates from the uterus prematurely. When this separation occurs before the baby is born, the baby is without adequate blood supply. Hypertension damages your smallest blood vessels, increasing the risk of this problem. Abruption is very rare but very serious, and can occur even without a history of hypertension. No test is available to predict an abruption, and it may occur without warning. When abruption starts, you have marked abdominal pain, often with vaginal bleeding. If you have these symptoms, go to the nearest hospital as quickly as possible. If the pain is from something minor, that is fine. If an abruption is occurring, any delay could be tragic. Once at the hospital, an emergency cesarean section is done if vaginal delivery is not anticipated soon.

The Physical Exam

The purpose of the physical exam as part of a pre-pregnancy visit is to make sure there are no medical problems. Expect a complete physical, including an exam of your heart and lungs. Your physician does a pelvic exam to evaluate your uterus and to detect any tumors of the uterus or ovaries. Within the uterus, there may be fibroids or polyps that could complicate pregnancy. When tumors are noted, a complete evaluation with an ultrasound is done. If surgery is required, then obviously it should be done prior to your becoming pregnant. The exam also will include a Pap smear to see if your cervix is healthy. If that test shows a problem, it should be treated before you become pregnant.

Laboratory Work

The pre-pregnancy visit also includes a lab evaluation. Each physician has a battery of lab tests he or she orders if you are planning to start a family. This section covers the most common tests. If you have more or fewer tests, then ask your physician to explain the difference. This section addresses evaluation for rubella, diabetes, toxoplasmosis, chickenpox and AIDS.

Rubella, or German measles, feels much like a minor viral infection. You have flu-like complaints, with muscle pain, stiff joints, headache, swollen neck glands and a fever. A rash appears on your face and neck. While this infection is minor for an adult, if you are exposed in early pregnancy, rubella can cause such birth defects as hearing loss, growth retardation and heart abnormalities. (The chance your baby will have a birth defect is 25 percent if you become infected with rubella in the first trimester of pregnancy, and only 1 percent in the second and the third trimesters.) In order to avoid an unfortunate situation, a blood test is done to determine if you are already immune. If you are immune, there is no risk to a developing baby if you are exposed to someone with a rubella infection while you are pregnant. If the test shows you are not immune, you are given a vaccine. You should avoid getting pregnant for three months after having the vaccine. Most people use condoms during this waiting period. After this time, you are immune and not at risk in a subsequent pregnancy.

A blood glucose test screens for **diabetes**. If your glucose (sugar) level is high, a more involved test is done to diagnose diabetes. The importance of this information is explained in the section on diabetes earlier in this chapter. If you have diabetes, you are at higher risk of having a baby with a birth defect. The only way to lower that risk is to be the best possible condition and control at the time you become pregnant. Therefore, prior to pregnancy is the best time to detect this condition.

Toxoplasmosis is an infection that causes few problems in adults. Like rubella, an infection in the early stages can cause birth defects, but for toxoplasmosis there is no vaccine. The complications of toxoplasmosis for the infant include visual problems, hearing loss, mental retardation and seizures. If a blood test shows you are immune to toxoplasmosis, there is no risk to a baby during pregnancy. If you are not immune, you need to avoid exposure to this infection. Toxoplasmosis is transmitted through contact with cats, raw meat and garden soil where a cat left droppings. The main risk with cats involves the litter box. If you have a cat and are not immune to toxoplasmosis, you should have another person change the litter box. If you must change the cat's box, you should wear a mask and wash your hands thoroughly afterward.

Chickenpox is a common childhood disease that causes a pronounced rash, fever and general body pains. If you have not had chickenpox, you are tested for immunity. Many adults do not remember having had this infection but are immune when tested. If you are at risk for chickenpox, you may now have a new vaccine. If you are exposed and are not immune, there is a 5-percent chance that your baby may have birth defects, such as scars of the skin, short limbs and mental retardation. If you work in a school, child-care center or hospital, you should discuss this test and the vaccine with your physician. Currently there is not a standard for vaccination in this situation, as the vaccine has only recently been released. It is being used widely by physicians caring for children. Chickenpox is a prevalent problem in most neighborhoods at some point. It is reasonable to be tested regardless of your occupation if you do not remember having had chickenpox in the past.

AIDS is a life-threatening problem that lowers your ability to fight off infection. It is becoming more common among women, who acquire it most often through having intercourse or through having intercouse or injecting themselves with drugs. The AIDS virus can be transmitted to a baby during pregnancy, at birth or with breast-feeding. The transmission rate is 30 percent. A baby with AIDS usually dies at a young age. In order to avoid this tragic outcome, you should be tested for this virus before you try to become pregnant. If you have the virus that causes AIDS, then you need to be completely educated before deciding if you want to get pregnant. Many women with AIDS choose not to have children when they learn what could happen.

Healthy Habits

Much of what you can do to prepare for pregnancy does not involve testing at a doctor's office. Keeping fit, eating well and avoiding unhealthy situations can help you have a healthy baby.

Exercise is very good for you and the baby during pregnancy. It is best to already have an exercise routine before becoming pregnant. The ideal exercises are low-impact and give a cardiovascular workout. The exercise also should be fun, convenient and inexpensive. Try to avoid things that require a great deal of coordination, as your center of gravity changes as pregnancy progresses. Consider walking, swimming and low-impact aerobics. With any exercise in pregnancy, do not push yourself to exhaustion. Also, avoid allowing your body to overheat or become dehydrated. It is important not to use a sauna or whirlpool, as these tend to raise your temperature too high and increase your baby's risk of brain damage.

In anticipation of being pregnant, avoid drugs and alcohol. If you smoke, stop. For common medical problems, your doctor can give you a list of over-the-counter medications that are safe in pregnancy. Try to limit your use of medicines to those on such a list. If you take prescription medication, make sure your doctor is aware you are trying to get pregnant. Some conditions require that you continue medication while pregnant. These issues are addressed at your pre-pregnancy visit.

To not wear a seat belt while pregnant is a mistake. If you are in a car accident, your greatest risk is being thrown out of the car. In order to lower this risk, you must wear your seat belt. A common excuse for not wearing a seat belt during pregnancy is that the baby will be harmed. In fact, if you do not wear a belt, you can be thrown against the steering wheel and possibly crush the baby. More likely, you will be injured from being thrown from the car. The resulting injuries are the main cause of damage to babies. The statistics support that babies survive more frequently when you wear your seat belt.

EXERCISES TO HELP YOU PREPARE FOR PREGNANCY

🪶 *Walking one mile per day (this is my favorite to suggest)*
🪶 *Swimming twenty minutes per day*
🪶 *Doing low-impact aerobics*
🪶 *Bicycling*

Prenatal Vitamins

The use of prenatal vitamins is common during pregnancy. They should be started one month before you want to get pregnant. Folic acid (folate) in prenatal vitamins lowers the chance the baby will have a problem in the development of its spine or head. There normally needs to be 400 micrograms (0.4 mg) of folic acid in the prenatal vitamin. If you have a family history of a baby with a birth defect involving the head or spine, then you should take 4 mg of folic acid per day while attempting to conceive. It is important to avoid large doses of multivitamins while trying to conceive.

How to Increase Your Chances of Becoming Pregnant

Getting pregnant can normally take up to a year, with an average time of four months. Therefore, if you do not get pregnant at first, try not to worry, and keep trying. If you are not pregnant after 12 months, you should see your doctor.

To help yourself become pregnant, avoid the use of lubricants when having intercourse. Most lubricants are harmful to sperm, and many are designed to kill sperm. After your partner ejaculates, rest on your back with a pillow under your bottom for 10 minutes. This position keeps the sperm against the cervix, which is the "door" to your uterus. Also, your partner should stop thrusting after ejaculation, as the penis acts like a plunger, pushing sperm out of the vagina.

The best time in your menstrual cycle to get pregnant is 14 days before the start of a period. That is the day of ovulation, when an egg is released from the ovary. If you have a 28-day cycle, then that will be day 14 of the cycle. Day one of a cycle is the first day of the period. With a 30-day cycle, the best time will be on day 16. To ensure a ready supply of sperm when the egg is released, you should have intercourse the day of – as well as the days before and after – ovulation.

Conclusion

While this chapter offers many serious topics to consider, most women do not have to worry about these problems. The goal of this chapter is to help you understand why certain tests are done before you become pregnant. Also, you now should know about special problems that require attention before pregnancy. With this knowledge, you should better understand your doctor's advice. Again, use this information to approach pregnancy with more confidence and comfort.

Additional Resources

Books

- **Before You Conceive: The Complete Pre-pregnancy Guide,** *John R. Sussman, M.D., and B. Blake Levitt,* Bantam Doubleday Dell, 1989.

- **Planning for Pregnancy, Birth and Beyond,** *American College of Obstetricians and Gynecologists,* Signet, 1997.

Organizations

- **March of Dimes Birth Defects Foundation**
  National Office
  1275 Mamaroneck Avenue
  White Plains, NY 10605
  (888) MODIMES (663-4637)

- **The American College of Obstetricians and Gynecologists**
  409 12th Street S.W.
  PO Box 96920
  Washington, DC 20090-6920
  ACOG Resourse Center: (202) 863-2518
  Fax: (202) 484-1595
  http://www.acog.org

Internet Sites

- **http://www.noah.cuny.edu/pregnancy/march_of_dimes/ pre_preg.plan/prepreg.html**
  This information about pre-pregnancy planning is part of the New York Public Library's "Ask NOAH About" series.

- **http://www.noah.cuny.edu/pregnancy/march_of_dimes/ genetics/gcbooklt.html**
  This "Ask NOAH" site reviews genetic counseling.

- http://www.noah.cuny.edu/pregnancy/march_of_dimes/
  substance/alc&preg.html
  This "Ask NOAH" site explains the impact of alcohol on pregnancy.

- http://www.modimes.org/pub/diabetes.htm
  This "Diabetes in Pregnancy" information sheet is part of the March of Dimes' public health information, prenatal series.

- http://www.modimes.org/pub/rubella.htm
  The March of Dimes reviews rubella's impact on pregnancy.

- http://members.aol.com/midwifery/
  This site of Midwifery Today, Inc., offers information on birth and midwifery.

- http://siteguider.com/preparing.html/
  BabyZone's "Preparing for Pregnancy and Parenthood" area offers fun and helpful articles, checklists and links.

CHAPTER TWELVE

FIRST TRIMESTER

Creating a New Life

*P*regnancy is the most challenging physical, emotional and spiritual transformation a woman can experience. Besides the obvious body changes, such as a progressively protruding abdomen, you will invariably experience more mood swings, find yourself daydreaming more than usual and wonder how you could have become so forgetful. You may also be confronted with such difficult issues about how the pregnancy and child will affect the relationship you have with your partner. In the balance, you will delight when you hear the heart beating for the first time, and thrill at the first glimpse of your new baby on ultrasound. You will also certainly experience a new level of intimacy with your partner.

> " When I was newly pregnant, my driving really suffered. My mind would wander, and so would the car — right into the next lane."

This chapter discusses the first fourteen weeks of pregnancy, including weight-gain recommendations, normal fetal development, genetic testing and possible problems. The information here should help you realize the importance of visiting your physician early in the pregnancy to make sure this critical stage goes as well as possible. Your baby is developing from a small ball of cells into a recognizable person during these weeks, and early prenatal visits help to make this transformation as smooth as possible. You want to give your child a healthy start in life, and taking great care of yourself during pregnancy is the best way to do this.

When You're Suspecting You're Expecting

HOW TO KNOW YOU ARE PREGNANT

The best indicator of pregnancy is **amenorrhea**, the absence of your periods. If you are of reproductive age and sexually active (regardless of what method of birth control you use), you should consider the possibility that you might be pregnant if you miss a period. If your periods are normally regular, skipping one is an especially good indicator of pregnancy.

When your period is more than three days late, you can check a home pregnancy test with an early-morning urine sample. Consumer Reports magazine rated home pregnancy tests in 1997, reporting that Answer and Clearblue Easy were the most sensitive and easiest to interpret. The tests work by detecting a hormone made by the placental tissue called human chorionic gonadotropin (HCG). The **placenta** is tissue that connects the baby to your uterus and provides your baby with nutrients. It is also called the "afterbirth" since it comes out after you deliver the baby. Most home pregnancy tests today are sensitive enough to detect a pregnancy by the first day of a missed period. If the test is negative, repeat it in one week if you still have not had a period. In the meantime, assume you are pregnant and do not drink any alcohol or use drugs. Contact your doctor immediately if you take prescription medications and ask if they are safe to use in pregnancy.

" I suspected I was pregnant again right away because I got that familiar funny taste in my mouth and I fell asleep on the couch two nights in a row!"

Early in pregnancy, you may also experience nausea and vomiting, breast enlargement and tenderness, headaches, menstrual-like cramps and bloating, and fatigue.

WHEN TO SEE THE DOCTOR

In general, it is wise to see your doctor for your first obstetric visit before you have missed two periods. You should ask to be seen very early if you have serious medical problems such as diabetes or hypertension, take prescription medication, have a complicated prior pregnancy history, or are at risk for an ectopic pregnancy (see section below). You should also be seen early if you have pain unrelieved with Tylenol, are throwing up everything you eat or drink, or are bleeding like a period.

At your first visit for pregnancy, expect to have a complete physical exam. Blood and urine samples are taken for analysis. You learn your due date as well as basic information about such topics as diet and exercise in pregnancy. Frequent, small meals are best tolerated during the first trimester; they help you avoid nausea by keeping your blood sugar constant and not overwhelming your system with too much food. For exercise, you should try to walk ½ mile per day, but you may have tremendous fatigue during this time. Do not push yourself too hard. Once you are at week 20, you should increase your walking routine.

" My first OB visit was pretty uneventful. Just a few questions. I really was excited."

" While I exercised, I noticed throughout the pregnancy that I got very winded. I couldn't do the aerobic capacity I was used to."

You return every four to five weeks during the first trimester for follow-up visits. At the week-12 visit, you can usually hear your baby's strong, rapid heartbeat with a special Doppler device. This is a wonderful visit for your partner to attend. Hearing your baby for the first time is very special; it is also important because it tells you that the baby is doing well. Your chance of miscarriage is reduced from about 15 to 20 percent to between 3 and 5 percent once you hear the heartbeat.

HOW TO CALCULATE YOUR DUE DATE

Pregnancy in humans lasts 280 days, measured from the first day of your last menstrual period (LMP). The LMP, when known with certainty in a woman with regular menstrual cycles, is the most reliable way to estimate the age of your pregnancy. The age of the pregnancy is referred to as the **gestational age**, and your due date as the **estimated date of confinement** (EDC). You are due at a gestational age of 40 weeks. You are pregnant only 38 weeks, since we include the two weeks from the first day of your period until ovulation in the 40 weeks. It is critical that your due date be accurate because decisions may need to be made later in your pregnancy based on this information. Using a formula called Nagele's Rule, the EDC is calculated by subtracting three months from the LMP and adding one week. The lenght of your pregnancy is described in weeks, not months.

If you are unsure when your last menstrual period began, your doctor estimates the gestational age with other clinical tools. The size of your uterus on early pelvic exam, the date when the baby's heartbeat is detected, and the date you first perceive movement all give helpful information to date your pregnancy. Ultrasound in the first half of pregnancy is also an extremely accurate tool for assessing fetal age, and it gives invaluable information about fetal anatomy as well. Most women today receive at least one ultrasound during pregnancy.

" During my first pregnancy, I took healthy eating to the extreme. I remember I wouldn't eat a maraschino cherry because it had red food coloring in it!"

The Food Factor
HOW MUCH WEIGHT YOU SHOULD GAIN

During pregnancy, food should be considered medicine. The goal of healthy eating is to maximize your and your baby's health by achieving appropriate weight gain with optimal intake of nutrients.

Many women ask the question, "Is my weight gain normal?" at some point during pregnancy. The answer depends in part on what your weight was before you got pregnant. If you are underweight, you should gain more than average; if you are overweight, it is best to gain less. Note that weight loss by severely restricting calories – even if you are obese – is **never** recommended in pregnancy.

During the first trimester, recommended weight gain is three to six pounds. If you have significant nausea and vomiting in early pregnancy, you may lose weight during the first trimester. This weight loss does not harm the baby since your system can provide what the baby needs at this early stage. Many women lose weight or do not change their weight during this time and have normal babies.

The **body mass index (BMI)** is a simple method for assessing your percentage of body fat. It is more accurate than calculating the ideal body weight because it takes your body density into consideration. Use the formula below to find your BMI.

HOW TO CALCULATE
YOUR BODY MASS INDEX (BMI)

❧ *First divide your height in inches by 39.4 to convert to meters.*
Example: 5' 3" = 63"; 63 ÷ by 39.4 = 1.59.

❧ *Square the meters by multiplying it by itself.*
Example: 1.59 x 1.59 = 2.52.

❧ *Divide your weight in pounds by 2.2 to convert to kilograms.*
Example: 120 pounds ÷ by 2.2 = 54.54 kilograms.

❧ *Divide the kilograms by the height in meters squared.*
Example: 54.54 ÷ by 2.52 = 22.

The National Academy of Sciences recommends the following weight gain in pregnancy based on your prepregnancy BMI classifications:

BMI	Total Weight Gain (lbs.)	Rate (lbs./month from 14 weeks)
Underweight (<19.8)	28-40	5.0
Normal weight (19.8–26.0)	25-35	4.0
Overweight (26.1-29.0)	15-25	2.6
Obese (>29)	15	2.0

The above figures are for singleton pregnancies, not twins or triplets. If you are pregnant with twins, talk to your doctor about a nutrition consultation.

WHERE THE WEIGHT GOES

In an average woman, 60 percent of the weight gained during pregnancy comes from the growth of the uterus and breasts, increased blood volume, retained water, and fat (the water accounts for about a quarter of the total weight gain). The baby, placenta and amniotic fluid account for the other 40 percent. Most of the weight you gain in the first half of pregnancy is not from the baby, but changes to your body. Fetal growth accounts for most of the weight gain in the second half of pregnancy.

HOW TO FIGURE THE NUMBER OF CALORIES YOU NEED

The daily calories required to meet your energy needs and achieve appropriate weight gain are estimated by multiplying your ideal body weight in kilograms by 35 and adding 300 calories to the total.

STEP 1:	Find your ideal body weight in pounds
	For women: 100 + (4 x [height in inches minus 60])
Example:	At 5'7", your ideal body weight in pounds is 128. 100 + (4 x [67 – 60]) = 128

STEP 2:	Convert to kilograms
	Divide your ideal body weight in pounds by 2.2. Example: 128 lbs. ÷ 2.2 = 58 kilograms

STEP 3:	Multiply by 35
Example:	58 kilograms x 35 cal/kilogram = 2,030 calories

STEP 4:	Add 300 calories
Example:	2,030 cal + 300 cal = 2,330 calories

Thus, for a woman of any weight who is 5'7" tall, the suggested intake per day during pregnancy is 2,330 calories. Adjustments may be necessary if you are either extremely sedentary or active. If counting calories sounds like a hassle, you are right, it is. But the effort you make and discipline you employ now will pay off during and after your pregnancy. If you prevent excessive weight gain, you will have fewer problems with back pain, heartburn, leg swelling, and labor, to name a few. It is not ideal for the developing baby if you start your pregnancy underweight and gain too little, or obese and gain too much. You have an easier time returning to your prepregnancy weight if you are careful about weight gain in pregnancy.

WHAT YOU SHOULD KNOW ABOUT VITAMIN & MINERAL SUPPLEMENTS

If you eat a balanced diet consisting of a variety of fruits and vegetables, protein, dairy products and whole grains, routine vitamin supplementation is not necessary. The average woman, however, does not eat a healthy diet every day. Daily prenatal vitamin supplements help to ensure that you get the vitamins you need. With the exception of folic acid — the recommended daily allowance of which is more than doubled in pregnancy — most vitamin allowances in pregnancy are only slightly increased. Too much vitamin A, in fact, can cause birth defects.

Except for iron, mineral supplementation is not required, either. Because of monthly menstruation, your iron stores may be less than optimal when you get pregnant, and it is difficult to consume adequate iron by diet alone. The additional iron is necessary for red-blood-cell production for you and the baby. Your red blood cells carry oxygen to your body, including to the baby through the uterus. The National Academy of Sciences recommends a daily dose of 30 mg of ferrous iron (available separately or in prenatal vitamins). For maximum absorption, take iron between meals or at bedtime, if you can tolerate the possible upset stomach. Iron supplements come in many formulations, and you should ask your doctor to recommend another one if you are having a problem with indigestion or constipation. Avoid taking iron and calcium at the same time as the calcium reduces the iron absorption. Calcium requirements are increased during pregnancy by one-third and are obtained by eating additional dairy products such as low-fat cheese, milk and yogurt.

WHEN YOU SHOULD SEE AN EXPERT

In certain situations, you should consult with a nutritionist during pregnancy. These include if you are diabetic, lactose-intolerant or vegetarian; have phenylketonuria or a hemoglobinopathy such as sickle-cell disease; take seizure medication; or are pregnant with twins.

Many excellent books have been written on the subject of nutrition in pregnancy, and some of these books have detailed recipe sections. Please see the reference section at the end of this chapter for further information.

When Morning Sickness Strikes

WHO GETS IT?

You can expect to experience some degree of nausea and vomiting – or "morning sickness" – during pregnancy. This unpleasant part of pregnancy occurs in up to 90 percent of women. You may find it a minor annoyance – perhaps your nausea upon awakening abates with a few bedside crackers. At the other extreme, you may have nausea and vomiting so severe that your quality of life and ability to work are affected. Morning sickness is traditionally considered a problem of the first trimester, but many women have nausea and vomiting several weeks into the second trimester, and a few may vomit up until the time of delivery. Nausea and vomiting can also be due to other medical conditions unrelated to pregnancy, such as appendicitis and thyroid disease, so be sure to discuss your past medical history and symptoms with your doctor.

" I had morning sickness with my first pregnancy, but I was so excited that I didn't care what was happening to me as long as it was pregnancy-related."

WHAT CAUSES IT?

The cause of morning sickness is not well-understood. It is more common with twins or triplets. Elevated hormone levels enhance your sense of smell, and you may experience a bad taste in your mouth. The hormone progesterone relaxes the muscles in your digestive tract and slows the movement of food through your system. The hormones of pregnancy (HCG and progesterone) rapidly increase in early pregnancy, peak at weeks 8 to 10, and then decline to almost non-pregnant levels by week 12. It is with the peak hormone levels at weeks 8 to 10 that you feel the worst, because your intestinal tract is virtually paralyzed. Your food can hardly get past your stomach, and you feel sick. At week 12, when the hormone levels are lower, your intestines work more normally, and you feel much better. While your stomach is "paralyzed," you must eat a small amount of food every hour. You must never let your stomach get empty or too full.

WHEN THE PROBLEM IS SERIOUS

Severe vomiting causing dehydration, weight loss and disturbance of body salts is known as **hyperemesis gravidarum**. If diagnosed with this condition, you are given IV fluids, salt replacements and anti-nausea medication, frequently in the hospital. In severe and prolonged cases, you are given food through an IV, with supplements of vitamins, sugars and proteins.

HOW TO COPE

The following is a list of suggestions and home remedies you can experiment with for relief of morning sickness:

- ❧ *Keep a diary of symptoms, and try to identify and avoid triggers.*
- ❧ *Stay cool and air-conditioned, as hot, humid weather makes nausea worse.*
- ❧ *Eat frequent small meals, with foods you crave, like dill pickles.*
- ❧ *Avoid touching or smelling food while it is prepared.*
- ❧ *Drink ginger products like ginger ale or pickled ginger.*
- ❧ *Avoid loud environments.*
- ❧ *Rinse your mouth with fresh lemon juice and water.*
- ❧ *Avoid strong smells, such as pet litters and food, diaper changes (see if your partner will take over or consider hiring home help), coffee, and gas stations.*
- ❧ *Use Emetrol, an over-the-counter anti-nausea medication.*
- ❧ *Apply accupressure wristbands called Sea-bands.*
- ❧ *Keep crackers at your bedside to nibble on before you get out of bed.*
- ❧ *Eat a protein-rich snack, such as cottage cheese or peanut butter before bedtime.*
- ❧ *Search the Internet for suggestions, and ask friends and relatives for ideas.*

Your doctor can also prescribe medications for you if you are still having problems.

Zygote, Embryo, Fetus: How Your Baby Develops

Fertilization of the egg by sperm occurs within 24 hours of intercourse. This union forms what is known as a **zygote**. The zygote begins to divide as it travels through your fallopian tube toward the uterus where, by the seventh day after fertilization, the zygote implants in the uterine lining (one week before you have even missed a period!). In this part of the chapter we will highlight the development of the **embryo** (so called during the fourth through the eighth weeks of development) and **fetus** (starting at nine weeks of development). Remember, the length of pregnancy is considered to be 280 days, or 40 weeks from the first day of your last period.

WEEKS 5 AND 6

By the time your period is one week late, the embryo has formed into three different layers that will each specialize into all the different tissues and organs of the body. The period during which all major organs form is called **organogenesis** and occurs between weeks 5 and 10 of pregnancy. This is the time when the embryo is most vulnerable to factors interfering with development. Most birth defects find their origin during this critical period. Beyond the first 12 weeks, organs still can be damaged, but at this point at least they are all present. (See "What Can Harm the Baby?")

The brain and spinal cord begin to develop during the fourth week, making the nervous system the first organ system to appear.

Blood vessels in the tissue that is developing into the placenta establish contact with the baby's circulation through the umbilical cord. When the baby's heart begins to beat in the sixth week of pregnancy, the placenta supplies the embryo with nutrients and oxygen.

If you have an ultrasound at this time (and up to 12 weeks), the crown-rump length (CRL) determines the age of the embryo. The CRL is the measurement from the top of the head (crown) to the buttocks (rump) and is recorded in millimeters. At 6 weeks, the embryo is 4 mm long (less than 2 inches).

WEEKS 7 AND 8

By the beginning of the seventh week, the arms and legs appear as paddle-shaped structures. The gastrointestinal tract starts to form by the eighth week. This includes the stomach, intestines and liver. During this time, the eyelids develop.

WEEKS 9 AND 10

Fingers are distinct by the ninth week, and toes by the tenth. Individual vertebrae that make up the backbone are identified at 10 weeks.

WEEKS 11 THROUGH 13

At this stage, the head makes up about half of the baby's total length, and the face takes on a human appearance. The CRL is around 5 cm, or 2 inches. The kidneys begin to produce urine at 13 weeks. The genitalia have male and female characteristics but still are not fully formed; thus, gender cannot be identified on ultrasound in the first trimester.

What Can Harm the Baby

Fortunately, the list of medications, chemicals and other things that are known or suspected **teratogens** – substances that cause abnormal development – is relatively short. They include: alcohol, aminopterin, androgenic hormones (testosterone), anesthetic gases, busulfan, coumadin (a blood thinner), DES, vitamin A, lead, mercury, organic solvents (such as paint and dry cleaning chemicals), anticonvulsant medication (such as valproic acid, trimethadione and phenytoin), tetracycline, thalidomide, PCCs and PCBs, hyperthermia (such as from hot tubs) and high-dose radiation. However, 65 percent of human malformations occur for unknown reasons.

" I gave up baths during pregnancy and took showers instead. Soaking in a tub of lukewarm water just wasn't worth it to me."

The timing of the exposure, the dose and the genetic susceptibility of the fetus all play a role in determining whether the exposure to medication or another teratogen will result in death of the baby, a malformation (i.e., spina bifida), abnormal growth, or dysfunction of an organ like the liver, brain or heart. Exposure in the first eight weeks of pregnancy usually either causes no problems with the baby or leads to miscarriage. It is an all-or-nothing effect at this early stage. Exposure from weeks 9 to 15 is more likely to stunt growth or affect organ function.

If you are taking prescription medications and are planning a pregnancy, ask your doctor if you should continue to take them. Alternatives are usually available. If your pregnancy is unplanned, it is best to call and speak to your doctor's office immediately about the medications you are taking, including over-the-counter medicines. Many medicines on the market have not been tested in pregnancy, and your decision to continue them should be based on why you use it, what happens when you do not, and risks to the fetus. Talk with your doctor about this risk.

WHAT CAN I TAKE?

The following over-the-counter medications are considered acceptable to use in pregnancy. It is probably a good idea to avoid all medications unless you really need them.

Tylenol and Tylenol Sinus	Immodium AD
Dimetapp	Kaopectate
Chlor-trimeton	Colace
Afrin nasal spray	Metamucil
Ocean nasal spray	Citrucel
Robitussin cough syrup, plain or DM	Fibercon
	Milk of Magnesia
Chloraseptic spray or lozenges	Senokot
Cepacol throat lozenges	Dulcolax
Emetrol	Anusol HC
Gas-X	Preparation H
Tums	Tucks
Rolaids	0.5% hydrocortisone cream
Mylanta	Caladryl lotion
Maalox	Benadryl

How Abnormalities Can Be Detected

All parents wonder during pregnancy if their baby is normal. Approximately three percent of infants born alive have a major birth defect such as Down's syndrome, cleft lip or cystic fibrosis. Some conditions are obvious at birth, while others may not manifest themselves until later in life. Birth defects can be due to teratogens as discussed earlier, an abnormal number of chromosomes, single or multiple chemical defects in a particular gene or genes, or a combination of the above. Chapter 11, "Pre-Pregnancy Consult," provides more information on this topic, but we also review it here.

You should inform your doctor of any family history of birth defects, mental retardation, hemophilia, Down's syndrome, muscular dystrophy, cystic fibrosis or neural-tube defects (such as spina bifida). Your doctor may recommend a visit with a genetics counselor who can review your family history and help determine if specialized testing is warranted. Some birth defects, for example, are best evaluated with a highly detailed ultrasound scan. You may also be relieved to find that your own baby's risk is so remote that you feel comfortable declining further investigation.

SCREENING FOR GENETIC PROBLEMS

Genetic screening in the form of maternal blood tests is routinely offered to pregnant women of certain ethnic groups who are at risk for carrying genes for **recessive** conditions. This testing can be done before you are pregnant. In these types of diseases, a child can be affected only if both parents pass on the gene. Therefore, if you test negative, your child cannot have the condition even if the father carries the gene. African-Americans should be screened for sickle-cell disease; Ashkenazi Jews should be screened for Tay-Sachs disease; Italians and Greeks for beta-thalassemia; southeast Asians and Chinese for alpha-thalassemia; and northern European whites for cystic fibrosis.

ALPHA-FETOPROTEIN TESTING

All pregnant women are offered serum (blood) screening tests for neural-tube defects, and if under age 35, serum testing for Down's syndrome as well. (Women over age 35 represent a different category and are discussed separately.) These tests are scheduled at the very beginning of the second trimester, so you need to educate yourself about them now. Alpha-fetoprotein (AFP) is a protein made by the baby's gastrointestinal tract and liver. Between 15 to 20 weeks of pregnancy, your blood is tested for AFP. Elevated levels suggest the possibility of a neural-tube defect such as spina bifida (a spinal-cord abnormality) or anencephaly (a condition where the brain does not develop). If the AFP results are low, you are at higher risk of having a baby with Down's syndrome (a chromosome problem). If you have not had an ultrasound, one should be performed to check for fetal death, multiple gestation (twins, triplets, etc.) or incorrect pregnancy dates, all of which can explain an abnormal AFP. An ultrasound can also diagnose most types of neural-tube defects. If no explanation for an abnormal AFP is found on ultrasound, an amniocentesis is recommended to check the baby's chromosomes for Trisomy 21 (Down's syndrome). The amniotic fluid level is tested to see if it is indeed abnormal, or if the blood level was misleading. When you have the amniocentesis, a very detailed ultrasound is also done.

If the AFP is low, your risk of having a baby with Down's syndrome or Trisomy 18 (another type of chromosomal abnormality) is increased. The lower the result, the greater your risk that the baby has abnormal chromosomes. It is important to realize that this blood test is only a screening test; it is possible to have a normal baby even when your test result is abnormal (a false-positive test). Of all the tests that are done, the majority return normal, and this is very reassuring. Of the tests that return abnormal, 90 percent of these babies have no problems; we just have to do more testing to make sure. The purpose of the AFP test is to identify a group that is at higher risk than the general population for a particular condition. If you are found to be at high risk of having a problem with the baby, you may then opt to have further testing, which in the case of Down's syndrome, is an amniocentesis. These tests are considered diagnostic tests – they determine for certain if you have a fetus affected with Down's syndrome or other chromosome abnormality. Amniocentesis has traditionally been performed early in the second trimester (15 weeks), and is discussed in the next chapter.

The risk of having a chromosomally abnormal fetus increases with your age. At age 25, your risk of having a child affected with Down's syndrome is 1 in 2,500; and at 35, your risk is 1 in 385 for Down's and 1 in 204 for any chromosomal abnormality. At age 35, the risk of having an abnormal fetus is approximately equivalent to the risks associated with amniocentesis and CVS. For this reason, diagnostic tests are offered to women over 35 without waiting to do the screening AFP test. If the AFP test returns normal and you are over age 35, this does not rule out the possibility that you may have a baby with Down's syndrome.

CHORIONIC VILLUS SAMPLING

Why CVS is Performed

CVS is a prenatal diagnostic test performed between weeks 9 and 12 to obtain fetal placental tissue for chromosome analysis. The advantage of CVS over amniocentesis is that it allows earlier detection of an abnormal pregnancy. With the information that the baby's chromosomes are abnormal at an early stage of the pregnancy, you have the option to terminate the pregnancy when the procedure is more private and less risky.

You are offered CVS (or amniocentesis) if you will be over age 35 at delivery, have had a previous child with a chromosomal abnormality, gave birth to a stillborn child, or more uncommonly, if you or your husband have a chromosomal abnormality.

What to Expect During CVS

With a CVS, placental tissue is obtained through cervical, vaginal or abdominal approaches. The route depends on the location of the placenta and the position and shape of your uterus, among other things. The most common approach to the CVS is through your cervix. You are placed in the same position as for a Pap smear, with a speculum in the vagina. Your cervix is made sterile with Betadine solution, and then a small metal instrument is passed through your cervix and into the uterus. The instrument is followed the entire time with the ultrasound. A sample of the tissue that surrounds the baby – the future placenta – is obtained. This tissue has the same chromosomes

324 🦢 Newman / Stevens

as the baby. The instrument is removed, and the tissue is sent to the lab to be cultured for two weeks. You should have the results within three weeks. When the test is over, you may have some cramping and spotting. Your risk of having a miscarriage is 1 in 100. The safety of CVS and amniocentesis are very similar in experienced hands. With CVS there is a 1-in-3,000 risk of causing defects to the baby's limbs.

When Pregnancy Ends in Miscarriage

Miscarriage is the spontaneous loss of a pregnancy before 20 weeks. If all pregnancies are counted, miscarriage occurs in approximately 50 percent, an astoundingly high figure. The majority of these miscarriages occur before you are late for your period and you even know you are pregnant. If you only consider pregnancies that result in a late period, the risk of miscarriage is 15 to 20 percent. As you get older, your risk of having a miscarriage increases. Women over 40 have a 26-percent chance of a miscarriage – double that of a 20-year-old.

" I wanted to know why the miscarriage happened, and the doctor couldn't give me a specific answer. That was hard for me."

WHAT CAUSES MISCARRIAGE?

The majority of miscarriages occur in the first trimester (first 13 weeks). Of these, 70 percent are due to chromosomal abnormalities, such as Down's syndrome. With these problems, the young fetus stops developing, and a miscarriage occurs. If the baby continues to develop, you will have a baby born with a birth defect due to chromosome problems.

If you have had three or more miscarriages in a row, you have experienced what is known as **recurrent** or **habitual abortion**. There may not be a special reason for these losses, and your risk with your next pregnancy may still be 15 to 20 percent. If you have never carried a child to term and have had two or more miscarriages, your chance of having a successful pregnancy with your next pregnancy is only 55 to 60 percent. If you have had three miscarriages in a row, or two miscarriages and no children, you should speak with your doctor about special testing.

GENETIC ABNORMALITIES

Of all couples who have experienced recurrent miscarriage, 3 to 8 percent have a genetic abnormality that they pass on through their eggs and sperm. To determine if you and your partner have this problem, your blood is tested to see if your chromosomes are normal. There can be a problem with one of your chromosomes that causes each pregnancy to stop developing and result in a miscarriage. If you have ever had a malformed, stillborn or mentally retarded infant, or if you have a family history of such problems, having your chromosomes tested is especially important.

ENVIRONMENTAL FACTORS

Alcohol consumption, cigarette smoking and heavy coffee consumption have all been linked to miscarriage. While the definition of "heavy" is vague, it is best to consider more than one cup of coffee per day too much during pregnancy. If you are trying to conceive and have had one or more miscarriages, avoid alcohol, tobacco and caffeine. Exposure to anesthetic gases also is associated with pregnancy loss in the first trimester, so you should avoid general anesthesia early in pregnancy. If you work in an operating room or dentist's office and have had more than one miscarriage, talk to your doctor. A dry-cleaning agent called tetrachloromethylene also is associated with miscarriage. Wearing clothing that has been dry-cleaned is considered safe, but be careful if you work in dry cleaning.

HORMONAL FACTORS

Hormonal factors can cause recurrent abortions or miscarriages. Uncontrolled thyroid disease or diabetes mellitus may play a role in miscarriage. Another suspected cause is luteal-phase deficiency. The luteal phase refers to the two weeks of the menstrual cycle after ovulation (the two weeks before your period). During this time, the ovary makes progesterone that prepares and sustains the endometrium of the uterus to support a developing baby. Inadequate production of progesterone may cause a miscarriage. To determine if you have a luteal-phase deficiency, your doctor performs an endometrial biopsy just before you have a period or draws a blood sample to test the level of progesterone on day 21 of your cycle. Luteal-phase deficiency is treated with vaginal progesterone suppositories. These suppositories are used from the time you ovulate until you either have a period or are 12 weeks pregnant. At that point, the uterus is no longer dependent on progesterone for support, and your risk of having a miscarriage is much lower.

UTERINE ABNORMALITIES

Approximately 12 to 15 percent of women with recurrent miscarriages have an abnormality of the uterine cavity, such as fibroids or polyps. These problems may prevent normal attachment of the baby to the uterus or shrink the cavity's size and limit space for fetal growth. Many of these conditions are diagnosed with an ultrasound. Surgical removal of the fibroid or polyp offers improvements in term of delivery rates.

IMMUNE-SYSTEM ABNORMALITIES

Abnormal immune responses may be the cause of early pregnancy losses. One of these, the anti-phospholipid syndrome, results in abnormal blood clotting. With anti-phospholipid syndrome, you miscarry later in pregnancy, near weeks 12 to 20. A blood test is done to diagnose this problem. If it is present, you are given steroids and a blood thinner called heparin to lower your risk of having another miscarriage.

THE WARNING SIGNS

Light vaginal bleeding for a few days early in pregnancy is not uncommon. You may experience mild pelvic cramps as your uterus grows. However, vaginal bleeding that continues more than 48 hours, requires more than three small sanitary-pad changes per day or is accompanied by painful cramps is concerning. You should also be concerned if the "pregnant feeling" you had — breast tenderness, nausea, bloating — goes away suddenly. You should call your doctor's office if you have any bleeding during the first trimester.

"I HAD A MISCARRIAGE"

I had a miscarriage after my first baby. I knew I had a problem because I was bleeding. But I just sensed there was a problem because my whole body felt sick, like something was not right, like I had a bad bug. And there was no morning sickness like with my first baby.

The bleeding continued, and it started to change color. My doctor's office had a sonographer, so they told me to come in.

So sure enough, the ultrasound showed an empty sac. I really felt OK; it wasn't until later that I had one little outburst by myself. And it was because I went into the room, the baby's room. And I just had a little cry to myself. But other than that, I couldn't wait to come home and grab the kid I was fortunate enough to have. Maybe if I had lost my first one, it would have been different, but I had a kid to come home to. So it wasn't as tragic for me. But I felt for girls who had been trying and didn't have one.

BLOOD TESTING

In order to evaluate whether your pregnancy is heading toward a miscarriage, your doctor may check blood levels of a placental hormone called HCG (human chorionic gonadotropin). This hormone level should increase over two days by at least 66 percent. If it does not, your pregnancy is considered at high risk for either a miscarriage or ectopic pregnancy. If the levels are decreasing, there is a good chance you are about to have a miscarriage. In addition to the blood test for HCG, a vaginal ultrasound is done to look for characteristics of a normal pregnancy. A small sac in the uterus is seen with a vaginal ultrasound when you are between 4 and 5 weeks pregnant, and an embryo with a heartbeat at 6 weeks. If these are not present, you may not be as far along in pregnancy as originally thought, or you may have a pregnancy that will inevitably miscarry.

TYPES OF MISCARRIAGES

There are three types of miscarriage: missed abortion, incomplete abortion and inevitable abortion. A **missed abortion** is when the baby has died and you have no idea there is a problem. In this situation, you come in for a routine visit, usually for your ultrasound, and find out that the baby has died already. You may have noted an abrupt decrease in breast tenderness and nausea a few days before the visit. This is one of the most emotionally painful experiences we share with women in the office, because everyone comes in for the ultrasound exited about seeing their baby for the first time. This is another reason to have your partner there for the ultrasound visit, as you need the support of your family, friends and physician if this unfortunate event occurs.

With an **incomplete abortion,** you have passed a portion of the pregnancy tissue, but not all of it. Your uterus continues to cramp and bleed until the remaining tissue is removed with a D&E.

With an **inevitable abortion,** you have spotting and cramps, but have not passed any tissue. On exam your cervix may be dilating, with tissue present at the opening. On ultrasound the baby is dead. You are without a doubt going to have a miscarriage. You can wait for a spontaneous miscarriage or schedule a D&E.

OUTPATIENT D&E OR "NATURAL" MISCARRIAGE

If you find out that your baby has died, you can wait for the miscarriage to occur or you can schedule a D&E. D&E stands for dilation and evacuation, and refers to the dilation of the cervix and evacuation of the pregnancy tissue. A D&E is an outpatient surgical procedure. You are either put to sleep with general anesthesia, or you can have an epidural or spinal. Your feet are placed in stirrups, and a speculum is inserted into your vagina. The vagina and cervix are made sterile with Betadine. The cervical canal is dilated with metal probes, and the pregnancy tissue is removed with a suction tube or by scraping the lining with a sharp instrument. After this procedure, you will have mild to moderate cramps and spotting for a few days.

If you have a D&E, you should wait at least two normal menstrual cycles before trying to get pregnant again. You should use condoms during this time. By waiting, you allow the lining of the uterus to repair itself and be ready to accept a baby when the time comes.

If you decide to forgo the D&E and wait for a natural miscarriage, you need to know what to expect. You start having cramps in your lower abdomen that get progressively worse. Your vaginal bleeding gets heavier than a period. Both the pain and bleeding reach a high point, and then you should pass some tissue. If the pregnancy is very early, the tissue looks like ground beef. If the pregnancy ends a few weeks later, you may see a small baby within a water-filled sac in addition to this other tissue. Once the pregnancy material passes, your bleeding and cramping should rapidly decline. If they do not, you may still have some tissue within the uterus that is not coming out. In this situation, you still need to have the D&E. Since a natural miscarriage involves so much pain and bleeding, and because there is no guarantee of avoiding a D&E, most women choose to schedule a D&E.

HOW TO HANDLE THE EMOTIONS

Although every woman reacts differently, for many, the loss of a pregnancy is an emotionally devastating event. You may have found yourself frequently thinking about the future with your new child. You had dreams of enjoying this boy or girl, playing in the yard and watching your youngster grow. You may have made plans for decorating the nursery, breast-feeding and working part-time.

The loss of a baby to miscarriage is as real as the loss of a 2-month-old, and you need to give yourself time to mourn. You do not just "get over" the pain. Also, it is not a good idea to get pregnant right away just to avoid grieving over a miscarriage. Allow yourself time to work through the pain of the loss before moving forward with your

" The miscarriage was the worst thing that had ever happened to me. I was disappointed beyond belief. I was just so sad, and well-meaning people said many insensitive things that didn't help a bit. I wanted to hide out for a while."

> *"The pain of my grief was intense. I couldn't believe how much my heart ached. A counselor helped me to understand that I wasn't crazy for missing my baby."*

plans. The number of women who start sharing their stories of having had a miscarriage and then a normal pregnancy will impress you. This natural support system is very helpful, so allow your friends and neighbors to share with you and comfort you at this very difficult time. Talk about your feelings with your partner and close friends. Consider seeking counseling if the normal blues that come with disappointment and loss progress to problems with sleeping or eating, feeling hopeless about the future or recurrent crying spells — signs that you may be depressed. Look in the phone book or ask your doctor for local organizations and support groups available to you.

When You Have an Ectopic Pregnancy

WHO IS AT RISK?

An ectopic pregnancy is a potentially life-threatening condition where the pregnancy implants outside the uterus. Ninety-five percent of ectopic pregnancies occur in the fallopian tubes, but ectopic pregnancy can also occur in your abdomen, cervix or ovary. You are at an increased risk of ectopic pregnancy if you have a history of the following: prior ectopic pregnancy, current use of an IUD, prior infection of gonorrhea or chlamydia, any surgery on your fallopian tubes, endometriosis, or infertility treatment.

WHAT TO WATCH FOR

During the first four to eight weeks of your pregnancy, you should be concerned if you have persistent pelvic pain. This pain is especially worrisome if it is off to one side of your abdomen. If you have risk factors for ectopic pregnancy, you should be especially vigilant early in your pregnancy and schedule an appointment with your doctor as soon as you learn you are pregnant.

WHAT YOUR DOCTOR DOES

If your doctor is concerned about the possibility of an ectopic pregnancy, he or she follows your blood level of the hormone HCG (human chorionic gonadotropin). The placenta makes this hormone, and it doubles every two days in almost all normal pregnancies. As previously indicated, an abnormal increase in the level of HCG suggests that you have an ectopic pregnancy (or that you are going to have a miscarriage). Your doctor also performs a vaginal ultrasound. If your HCG level is 2,000 or more and no pregnancy is seen in the uterus, you may have already miscarried, or you may have an ectopic pregnancy. It is very frustrating to wait the week or two it may take to determine whether your pregnancy will go to full term, end in a miscarriage or be an ectopic. Trust that your physician is working hard to get you an answer as soon as possible.

HOW YOU ARE TREATED

Laparoscopic surgery

If you have an ectopic pregnancy, your doctor will discuss treatment options with you. One option is surgical removal of the ectopic pregnancy using the laparoscope. This instrument inserted through your umbilicus and into your abdomen. If your fallopian tube has ruptured and is bleeding heavily, the fallopian tube is removed. If the tube is swollen but not ruptured, it is cut open, and the ectopic pregnancy tissue is removed. The tube heals on its own over the next few weeks. If this surgery is done through the laparoscope, you can go home the same day. In rare cases, small fragments of pregnancy tissue may continue to grow after surgery. When this occurs, the medicine Methotrexate (see below) is used to remove any remaining tissue.

Non-surgical treatment with Methotrexate

Depending on the size and location of the ectopic pregnancy, and your medical history, you may be treated with Methotrexate, avoiding the need for surgery. Methotrexate has been used for decades in the treatment of cancers and recently has been used for the treatment of ectopic pregnancies. Treatment with Methotrexate involves giving you a single dose of the medication and then monitoring you closely with a series of weekly blood tests to make sure it works. There remains the risk of your tube rupturing, and emergency surgery is still a small possibility. Most research to date reports Methotrexate is 90-to 95-percent effective in treating ectopic pregnancies without the need for surgery. Many physicians do not use this method due to the risk that you could bleed internally at home if your tube ruptures while you wait for the medicine to work.

After ectopic pregnancy, your chance of having a normal pregnancy within the uterus is 80 percent with your subsequent pregnancy. There is no difference based on how your ectopic was treated, either with surgery or Methotrexate.

You may wonder if by using Methotrexate or having surgery to remove an ectopic pregnancy, you are having an abortion. You are not; you are simply saving your life in a situation where the baby has no chance to live. An ectopic pregnancy is in an abnormal location where the baby cannot grow to term, and the pregnancy cannot be relocated to the uterus. If you do not remove the ectopic pregnancy, you are at risk of having your fallopian tube rupture, and you could bleed to death.

Conclusion

Making it through the first trimester of pregnancy is very special. When you get through this time without experiencing a miscarriage or ectopic pregnancy, your chance of having a healthy, full-term baby is great. The tremendous fatigue and nausea of early pregnancy begin to go away as this trimester concludes. You build an emotional bond with your new baby that is cemented when you see the ultrasound images. Good luck and on to the second trimester!

Additional Resources

Books

- **Belly Laughs and Babies: A Heartwarming, Humorous Collection of True-Life Stories from Pregnancy, Childbirth and Crazed New Parenthood,** *Mary Sheridan,* Laughing Stork Press, 1997.

- **Eating Expectantly: A Practical and Tasty Approach to Prenatal Nutrition,** *Bridget Swinney and Tracey Anderson,* Meadowbrook Press, 1996.

- **Surviving Pregnancy Loss: A Complete Sourcebook for Women and Their Families,** *Rochelle Friedman and Bonnie Gradstein,* Citadel Press, 1996.

- **How to Survive the Loss of a Love,** *Melba Colgrove, Harold H. Bloomfield and Peter McWilliams,* Prelude Press, 1991.

- **Ectopic Pregnancy: Diagnosis and Management,** *Isabel Stabile,* Cambridge University Press, 1996.

Organizations

- **March of Dimes Birth Defects Foundation**
  National Office
  1275 Mamaroneck Avenue
  White Plains, NY 10605
  (914) 428-7100
  (888) MODIMES

Internet Sites

- **http://ificinfo.health.org/brochure/eatpreg.htm**
  The International Food Information Council Foundation and the March of Dimes Birth Defects Foundation present this information on healthy eating during pregnancy.

- http://www.modimes.org/pub/prenatal.htm
  The March of Dimes Birth Defect Foundation makes information available here on such topics as alpha-fetoprotein screening, chorionic villus sampling, drinking during pregnancy, and stress during pregnancy.

- http://www.hygeia.org
  The Hygeia Web Site, presented by a board-certified obstetrician-gynecologist, features a monthly journal on pregnancy and pregnancy loss, related poems, a Visitors Contribution Area, registries for caregivers and people who have experienced pregnancy loss, resource lists and more.

- http://www.en.com/users/nmarino/loss.htm
  This page, put together by a mother who wanted more information after her miscarriage, offers answers to frequently asked questions on miscarriage and pregnancy loss, information on how to help someone who has experienced a miscarriage, links to online pregnancy loss groups and more.

- http://www.pinelandpress.com/support/miscarriage.html
  This comprehensive resource for pregnancy loss refers you to related computer bulletin boards, news groups and web sites, and an annotated book list.

CHAPTER THIRTEEN

SECOND TRIMESTER

Looking Pregnant & Feeling Great

ow that you have made it through the first trimester, you can relax and enjoy being pregnant. The second trimester is the best part of pregnancy for most women. The greatest risk of a miscarriage is behind you, and the fatigue and nausea are on their way out, too. When you feel your baby move for the first time, you experience one of the most wonderful feelings any person can ever have. You are at the most comfortable stage of pregnancy, since you are not as large as you are going to be during the third trimester. During the second trimester, try to avoid eating too many sweets, and start a mild exercise routine.

The second trimester of pregnancy begins during the fourth month of fetal life. Counting from the beginning of your last menstrual period, this is around the 15th week. It ends at the end of the sixth month, at around 26 weeks.

What You Should Do

CHOOSE A CHILDBIRTH CLASS

Register for prenatal classes during the second trimester. In many communities, the classes fill up quickly and may not be available if you wait until the third trimester to register for them. Classes are usually offered by the

" During the second trimester, I felt great. The tiredness went away, and I got a lot more energy. And then the movements started, which got me really excited. I heard the heartbeat on a regular basis. A lot of exciting things happened."

hospitals in your area. Your doctor can give you a list of places that offer prenatal classes. Several national organizations also provide classes in most towns. These include groups that teach "natural" childbearing, such as the Lamaze and Bradley methods. In their strictest form, these "natural" methods are designed to avoid as much medical intervention as possible and teach relaxation techniques to help you make it through labor without medication. Most prenatal classes offered at local hospitals combine some of the teachings from these "natural" methods with education about methods of monitoring your baby and pain control during labor. In these classes, you are educated about available pain medications, monitoring and epidural techniques that help during labor. It is important to consider what you want to get out of the classes before you register for them.

FIND A DOCTOR FOR YOUR CHILD

You should determine who is going to take care of the baby after he or she is born. Some families prefer a pediatrician to take care of the baby; others use a family physician. Check with your insurance company to see which physicians are on your "list." Try to select a physician who is close to your home. When you have a sick child, you will not want to travel far. It is a good idea to check about the office policies in the practices that you are considering. Ask what hospitals they go to and how they handle emergency calls. Find out their policies about calling in prescriptions. Some offices allow you to meet with the physician while you are pregnant to see if you like him or her. In any case, make sure you have someone designated to care for the baby after delivery. Then inform your obstetrician of your choice.

" A friend of mine forgot to tell her insurance company that she was pregnant by the deadline, so her delivery was not covered. I made sure that didn't happen to me!"

CHECK IN WITH YOUR EMPLOYER, HOSPITAL AND INSURER

During the second trimester, is the time to inform your co-workers about your plans to be away from work. This advance notice allows them time to adjust their expectations about your future workload, reducing later stress for you and them. You should choose the hospital where you plan to deliver and pre-register with that hospital. Check with your obstetrician to make sure he or she covers the hospital where you plan to deliver.

" My insurance company – which was supposed to cover maternity at 100 percent - made us prepay the deductible and would only refund it if I stayed in the hospital less than 24 hours."

You also should inform your insurance company that you are pregnant and when you are due. Confirm with your insurance company that the hospital you have chosen is fully covered by your insurance plan. In some areas of the country, insurance plans are severely limiting women's choices in terms of which physicians they can see and which hospitals they can go to. This is usually a sign of a lower-quality insurance plan, and you need to speak with your employer if this is happening in your plan. Each year, companies reevaluate their contracts with insurance carriers, and if employees complain about loss of freedom of choice, changes usually occur.

Make sure that you are "pre-approved" by your insurance company for your delivery. Make sure you also understand their policies concerning the length of time you can stay in the hospital after the baby is born.

EXERCISE

If you have not begun already, the second trimester of pregnancy is a good time to get into an exercise routine that you can continue throughout the rest of your pregnancy. Studies show that exercising regularly during pregnancy helps you have an easier delivery and reduces your chance of delivering by cesarean section. Exercise also helps you have fewer problems with backache, constipation, depression and fatigue.

You should try to pick an exercise that is safe and not too strenuous. Exercises where you can fall and hurt yourself or the baby should be avoided. Common sense should prevail throughout pregnancy – avoid snow skiing, water skiing, surfing and bungee jumping, for example. If you are in doubt about a particular activity, ask your physician. Walking, swimming and low-impact aerobics for pregnancy are recommended.

GUIDELINES FOR EXERCISE IN PREGNANCY

Here are some guidelines to follow while doing any exercise during pregnancy.

- 🦌 *Drink plenty of fluids before and after exercise to avoid dehydration.*
- 🦌 *Keep your heart rate below 140 beats per minute.*
- 🦌 *If you are doing a vigorous exercise, rest after 15 minutes.*
- 🦌 *Avoid exercise in the supine position after the fourth month (i.e., sit-ups flat on your back).*
- 🦌 *Avoid exercise that involves taking a deep breath and bearing down (called the Valsalva maneuver).*
- 🦌 *Do not exercise if you have a fever.*
- 🦌 *Keep your temperature below 101 degrees.*

Remember to exercise the pelvic-floor muscles also. Most women have heard of Kegel exercises but rarely practice them. Kegel exercises involve contracting the pelvic-floor muscles, holding the contraction for a few seconds and then repeating this several times a day. You can identify these muscles by trying to stop your flow of urine in midstream. (Do not make a habit of this; just try it to identify the muscles.) Another way is to put one or two fingers in the vagina and try to use the vaginal muscles to "grip" them. If you are still having difficulty doing Kegels, your doctor should be able to teach you how to do them or make sure you are contracting your pelvic-floor muscles correctly. Doing these exercises regularly helps promote the tone and elasticity of the pelvic floor. Toned pelvic-floor muscles help you during delivery and are easier to get back in shape afterward.

What is Happening With the Baby

During the second trimester, your baby really begins to grow. By the beginning of the second trimester, the baby has all of the physical features of a full-size baby. Boys are distinctly different than girls. During this period, the organs that formed during the first trimester begin to function.

While the baby has all the organs of a newborn, these organs are not mature enough to support the baby if he or she were to be born at this point. The baby has almost no chance of surviving if born prior to 24 weeks. A baby who does survive birth before 24 weeks has a 90 percent chance of having severe mental retardation and cerebral palsy. From 24 to 28 weeks, the baby has a greater chance of survival and a lower risk of having cerebral palsy. Each week is critical during the second trimester in terms of the baby's development and maturity. Getting through the second trimester without delivery needs to be a very high priority for everyone involved – you, your spouse and family, your physician and your co-workers.

" When I was expecting, I sat out during our annual ski trip and went shopping instead."

❧

" I wanted to know what was going on in there with my baby. I studied books like 'A Child is Born' for week-by-week photos."

BY WEEK 15

By the 15th week, the baby is 7 inches long and weighs about 4 ounces. His or her head is large compared to the body, the skin is transparent and the bones are distinct and calcified. The baby is able to move around within the amniotic sac, however, you may not feel this movement yet since the baby is still small and not hitting against the side of the uterus. You may feel a slight "fluttering" at times, but feeling distinct movement is rare. The baby is developing sucking and swallowing reflexes. By the 18ᵗʰ week, the baby is big enough to kick or hit against the side of the uterus, and you may feel distinct movements. Do not be alarmed, however, if you do not feel the baby move until week 21 or 22. Some women expect to be able to feel the baby move every day. However, remember that the baby is changing its position all the time. You may be able to feel the baby one day and not the next. Consistent movement does not usually happen until after 24 weeks.

> *" I could see the baby 'swimming' from side to side on the ultrasound, but I couldn't yet feel a thing."*

BY WEEK 20

By 20 weeks, the baby is 10 inches long and weighs between 8 ounces and 1 pound. The eyelids are still fused closed. The skin is less transparent and begins to be covered with fine hairs called **lanugo**. A white, fatty substance called **vernix** sticks to the skin. This vernix provides a protective covering for the skin during the rest of the pregnancy and can be seen when the baby is born.

BY WEEK 24

By around 24 weeks, the baby is 13 inches long and weighs about 1½ pounds. The fingernails are forming, and the eyebrows and eyelashes are distinct. The skin is red because of increased blood flow beneath it. The skin is also very wrinkled. At this point the baby has little body fat. The baby's movements are now distinct and can sometimes be seen by looking at your abdomen. The baby can suck his or her thumb and can hear the sound of your voice.

BY THE END OF THE 2ⁿᴰ TRIMESTER

By the end of the second trimester, the fetus looks like a miniature baby. Your baby is referred to as a fetus from the end of the eighth week until delivery. A head of hair is developing. The baby begins to use his or her lungs to move fluid in and out. The baby swallows amniotic fluid. The way your baby gets nutrients is through the umbilical cord, which is attached to your uterus with the placenta.

Nutrients do not come from the baby's stomach, as occurs after birth. Amniotic fluid that the baby swallows is absorbed into the baby's bloodstream as water. The blood goes to the baby's kidneys, where urine is produced. The urine is stored in the bladder and then released as more amniotic fluid when the baby urinates. The eyes open for short periods of time. While the organs are all working at this point, they are still immature and cannot sustain their own function for long.

How Your Body Changes

Many changes occur to your body during this part of pregnancy. All of these changes are in response to your hormones and the growth and development of the baby. There are also certain new symptoms that you may notice. In general, however, you should feel good most of the time during this period of your pregnancy.

One of the most obvious changes is the growth of your abdomen, which is directly related to the growth of the baby. You are no longer able to wear your normal clothes and should start wearing maternity outfits. By 16 weeks, you have a little "pot-belly." By 20 weeks, the top of the uterus should be at the level of the belly button. Do not wear tight-fitting clothes as they can compress your blood vessels, reducing the blood flow to the baby.

Toward the end of the second trimester, you may develop stretch marks on your abdomen as your skin stretches beyond its normal elasticity. Some women are affected more than others. There is a genetic component to how prominent the marks become. It is a good idea to keep your skin lubricated with a good moisturizer; however, some stretch marks are unavoidable.

You may develop a dark line in the skin between the navel and the pubic area. This is called the linea nigra or dark

" I remember that in-between time when I was too big for my regular clothes but felt funny wearing maternity clothes. At least the maternity clothes announced that I was pregnant, not just gaining weight."

Second Trimester: Looking Pregnant & Feeling Great

line. It persists until a few weeks after delivery and then becomes less prominent.

CHANGES IN YOUR SKIN, HAIR & NAILS

You also may experience other skin changes. Some women notice that their skin is more oily than usual, while others develop acne again. Try to keep your skin clean with gentle soap and water. You may notice that your nails and hair begin to grow faster. This is due to the hormonal changes and the vitamins in your diet. Remember that each person is different and not all of these changes occur in everyone. In fact, some women report that their hair is thinner and falls out more, sometimes in clumps.

The breasts also undergo some dramatic changes during the second trimester. They continue to enlarge throughout this time. The tenderness that is common during the first trimester should improve significantly. You may have to change your bra size twice during the second trimester.

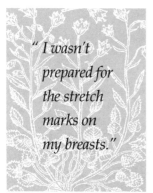

" I wasn't prepared for the stretch marks on my breasts."

From around 20 weeks on, you may notice a yellowish liquid coming out of the nipples from time to time. This is called **colostrum** and is produced throughout the rest of the pregnancy to be your baby's first food. Toward the end of the second trimester, the nipples and the skin around them darken. The areola begins to get larger.

HORMONES AND THE VAGINA

The vagina also responds to the increased hormones during the second trimester. Most women notice an increase in vaginal secretions. You may need to wear a mini-pad to protect your undergarments. The discharge should not itch, or have a strong odor, or contain blood. If you have a discharge that itches, burns, has a bad order, or is frothy or bloody, contact your physician to make sure that you do not have a vaginal infection that needs treatment.

Common Aches and Pains
ABDOMINAL PAIN – NORMAL OR NOT

As the uterus begins to grow rapidly, you sometimes have some pain that is caused by stretching of the ligaments that support the uterus. This is called **ligamentalgia,** and it can be quite painful at times. This pain is worse with movement and is relieved by bending slightly at the waist. There is nothing you can do to prevent ligamentalgia, and the more children you have, the worse the pain. No one knows why this happens, but you can expect to have much more abdominal discomfort during your second pregnancy than you did with your first. Bed rest does not help since the uterus is going to grow regardless, and the growth of the uterus is the reason for the pain. The pain ranges from a dull ache to a sharp stabbing sensation on the sides of the uterus. This pain should not be in the middle of your abdomen and you should not have nausea with it. At times, it is difficult to know if this pain is premature contractions. The best way to know is to have your obstetrician check your cervix; if it is dilating you probably are contracting, and if your cervix is normal you probably have ligamentalgia. Tylenol and rest help to reduce the discomfort for a short while. It is very important to always communicate with your doctor whenever you have abdominal pain in pregnancy.

COPING WITH VARICOSE VEINS

Varicose veins may develop during the second trimester. These are caused by a partial obstruction of blood flow from the lower legs up into the abdomen. There is a genetic component to these also. If you begin to develop varicose veins, or if you know that your are predisposed to getting them, try to avoid prolonged standing. A brisk walk helps reduce varicose veins, as it improves the tone of the muscles in your lower legs. These muscles must be strong to help get blood out of your legs and past your uterus to reduce the stress on the veins of your legs. If you must stand for long periods of time, invest in a good pair of support hose. Special maternity hose made with extra elastic are available at most maternity shops. Try to wear comfortable shoes, and avoid high heels during the rest of the pregnancy.

HOW TO HANDLE HEMORRHOIDS

Hemorrhoids may also become a problem. These are caused again by the partial obstruction of blood flow by the uterus as it grows. The problem is made worse when you have hard stools and strain during bowel movements.

While they can be quite painful, hemorrhoids are rarely dangerous. If they bleed, they should be checked by a physician to make sure there is not another cause for the bleeding. If you develop hemorrhoids, use a mild stool softener to prevent constipation and eat a high-fiber diet. You should drink enough fluid to keep your urine clear and not dark yellow, walk ½ mile per day and have a glass of Citrucel or Metamucil each day. By doing these three things, you reduce your chances of having problems with hemorrhoids. If the problem persists, over-the-counter preparations like Colace can be useful. Check with your physician if your hemorrhoids are persistent or very painful.

ENERGY AND SEXUALITY

During the second trimester, along with decreased nausea you also should have increased energy. The fatigue that was common in the beginning should improve. However, you should still get eight hours of sleep at night and try to rest at least twice a day.

" I felt invincible during the second trimester. I finished my master's thesis, traveled a lot, and in general felt like 'the little engine that could.'"

Some women notice an increase in sexual energy during this part of the pregnancy, while others notice a decrease. Make sure that you discuss how you feel with your spouse, as he may be feeling uncomfortable about the changes. If you desire more sexual activity, let him know it is safe to have intercourse at this point in pregnancy. Some men are afraid they will hit the baby with the tip of the penis during intercourse; reassure your partner that this does not occur. The baby is well protected by your cervix. If you have a decreased desire for intercourse, let your partner know you love him, but at this time the changes of pregnancy have made you less desiring of intercourse. You may feel a great need simply to be held, and it is important to communicate your needs. If your husband expresses a strong need to have intercourse, ask him to be patient, or consider masturbation with or without your participation as a healthy option.

Nourishing That New Life
EATING WELL FOR BOTH OF YOU

Your diet changes in response to your increased appetite during this part of the pregnancy. You feel hungrier and want to eat more. Most recent studies suggest that the second trimester is the most critical time to eat correctly so your baby has the proper nutrients to grow and develop. You should gain around 10 pounds during the second trimester. By 20 weeks, you should have gained 8 to 9 pounds from the beginning of the pregnancy.

Eat a well-balanced diet. Avoid simple sugars (sweets) and foods that are high in fat. Try to eat foods that are high in fiber to counteract the sluggishness of the bowels that is part of pregnancy.

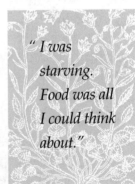

" I was starving. Food was all I could think about."

Drink one or two glasses of low-fat milk a day to help get extra calcium. The baby's bones are growing and calcifying. It is important to get extra calcium in your diet. If you cannot tolerate milk, drink calcium-fortified orange juice. You can also use a calcium supplement by taking a couple of Tums per day. Tums are calcium carbonate tablets and are a good source of calcium.

DEALING WITH DIGESTIVE DIFFICULTIES

Toward the end of the second trimester, you may begin to have significant problems with heartburn and gas. These problems result from the slower emptying of the stomach that occurs during pregnancy. Try to allow time for your stomach to empty before lying down at night – which means no midnight snacks. If you experience heartburn, you can try a liquid anti-acid like Maalox or Riopan. If these are ineffective, your physician may recommend you try different medications like Zantac or Pepcid. The liquid anti-acids give quick relief, and Zantac is used to reduce future attacks. If you take Zantac you should stay on it every day. It works over time and should not be taken only when you feel pain. Some women also carry around rolls of Tums to help with heartburn.

Other Second-Trimester Changes

You may feel warmer than usual, and your body temperature actually is going up. In general, you may be ½ to one degree warmer than usual. This elevation of your body temperature is due to the increase in metabolism that occurs in pregnancy. This may be the only time in your relationship with your husband where you think the room is too hot and you need to turn up the air conditioner.

Finally, you may notice significant emotional changes. Some women feel great and bask in the excitement of the pregnancy. Others may feel emotionally unbalanced, happy one minute and crying the next. Make sure that you have someone you feel close to in whom you can confide. Some women enjoy looking and feeling pregnant. Others do not like the way they look or feel during pregnancy. There is no right or wrong way to feel. Discussing your concerns help you cope with your feelings.

Special Tests: How and Why

Some special tests are typically done during the beginning of the second trimester. These include an ultrasound, amniocentesis and the alpha-fetoprotein test. We will discuss the use of each of these tests and what information you gain by having them done.

ULTRASOUND: A NON-INVASIVE SCREENING TEST
How It Works

Ultrasounds have been around for over 20 years, and studies have shown no significant risk to the developing fetus. There are no X-rays involved. To get the pictures, high-frequency sound waves are transmitted into the abdomen and reflect back to the machine. This is similar to sonar used on boats and submarines to "look" underneath the water. The pictures obtained with modern ultrasounds are quite astonishing: Hands, fingers, arms and legs are easily seen. Sometimes even external sexual organs can be seen clearly on these early scans.

" During ultrasound, our baby seemed to wave at us. Then she sucked her thumb."

What to Expect

Some physicians give you pictures of the baby for your family to see and to save in a scrapbook. Some offices even videotape the session for you. You may need to bring a blank videotape with you to get a copy, so ask what you should do when the ultrasound appointment is made. A trained ultrasound technician performs the scan, which takes place in a darkened room set up for this purpose. You lie on your back on an exam table, and the technician spreads a bit of gel on your abdomen to help the transducer glide smoothly. (If you are lucky, this gel has been warmed.) Then as the technician moves the instrument painlessly across your belly, you watch on a black-and-white screen as your baby becomes visible. You may not know what you are seeing at first, but the technician points out organs and bones, hands and feet, face and spine. Many women say they first bonded with their babies during that first glimpse via ultrasound. This ultrasound appointment is a great time to bring your spouse, as most men find this a fascinating visit. With this early ultrasound, the baby is so small you can see the entire body on the screen. If you have an ultrasound later in pregnancy, you only see a part of the baby at a time, like the liver or the leg, but not the entire body at once.

What Ultrasounds Can Detect

Many physicians order an ultrasound (also called a sonogram) in order to confirm the due date, rule out twins, and make sure there are no obvious malformations of your uterus or the baby. This sort of ultrasound is commonly done at the beginning of the second trimester.

Unfortunately, sometimes things are found or seen on the ultrasound that may indicate a problem. Abnormalities occur in 2 to 4 percent of all pregnancies. These may be minor findings like a small cyst in the kidney that just requires a follow-up scan. Sometimes, however, more serious problems such as heart defects are identified that require immediate attention or further studies. Make sure you discuss any abnormal findings carefully with your physician. And remember that a normal ultrasound does not guarantee that there is no problem with the baby. Some abnormalities are not easy to identify on early ultrasound.

Placenta Previa

A common problem that is seen is a placenta that covers the opening of the cervix where the baby later needs to pass. This is called a **placenta previa**. In many cases, just the edge of the placenta is covering the cervix. These are called "marginal" previas. As the uterus grows, it pulls up and away from the cervix, and most of these marginal previas resolve as the pregnancy progresses. Sometimes the center of the placenta is directly over the cervix. These are called "central" previas. These are more dangerous as the chance that they will persist to term is greater.

The problem with a placenta previa is that if it persists to term, it bleeds as the baby drops down into the birth canal. There is no safe way for the baby to be born vaginally if a previa persists, so cesarean section becomes necessary.

Most of the time a previa does not cause any problem during the second trimester. Previas usually only bleed or cause problems during the third trimester. Even so, some physicians recommend that their patients with placenta previa refrain from vaginal intercourse until a follow-up ultrasound is performed. Some physicians consider a previa seen on ultrasound at 14 or 16 weeks a normal finding, and unless there is vaginal bleeding, they do not restrict your activity. Discuss this with your physician if you are told you have a placenta previa so you know what to do.

Uterine Fibroids

Another common finding are uterine **fibroids**. Fibroids are smooth-muscle tumors of the uterus. They are more common after age 30. You can have one or multiple fibroids, and the tumors can be big or small.

Most fibroids do not cause problems during pregnancy; however, as the uterus grows, fibroids can also grow. Sometimes they grow rapidly during pregnancy and cause significant pain. Fibroids smaller than 5 centimeters rarely cause problems. In addition to being painful, large fibroids also are associated with premature labor. Your physician may perform follow-up ultrasounds to see if the fibroids are growing. Bed rest and more frequent visits to check for signs of premature labor are commonly prescribed.

Problems With the Baby

Occasionally, major malformations in the baby are seen or suspected. Special high-resolution ultrasounds are performed to better define these problems. Also, a consultation with a specialist called a **perinatologist** may be ordered. A perinatologist helps you and your physician determine the proper course of action or treatment needed when major malformations are identified. It is not unusual for a problem to be suspected by your physician only to find out on follow-up that there is no significant problem.

AMNIOCENTESIS: WHEN YOU NEED MORE INFORMATION

What It Is

An amniocentesis is ordered to evaluate suspected problems. This procedure is usually done during the beginning of the second trimester. In this simple test, a needle is used to remove a small amount of the amniotic fluid for analysis. The test is used to accurately detect genetic disorders and spinal cord problems.

" The Level II ultrasound was so detailed, I actually recognized my daughter after birth from her profile on ultrasound. I saw every bone, every finger and toe – all blessedly perfect."

Who Gets An Amniocentesis And Why

Amniocentesis is most commonly performed in women who are at increased risk of having a baby with a genetic problem. These women may be over the age of 35, or have a family history of a genetic disorder that can be detected by analysis of the amniotic fluid.

The amniotic fluid contains various chemicals and proteins released by the fetus. The fluid also contains skin cells shed by the baby. By removing the fluid and growing these skin cells in the lab, the DNA of these cells can be extracted and analyzed. The chromosome pattern and the sex of the baby are accurately determined. Certain genetic disorders are found by close analysis of the chromosomes. The fluid also contains other chemicals and proteins that aid in the diagnosis of many other metabolic and genetic disorders. The fluid is analyzed for a protein called alpha-fetoprotein (AFP). Elevated levels of AFP are found when babies have a neural-tube (spinal-cord) defect such as spina bifida. Spina bifida is a condition where there is an opening in the spine. Again, a consultation with a perinatologist is commonly requested.

How It Is Done

During an amniocentesis, an ultrasound is used to find a pocket of fluid around the baby. The skin of the abdomen is then made numb with lidocaine. A very long, thin, needle is then passed into the amniotic sac. The ultrasound is used to guide the passage of the needle into the amniotic sac without hitting the baby. About 20 cc (4 teaspoons) of amniotic fluid is removed and taken to a special genetics laboratory for analysis. The results may take up to two weeks to get back.

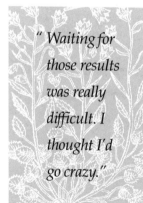

" Waiting for those results was really difficult. I thought I'd go crazy."

You may feel some cramping, like a strong menstrual cramp, during the procedure. You should plan on taking it easy the rest of the day after an amniocentesis. Most women can return to work within 24 to 48 hours.

What Are the Risks?

Most women do not have problems after amniocentesis. There are risks, however, including bleeding, premature rupture of the membranes, infection and miscarriage. The risk of miscarriage is less than 1 in 200. Because of these risks, an amniocentesis is only recommended when the chance of finding a problem is relatively high.

THE TRIPLE SCREEN: LOOKING FOR CHROMOSOME AND SPINE DEFECTS

What It Is

Another screening test that is offered during pregnancy is an AFP blood test. It is also called a triple screen. This test is performed between 14 and 21 weeks. A specimen of blood is drawn from your arm and sent to the lab for analysis. It is used to screen women who are otherwise not at increased risk for Down's Syndrome, Trisomy 18 and neural-tube defects such as spina bifida.

What It Detects

The test is known as a triple screen because the blood is analyzed for three things, the amount of alpha-fetoprotein (AFP), estrogen and human chorionic gonadotropin (HCG). The levels in the blood are then compared to expected levels. The results indicate either an increased risk that the baby has a chromosome problem or a neural-tube defect.

This test is a screening test, and if it returns positive you need additional testing to determine if a problem exists. If the risk of a chromosome problem is increased, you then have an amniocentesis, and if the risk of a spine defect is increased, you have a high-resolution ultrasound.

Increased Risk of Down's Syndrome

Your chance of having a baby with Down's syndrome increases as you get older. Most women over age 35 are considered at increased risk and are offered amniocentesis without first having the AFP test. The average risk of a women younger than 35 having a baby with Down's syndrome is around 1 in 700. Since most women having babies in this country are younger than 35, it stands to reason that most babies with Down's syndrome are born to women younger than 35 years old. This triple-screen test is used to see if women younger than 35 should have amniocentesis to check the baby for Down's syndrome. For more information about this testing, read Chapter 18 "Pregnancy After 35."

Increased Risk of Trisomy 18

Trisomy 18 is a chromosome defect similar to Down's syndrome but more severe and less common. In Down's syndrome there is an extra chromosome number 21, and in Trisomy 18 the extra chromosome is number 18. Babies with Trisomy 18 are usually severely mentally retarded and rarely live more than a year. These babies usually have cleft lips and heart defects.

Increased Risk of Neural-Tube Defects

Neural-tube defects occur in one pregnancy out of 1,000 in this country. Anencephaly and spina bifida are the two major types of neural- tube defects. **Anencephaly** is a condition where the baby's brain and skull do not develop properly. Babies who survive pregnancy and are born at term only live for a few days. Babies with **spina bifida** may have a mild defect and little handicap, or can be severely affected with paralysis of the lower extremities, loss of bowel and bladder control, and mental retardation.

What You Should Know

Most of these defects cannot be treated during pregnancy. Many women decide not to have the triple-screen test because they would not change anything if the baby did have a problem – in other words, they would not terminate the pregnancy. It is important to consider, however, that if your baby is known to have a spinal-cord defect before birth, this information may change how or where you are delivered. It may be better to have a cesarean section and a pediatric surgeon present at a hospital equipped to care for high-risk babies than to deliver vaginally at a community hospital and transfer the baby later on. Another advantage to the testing is the time it allows you and your family to prepare for the birth of a baby with special needs. Therefore, even if you would not consider abortion, there are other benefits to having these tests done. The decision, however, is yours.

Also keep in mind that even if your test result is abnormal, most likely there is nothing wrong with the baby. Further testing needs to be performed to rule out any of the above problems. Sometimes just a second sample of blood is obtained to confirm the previous result. Of the initial tests that return positive, only 1 in 10 has the suspected problem. The rest are normal. A normal test result does not guarantee that there are no problems, but it is reassuring to know that your risk is low.

What Can Go Wrong During the Second Trimester?

PREMATURE LABOR

There are a few problems that can occur during the second trimester of pregnancy. One of these is premature labor. Labor eariler than 24 weeks is rare. Many women begin to feel occasional contractions or tightening of the uterus after 20 weeks. If these are irregular, nonpainful and resolve with rest, they are most likely Braxton-Hicks contractions – "practice" contractions that do not mean you are in labor. Braxton-Hicks contractions are normal and may occur four to six times an hour. Normally, they subside if you lie down and drink a lot of fluid. If you experience contractions that become regular or are painful, you may be going into premature labor. You should report any contractions associated with an increase in vaginal discharge or spotting. If you are ever in doubt, contact your physician to be checked. It is better to be safe than sorry. Most of the time, if you are in premature labor, the contractions can be stopped. The sooner treatment is started, the easier it is to stop premature labor.

PREMATURE RUPTURE OF THE MEMBRANES

The membranes that surround the baby and hold the amniotic fluid may leak or rupture. This event is rare during the second trimester. If there is a small leak, the membranes may repair themselves, and the leak will stop. Notify your physician immediately if you think you may be leaking fluid. Complete rupture of the membranes is associated with premature delivery or miscarriage. Babies need to remain in the amniotic fluid in order for their lungs to develop normally. Before 24 weeks, their lungs are not developed completely, and their chance of survival is small. Luckily, premature rupture of the membranes is rare in the second trimester.

INCOMPETENT CERVIX

Another unusual problem that occurs during the second trimester is miscarriage due to an incompetent cervix. The cervix, a tough muscular ring, is responsible for holding the baby within the uterus until the end of pregnancy. The cervix is supposed to dilate only in labor or at the end of the third trimester. In some women, the cervix is not strong enough to stay shut during the second trimester. The pressure of the baby forces open a weak, or incompetent, cervix and leads to premature labor, premature rupture of the membranes or miscarriage. Typically, women with this problem present to their physician with mild contractions or no contractions, and everyone is surprised to discover that the cervix is already dilated. An incompetent cervix is more common in women who have had prior surgery of the cervix or multiple terminations of pregnancy. Sometimes the condition occurs because of congenital weakness of the cervix. Unfortunately, identifying an incompetent cervix rarely takes place during your first pregnancy. It is discovered once you have had painless, premature dilation of the cervix and miscarried or delivered a severely premature baby.

If you are suspected of having an incompetent cervix, a procedure called a cervical **cerclage** is performed in every future pregnancy. A cervical cerclage is performed after 13 weeks, once a normal ultrasound is obtained. The procedure is performed as an outpatient in the hospital. Anesthesia is used for the procedure, either general or spinal anesthesia. There are several different techniques, but most involve placing a suture or similar material around the upper part of the cervix to help keep it closed. This material is removed at the end of pregnancy to allow normal labor to occur. Most cervical cerclages are done through the vagina, and no cutting of the skin is necessary. If most of the cervix is missing due to previous surgery, there may not be enough of the cervix in the vagina to suture around. In this case, an abdominal cerclage is placed. This type of cerclage requires an incision on the abdomen. It is a bigger procedure and requires that you deliver by cesarean section.

Conclusion

The second trimester of pregnancy is a good time to get yourself and your home ready for a baby. The more you do now, the less you will need to do later. Make sure that you take time for yourself each day to relax, and try to enjoy this part of your pregnancy. As you become noticeably pregnant, those around you start to share in this very special event. You are nourishing a new life within your womb, and nothing compares to this. Use the information in this chapter to better understand some of the issues your physician is considering when you go for your visits. Now it is time to prepare for the final trimester.

Additional Resources

Books

- **Fit for Two: The Official YMCA Prenatal Exercise Guide,** *Thomas W. Hanlon,* Human Kinetics, 1995.

- **Easy Exercises for Pregnancy,** *Janet Balaskas,* MacMillan General Reference, 1997.

- **Essential Exercises for the Childbearing Year: A Guide to Health and Comfort Before and After Your Baby Is Born,** *Elizabeth Noble,* New Life Images, 1995.

- **Which Tests for My Unborn Baby: A Guide to Prenatal Diagnosis,** *Lachlan De Crespigny and Rhonda Dredge,* Oxford University Press, 1996.

Organizations

- **National Organization of Mothers of Twins Clubs Inc.**
  P. O. Box 23188
  Albuquerque, NM 87192-1188
  (505) 275-0955
  (800) 243-2276
  http://www.nomotc.org

- **Lamaze International**
  1200 19th Street, NW, Suite 300
  Washington, DC 20036-2422
  (800) 368-4404
  E-mail: lamaze@dc.sba.com
  http://www.lamaze-childbirth.com

Internet Sites

- http://www.parentsplace.com/readroom/twinsmag/index.html
  This site, sponsored by Twin Magazine, provides a variety of information for families who have twins or are expecting twins.

- http://siteguider.com/
  The BabyZone site offers information about pregnancy, maternity, family planning, infertility, childbirth, parenting and babies, as well as birth stories, message boards and links to pregnancy-related sites.

- http://www.babycenter.com/refcap/631.html
  This section of the BabyCenter site's Resource Center answers your questions about the Bradley Method of husband-coached childbirth and offers links to other "natural" childbirth options.

CHAPTER FOURTEEN

THIRD TRIMESTER

Expecting Great Things

he third trimester of pregnancy is a very special time. You are constantly reminded of your baby's presence, and your attention is focused on the upcoming birth. This is what you have been waiting for over the last nine months.

The baby's movements have become very pronounced, and you probably cannot sleep well at night. The fatigue at this point becomes almost overwhelming. But you tolerate these problems when a kick or poke of the elbow reminds you – as if you could forget – that you are nurturing a living being within your womb. The bond between you and your baby is very powerful and long-lasting. Allow yourself the quiet time to relish this feeling. Like the many years of parenting ahead of you, the third trimester of pregnancy is made up of difficult parts and wonderful parts. In order to love parenting, you must relish the special times. This chapter can help you do this by explaining the changes occurring to you and your baby at this stage.

The third trimester covers weeks 28 to 40 (and beyond), or months seven to nine. This chapter covers how your baby is developing during this time; what to expect at your office visits, which become more and more frequent; and what special problems may occur, along with how they are detected and managed.

"I could feel the baby move before I was even conscious of being awake in the morning – unforgettable and very reassuring. Sometimes I snuggled up to my husband and let the baby wake him with little kicks and pokes."

What is Happening With the Baby?

> "We made the most of the last few weeks before we became parents. We saw a lot of movies, ate out several times and enjoyed being together – without having to pay a sitter!"
>
> 🐚
>
> " I'm very ready. I really want this to be over with."

At 28 weeks, the baby weighs 3 to 4 pounds (1 to 2 kilograms), and is 18 inches long. By 40 weeks, the baby is 6 to 8 pounds (3 to 4 kilograms), and 20 inches long. This rate of growth is the greatest of the entire pregnancy. In the first and second trimesters, the baby's organs form; in this third trimester, they simply grow larger.

The development of one very important organ, the brain, is incomplete at the beginning of the third trimester. The brain is the last of your baby's organs to fully form. Take good care of yourself during this stage so that your baby's brain is allowed to develop to its full potential. Do not drink alcohol and stay out of hot tubs or saunas, as these adversely affect brain development. Instead, you can help stimulate your baby's brain during this time by speaking to the baby, reading aloud and listening to pleasing music.

What Hurts and Why

Whenever we feel discomfort or pain, it is normal to suspect a problem. This is particularly true when the pain is in your abdomen and you are pregnant. However, there are normal discomforts that occur at this stage of pregnancy. These discomforts tend to occur earlier and more intensely with each baby you carry. The two most common are groin pain and pelvic pain.

GROIN PAIN

During the third trimester, you may notice sharp pains in your groin and in the middle of your symphysis pubis (pubic bone) when you walk. The hormones of pregnancy help loosen your joints and allow them to move more easily, and as you walk, this increased movement of the joints causes sharp pain, as if you had sprained an ankle. The advantage of continuing to walk through this discomfort is that the more your hip joints move now, the better they will move during labor, thus making a vaginal delivery more likely and safer.

ABDOMINAL PAIN

Other pains that occur at this stage are related to the larger size of the baby. As the uterus grows upward, you may feel a sharp pain under your right rib. This pain comes from the gallbladder, a sac that lies beneath your liver and is very tender to touch. The constant pressure of the uterus on the gallbladder – especially if the baby pushes in this direction – causes upper abdominal pain. Many women complain the baby's foot is under their ribs when they feel this pain, but their own gallbladder is the culprit. The pressure in your upper abdomen also causes you to feel short of breath and develop indigestion. For the indigestion you should start eating frequent small meals again. This is also a common time to need antacids like Tums.

PELVIC PAIN

Near the end of your pregnancy, you also may feel pain deep in your pelvis. It occurs as the baby's head descends from your abdomen into your pelvis. With the head in your pelvis, there is pressure on your bladder and the nerves in this region.

Pressure on the bladder results in the need to urinate very frequently, even throughout the night. As a result, you are probably not getting a good night's sleep, and you experience the fatigue and forgetfulness associated with this stage of pregnancy. One benefit of this frequent waking is that you become accustomed to a fragmented sleep pattern before the baby arrives, so the stress of caring for a newborn around the clock is lessened a bit. It is still very challenging, but possibly not as much

"I had to go to the bathroom a lot. And that's a pain at night when you try to rest. The last month, I couldn't really sleep anyway since I was so uncomfortable."

of a shock on your system. It helps to understand why you feel the need to urinate so frequently.

Pressure on the nerves within your pelvis creates pain that radiates through your buttocks down the back of your thigh. This pain, called **sciatica**, becomes severe for some women. There is no treatment to remove this pain other than to deliver the baby. To get some relief, take Tylenol, rest on your side or in knee-chest position and try to get into a pool to walk as often as possible. Walking in a pool helps by lifting the pregnancy from your pelvis into your abdomen, relieving the pressure from the nerves in the pelvis.

What Happens During Office Visits

During the early part of pregnancy, you visit your physician every four to six weeks. In the last trimester of pregnancy, the visits are more frequent. Frequent office visits allow us to more closely monitor the baby's growth. In the last three months of development, the baby is putting more demands on your body than at any other time during your pregnancy. If your uterus is unable to keep up with this demand, the baby lets us know there is a problem by not growing at the appropriate rate or by not moving a normal amount. In order to have these events evaluated in a timely manner, you must come into the office more frequently. During weeks 28 through 32, the visits are usually every three weeks; during weeks 32 to 36, they are every two weeks; and beyond 36 weeks, the visits are every week. The frequency of visits increases as the risk of problems increases with an advancing pregnancy. During these visits your weight, blood pressure and fundal height (size of your uterus) are measured. At one of your visits near your due date, your physician checks your cervix with an internal exam and feels the position of the baby. The purpose of this exam is to find out what your cervix feels like before you start labor, and to make sure the baby is positioned headfirst and not breech.

"In those last few weeks, life seemed to revolve around doctor's visits."

STEPPING ONTO THE SCALES

You can expect to gain 10 to 15 pounds during this stage. If you gain too much or too little, an ultrasound may be done to make sure the baby is growing appropriately. In order to gain the proper weight, you should be eating three meals a day and two healthy snacks. You should not eat sweets, as they cross the placenta and go to the baby. (This does not mean to avoid fruits, as their natural sugar is acceptable.) At this stage, the baby is mature enough to release insulin in response to sugar. Insulin acts like a growth hormone, and the baby can get large shoulders, which can hurt both of you during delivery.

"I was very sensitive about my weight. Once the doctor made a very mild comment, and I had to cry when he left the room."

CHECKING YOUR BLOOD PRESSURE

In monitoring your blood pressure, we are watching for a pressure above 140 for the top number (systolic) and 90 for the bottom number (diastolic). Elevated blood pressure is discussed later in this chapter.

MEASURING YOUR UTERUS

The fundal height is measured from your pubic bone to the top of the uterus. The length in centimeters should equal the number of weeks you are pregnant at the time of the visit. If there is a large difference, your physician will evaluate this with an ultrasound.

SCREENING FOR INFECTION

In many practices a culture of your vagina is done at week 36 to screen for Group B Streptococcus bacteria. If this bacteria is present in your vaginal canal, you receive antibiotics during labor to minimize the chance your baby will become ill just after birth with this potentially fatal infection.

LOOKING FOR POTENTIAL PROBLEMS

During these visits, your physician monitors for many potential problems. We will review the most common problems encountered during pregnancy. Once a problem is noted, special testing is done to see if the baby is doing well. The idea is to deliver the baby if there is evidence of too much stress occurring within your uterus. However, we do not want to deliver a baby too prematurely, as the baby's lungs may not be developed. The inability to breathe could cause more harm than the stress in your uterus. This gives you an idea of how there is an art as well as a science to the delivery of health care.

What Complications Can Occur at This Stage

While there are many problems that can occur during pregnancy, we are going to discuss the 10 most common: hypertension, poor fetal growth, excessive fetal growth, decreased fetal movement, diabetes, postdates, twins, herpes infection, early rupture of the membranes and preterm labor. Before describing these problems, let us discuss the various means available to make sure the baby is doing well. These include the fetal movement count, nonstress test, contraction stress test and biophysical profile.

How Your Baby's Well-Being is Monitored

The **fetal movement count** involves making note of the number of your baby's movements within a two-hour period. All women should do this starting at 32 weeks of pregnancy. If the baby is less active than usual, lie down on your left side in a quiet room, have a snack and rest your hand on your uterus. As you feel movements within your uterus or with your hand, count them. If you do not feel 10 movements within two hours, call your physician that day – do not wait until your next visit.

The **nonstress test (NST)** is the most common test used to assure your baby is doing well in the uterus. During a nonstress test, variations in the baby's heartbeat are evaluated for up to 20 minutes. The baby is doing fine if there are accelerations in the fetal heart rate of at least 15 beats per minute lasting 15 seconds, with two episodes of acceleration within the 20 minutes.

With a **contraction stress test (CST)**, the baby's heart rate is observed for decelerations while you have contractions. You must have three contractions during a ten-minute session in order to evaluate the baby. There should not be any decelerations to have a reassuring test. If there are fetal heart-rate decelerations, your physician must consider how premature the pregnancy is when deciding on the best management plan. If there are small decelerations and you are very early in the pregnancy, you may be put on bed rest and closely monitored. If you are near term, labor is induced or you are scheduled for a cesarean section.

A **biophysical profile (BPP)** evaluates the baby's well being through combining a NST with an ultrasound. During the ultrasound, your baby is observed for breathing movement, flexion and extension of the hand, arm or legs, and movement of the central part of the body. Also, the amount of amniotic fluid is compared to normal. Each of these five areas is given a score of two points if they are normal: NST, amniotic fluid level, breathing movements, flexion of the arm/leg/hand, and flexion of the central body. The ideal score is ten; the baby is doing well with a score of eight. With a score of six, the test is repeated within a day or two. With a score of four or less, the baby is delivered unless there is a compelling reason not to do so, such a severe prematurity.

Why You May Need Testing

Now that you are aware of the special tests used in pregnancy, let us discuss when they are needed. This is not an all-inclusive list, but it does cover the vast majority of reasons your pregnancy may need special testing. Please understand this is a general overview, and your particular case may need a different approach. This section is intended to give you a basic understanding of special problems. You must discuss your particular pregnancy with your physician to see how he or she feels about your progress.

HYPERTENSION

Hypertension is the elevation of blood pressure. During pregnancy, the pressure should remain below 140 systolic (top number) and 90 diastolic (bottom number).

When the blood pressure is elevated, there is greater risk the placenta may prematurely separate from the womb. When this separation

occurs prior to birth, the baby could die. This premature separation is called **placental abruption**, and it is very rare. If an abruption
occurs, you feel a great deal of constant abdominal pain. If you feel
this type of pain in the month or two before your due date, call
your physician immediately.

One problem related to elevated blood pressure is **toxemia (also
known as pre-eclampsia)**. Symptoms of toxemia include pain in the
upper-right abdomen, headaches and dark spots in front of your eyes.
Your physician checks your reflexes if your blood pressure is elevated,
as they are exaggerated with this condition. Your urine and blood are
tested to determine if you have toxemia, as the urine contains too
much protein and the blood test reveals a drop in platelets, (the blood
component that helps form normal blood clots).

If you have elevated blood pressure and no other problems, the
pregnancy is monitored with a nonstress test every week. If your pressure is high enough to need medication, the pregnancy is monitored
with a contraction stress test or a biophysical profile. During these
weeks of monitoring, you are to be on bed rest as much as possible.
Finally, if you are diagnosed as having toxemia, the pregnancy is ended
by induction of labor or by cesarean section. The treatment of toxemia
is to get the baby delivered. While this is occurring, you are also given
a special medication called magnesium sulfate. This medication prevents you from having seizures, which can occur with toxemia. It is
important for you to realize that while hypertension in pregnancy is
common, the complications of toxemia and abruption are not.

POOR GROWTH

Every time your physician measures the size of your uterus, your
baby is being screened for poor growth. If the size is more than three
centimeters below the number of weeks of the pregnancy, then poor
growth is suspected. In this situation, an ultrasound evaluation is performed. Other possible causes of a small uterus include reduced amniotic fluid, incorrect dating of the pregnancy or a normal variation. A
normal variation can occur if you have had several children, as you
tend to carry the pregnancy lower.

If your baby is not growing well, special testing is needed to make sure that continuing the pregnancy is safe. The special testing includes a biophysical profile or NST twice a week. If the tests show that your baby is safe in the uterus, you should take special care of yourself to help the baby get the needed nutrients. You should get plenty of rest, drink plenty of fluids and eat healthy meals. If you smoke, you must stop. If the tests show that your baby is under stress in the uterus, the baby is delivered by cesarean section or induction of vaginal delivery. Once the baby is noted to have poor growth, you have an ultrasound every three weeks to make sure the baby has grown during this time. If the baby is small but shows good interval growth over three weeks, the baby is probably fine. You still have the tests, but you should feel reassured by the growth.

EXCESSIVE GROWTH

Too much, rather than too little, growth of the baby is a more common problem. This is noted when the size of the uterus is three centimeters more than the week of pregnancy. When excessive growth occurs, the baby is measured by ultrasound. It is important to note that no method can perfectly determine the weight of a baby.

If the baby is large, one possible cause is diabetes of pregnancy (**gestational diabetes**). You are tested at 24 to 28 weeks for gestational diabetes, and this testing is included in the discussion of diabetes below. However, most women with large babies do not have diabetes. You can cause excessive growth by eating too many sweets, such as ice cream, cake, candy, sweetened tea and regular soda. As was noted previously, sugar from these foods crosses the placenta and causes the baby to release insulin, which creates excessive growth. You should avoid consuming foods with these added sugars and be aware of the sugar that occurs naturally in foods you eat. There are some sweets in fruit juices, for example, which are best managed in pregnancy by walking one mile each day. Walking burns off these natural sweets.

The danger of excessive growth relates to the safety of having a vaginal birth. During labor, a large baby may come down the birth canal without a problem. However, once the head is out, the baby's shoulders may get stuck behind the pubic bone. This is a true emergency, since the baby is not getting a full supply of oxygen at that point. This situation is called **shoulder dystocia**. Your physician must act quickly, cutting an episiotomy and having you pull your knees back as far as you can toward your shoulders to enlarge the vaginal opening. Even if dystocia does not occur, the shoulders of a large baby are more likely to cause a larger tear in the vagina. If a baby is felt to be 4,500 grams (9 pounds, 9 ounces) or larger, cesarean section is considered the safest method of delivery.

DECREASED FETAL MOVEMENT

Any time you think the baby is not moving as frequently as normal, you should be on alert. You start feeling the baby move near the start of the fifth month, at about 20 weeks. It is normal to feel movement for a few days and then feel none for a day or two from weeks 20 to 24. From 28 weeks until delivery, you should feel the baby move every day. If you note a decrease in the frequency of movements at this time, have something to eat and lie on your left side. Count the number of movements you feel over two hours. If there are fewer than 10, call your physician right away.

The one time you can expect some decline in fetal movement is just before you go into labor. Many women report that their babies do not seem to move as much as usual as they are going into labor. However, you still should have 10 movements over two hours.

DIABETES

Diabetes can be a problem you have prior to pregnancy, or it may develop only during pregnancy. Regardless of when it occurs, the problem with diabetes is that you do not produce enough insulin for your body's needs. If you have diabetes prior to pregnancy, it is very important to let your physician know that you are planning to get pregnant. Your sugar levels must be in very good control at the time of conception to avoid greater risk of birth defects. In fact, the only time you can affect the risk of birth defects that relate to diabetes is at the beginning of pregnancy.

Most women do not have diabetes before pregnancy. A few develop it during the second half of pregnancy. You are tested for gestational diabetes at 24 to 28 weeks by drinking a sugary liquid and having your blood sugar checked one hour later. This test is called the glucose screen, glucose-tolerance test or O'Sullivan's test. If the level is too high (over 135 in most offices), you must have a more thorough test. This test involves drinking a larger amount of the sweet drink and having your sugar level tested several times over three hours. If these results are too high, then you are diagnosed with gestational diabetes.

The management of diabetes is directed toward keeping your sugar levels in the normal range. You are counseled on a proper meal plan and the importance of regular exercise. When possible, your sugar levels are controlled just by eating properly and exercising. Sometimes, even if you eat well, sugar levels remain too high. In this situation, you are started on insulin.

If diet and exercise control your gestational diabetes, your baby is followed with weekly nonstress tests. If insulin is required, your pregnancy is monitored with either a nonstress test or a biophysical profile each week. These tests are started at 34 weeks.

If you have diabetes in pregnancy, you have a lot of work to do to monitor your sugar level. In addition, there is extra work involved in the monitoring of the baby. You may feel added concern and stress as a result, but try to realize that with proper management you should have a wonderful delivery of a healthy baby.

Because diabetes affects the size of your baby, it can also affect how your baby is delivered. The higher level of glucose in your blood crosses the uterus and placenta to the baby. The baby responds by releasing insulin, which acts like a growth hormone. The end result is a larger baby. Of particular concern are the baby's large shoulders, which could cause shoulder dystocia during a vaginal delivery. In a woman without diabetes, the chance of having shoulder dystocia during labor increases when the baby weighs more than 4,500 grams (9 pounds, 9 ounces). If you have diabetes, this risk starts to go up when the baby weighs more the 4,000 grams (8 pounds, 8 ounces).

In order to avoid the risk of shoulder dystocia, many physicians prefer delivery by cesarean section if the baby is estimated to weigh more than 4,000 grams. The main reason for avoiding trial of labor and vaginal birth is that you do not know if the baby's shoulders will fit through the birth canal until the baby's head is delivered – which is too late. Now you can better understand why a woman with diabetes is more likely to have a cesarean section than a non-diabetic woman.

POSTDATES

Postdates refers to a pregnancy that goes two weeks past the due date. Most physicians have a special evaluation of any pregnancy that goes one week past the due date, making 41 weeks the practical time to consider postdates. You may personally consider yourself postdates the day after your due date. Having survived the aches and pains for nine months, you may think that being pregnant one more day is too much.

As part of a postdates evaluation, the baby is evaluated with a biophysical profile, nonstress test or contraction stress test. Also, your cervix is examined to see if it is favorable for induction. A cervix that is thin, soft and partially dilated is considered favorable. When the cervix is thick, firm and closed, it is not favorable.

If the baby shows any signs of not doing well, you are admitted to the hospital for an induction of labor or a cesarean section. If the baby is doing well and your cervix is not favorable for an induction, you are asked to monitor fetal movements every day and return within one week. If the baby is doing well and your cervix is favorable for induction, then you and your physician decide whether to wait another week or proceed immediately with an induction of labor.

Just for your knowledge, labor should not be induced without a medical reason because an induction of labor carries more risks than naturally occurring labor. With an induction there is greater risk of fetal distress, infection, epidural use and cesarean section. While a cesarean section is safe with modern medicine, it still carries a much greater risk of infection, hemorrhage requiring a blood transfusion, and death compared to a vaginal delivery. So please understand that your physician is considering what is best for you and the baby when you are asked to wait another week – and not being cold-hearted to your suffering at this late stage of pregnancy.

When you are two weeks past your due date, most physicians in the United States induce labor regardless of the condition of your cervix. Going beyond 42 weeks of pregnancy carries a greater risk of fetal death, and therefore is avoided. If your physician suggests waiting more than two weeks past your due date, there should be a very good explanation, and you may think about getting a second opinion.

MULTIPLE PREGNANCIES

Twins are becoming more common. With the increased use of infertility drugs, many couples are facing the challenges of having twins or triplets. While having more than one child at a time can be doubly exciting, the situation also creates anxiety for a couple. Not only is there the concern of getting through the pregnancy, but also the concern of a special delivery and then the extra demands of caring for two children. My wife and I have three children, each three years apart, and they are a lot of work. I have a great deal of respect for parents of twins. Most major cities have support groups for parents of twins, and you should join one as soon as you discover you are having twins. Also, there is helpful information on the Internet (see the additional Resources at the end of this chapter).

During the third trimester of a pregnancy with twins, the main concern is avoiding premature delivery. Prematurity is the greatest risk to the babies. You should rest in bed as much as possible starting at 20 weeks. As physicians, we try to consider your other demands in life when we recommend measures to head off premature labor. If active contractions are not occurring frequently, you may stay out of bed, but avoid any nonessential activities. If you must work, then rest on your side for 30 minutes as soon as you come home. As much as possible, avoid prolonged periods of being on your feet. If you are having contractions or abdominal pain, call your physician immediately.

Starting at 34 weeks, your babies are monitored weekly with a NST to make sure they are doing well. Also, an ultrasound is performed every two to three weeks to assure appropriate growth and normal amount of amniotic fluid. Labor begins earlier than 40 weeks in many multiple pregnancies and most twins are delivered by 39 weeks.

HERPES

Active herpes infection is of special concern in the third trimester. Herpes is a viral infection obtained through intercourse. The infection causes periodic outbreaks of small, painful blisters on the labia. If you have an outbreak during labor, you are delivered by cesarean section to avoid exposing the baby in the birth canal during a vaginal delivery. If you have a cesarean section before the sac surrounding the baby has been broken more than four hours, your baby's risk of contracting herpes is minimal. If you have frequent outbreaks of herpes, antiviral medications such as Zovirax and Famvir are available to increase the interval between outbreaks. Taking the medicine improves the chance that you will not have an outbreak during labor.

PREMATURE RUPTURE OF MEMBRANES (PROM)

You are said to have premature rupture of membranes whenever your bag of water breaks before you have gone into labor. PROM is not a serious problem if you are within three or four weeks of your due date. In this situation, you can wait for labor to start on its own or have labor induced with intravenous Pitocin or a prostaglandin gel, which is placed into your vagina.

When PROM occurs more than four weeks before your due date, there is greater concern. The baby's lungs may not be fully developed, and the baby may require assistance from a ventilator to breathe after birth. Another major concern is the risk of infection within the uterus. This risk increases the longer the membranes are broken. These two concerns are addressed differently. You receive an injection of steroids to promote rapid maturation of your baby's lungs, and you take antibiotics to prevent bacterial infection.

PRE-TERM LABOR

Pre-term labor is the onset of regular contractions that result in a change in your cervix before you are due to deliver. Most women begin to experience tightening of their uterus just after 20 weeks of pregnancy. These Braxton-Hicks contractions can occur up to once every hour but usually occur two or three times a day. The difference between Braxton-Hicks contractions and pre-term labor is the contractions of pre-term labor are much more painful and result in changes of your cervix. At times the difference is difficult for you to determine, so always let your physician know if your routine contractions seem to increase in strength.

When you have strong contractions that result in a change of your cervix before 37 weeks, you are admitted to your hospital's labor and delivery department. Your doctor looks for any potential reasons for these contractions. Some common causes include a urinary tract infection, pelvic infection, twins, uterine fibroids, the presence of too much amniotic fluid, and dehydration. Frequently, there is no known reason a woman enters pre-term labor. Tests you can expect include a urine test, vaginal cultures and an ultrasound.

The treatment of pre-term labor initially involves giving extra fluids; you are asked to drink a lot, and sometimes you receive IV fluids. Also, sedated with a morphine injection to stop the contractions. At 35 or 36 weeks, these steps may be all that your physician takes to treat the pre-term labor. If you continue to contract, you may be allowed to deliver. If you are less than 35 weeks, additional treatment is available, including magnesium sulfate infusion through the IV. In this situation, you also may be started on steroids to stimulate maturation of the baby's lungs and an antibiotic to lower the risk of infection if the baby does deliver prematurely. These are general guidelines, and your physician will review a treatment plan with you at the time this is occurring. Also, a member of the nursery staff may visit you to explain what interventions your baby may need if born very premature. Knowing what to expect can help reduce your anxiety during this very stressful time.

Conclusion

The topics of special testing and special situations are covered in this chapter to help you understand them better if they happen to you. We do not cover them to make you nervous about your pregnancy.

This last trimester of pregnancy is a wonderful and exciting time. Your baby is growing larger and stronger, preparing for life outside your uterus. In the vast majority of pregnancies, the baby will deliver within the time frame of three weeks before to two weeks after your due date. In our next chapter, we discuss issues related to labor and delivery. Please be assured that your physician will be monitoring your pregnancy, and you can simply enjoy this time of growth and unique bonding with your baby, despite the physical discomforts of this stage.

Resources

Additional Reading

- **Your Pregnancy Month by Month,** *Clark Gillespie, M.D.,* HarperPerennial, 1995.

- **Pregnancy, Birth and the Early Months: A Complete Guide,** *Richard I. Feinbloom,* Addison-Wesley, 1992.

- **Water Fitness During Your Pregnancy,** *Jane Katz,* Human Kinetics, 1995.

Organizations

- **National Organization of Mothers of Twins Clubs, Inc.**
  P.O. Box 23188
  Albuquerque, NM 87192-1188
  (505) 275-0955
  (800) 243-2276
  http://www.nomotc.org

- **National Diabetes Information Clearinghouse**
  1 Information Way
  Bethesda, MD 20892-3560
  (301) 654-3327

Internet Sites

- **http://www.herpes.com/pregnancy.shtml**
  Herpes.com offers insight and information on giving birth when you have genital herpes.

- **http://pregnancy.miningco.com/**
  The Mining Company's comprehensive pregnancy site offers a week-by-week guide, advice on preparing for multiples and more. Click on the "complications" link to get detailed information on diabetes in pregnancy, pre-term labor, hypertension and other problems.

CHAPTER FIFTEEN

LABOR & DELIVERY

Preparing for the Big Event

The delivery of your baby is one of the most wonderful things that will ever happen to you. The miracle of birth – when a baby goes from living within your uterus to breathing air – is spectacular. I have delivered more than a thousand babies, and I am still moved by this event. You must be excited to know your baby will soon be in your arms. Also, you are probably looking forward to saying goodbye to the discomforts of pregnancy, and to getting your "old" body back – or at least one that is closer to what you remember!

If you are expecting your first baby, the excitement you feel must be overwhelming. With the second, third or fourth baby, you may notice less excitement. You are no doubt still greatly anticipating the birth of your baby, but you now know a little more about the word before delivery – labor. There is nothing wrong with the way you feel, as it is part of a natural maturation process that you go through as a mother. This same process helps you deal with the demands of caring for a newborn and raising children.

This chapter discusses the signs of labor, false labor, when to call your physician, stages of labor, vaginal delivery, cesarean section, and the postpartum period.

When Labor Begins
IS THIS "THE REAL THING"?

If you are pregnant for the first time, you may be greatly concerned that you will not know when you are in labor. Everyone has heard of a couple who had their baby in the car or even on their living-room floor. While the idea of delivering without your physician may be stressful, please realize that this happens very, very rarely. When in labor, you will not have to ask anyone; you will declare it emphatically.

After the twentieth week of pregnancy, it is normal to feel occasional tightening of the uterus, called Braxton-Hicks contractions. They occur a few times a day at first, then as you approach 36 weeks you may have them every 30 minutes. The key to Braxton-Hicks contractions is that very little pain is associated with them. You have a tightening of the uterus that is not too uncomfortable. Braxton-Hicks contractions do not generate force, so your cervix remains closed. If you are concerned about the amount of discomfort associated with these contractions, just ask your doctor to check your cervix. I feel strongly that my job as an obstetrician is to make your pregnancy as stress-free as possible, and a simple cervical exam can alleviate your fear of having pre-term labor.

" I was at home when I went into labor. I knew it was the real thing because I broke my water when I was taking a nap. "

With labor, contractions occur every 10 minutes or less, and the cramping in your abdomen is progressively more severe. If you are less than 37 weeks (more than three weeks before your due date), please call your doctor if you feel these pains regularly – say, more than every 30 minutes. Also, if you do not feel right about the abdominal pain that you are experiencing, make the call.

When you are within three weeks of your due date, the baby is ready for labor. You are in labor when contractions are three to five minutes apart, last 45 to 60 seconds and are so uncomfortable that you have a hard time speaking through them. Speak with your doctor at one of your visits near the end of pregnancy to determine when and whom you should call when labor begins. As a general rule, if this is your first baby and you live within 30 minutes of the hospital, you should wait until this contraction pattern has occurred for two hours. The chance your contractions will stop at that point is very slim. If this is not your first baby, you should wait only 30 minutes to one hour. Regardless, if you feel pressure in your vaginal area, call immediately.

In addition to regular contractions, other indications for which you should call your physician or midwife include vaginal bleeding of any type or a loss of fluid from the vagina. You may lose a large volume of amniotic fluid all at once, or a small amount over time. If you notice you are soaking a mini-pad every 30 minutes, you need to call your doctor.

When your water breaks and there are no contractions, your physician may ask you to wait at home before coming to the hospital, or he or she may ask you to come in right away. If you have a history of herpes, go immediately to the hospital for an evaluation of active infection. If you have an active infection, a cesarean section is performed as soon as possible after rupture of the membranes to minimize the risk of transmission of herpes to the baby. If you do not have a history of herpes, your physician or midwife will discuss his or her plans with you.

Your physician's concern over your staying at home is that the baby may lie on the umbilical cord since the cushion of amniotic fluid is gone. If this problem actually occurs, the blood supply to the baby is compromised. This situation is extremely unlikely, and therefore it is not unreasonable for your doctor to allow you to wait a few hours at home before coming into the hospital. I ask my patients to come in for a brief evaluation of the baby. If the baby is fine, I have you walk about freely, waiting for labor to start. For the majority of women, labor will start within 12 hours of rupture of the membranes. If it does not, then I stimulate the start of labor with medication called oxytocin (Pitocin), which stimulates the uterine muscles to contract. Occasionally, induction of labor with Pitocin is started as soon as you rupture your membranes, when or if your cervix is already opening.

FALSE LABOR: PAIN WITHOUT GAIN

If you experience false labor, you will not call it false at all. The pain and frequency of contractions are the same with false labor as with true labor. The only way to differentiate the two is to see if your cervix changes over a few hours. If thinning or dilation is occurring, you are in labor. If there is no change of the cervix, you are in false labor. The contractions hurt, but there is no force generated within the uterus. A comparison is a muscle cramp: your leg hurts, but the leg does not move. While false labor is like leg cramps, true labor is like running a marathon.

When Labor Begins too Early
SOONER IS NOT BETTER

If labor occurs earlier than three weeks before your due date, it is pre-term. The risk to the baby increases the farther you are from your due date. With pregnancies earlier than 20 weeks, a delivery is referred to as an abortion or miscarriage. Between 20 and 23 weeks, the baby has no chance for survival. From 24 to 28 weeks, there is a 10- to 30-percent chance of survival, with a 70- to 90-percent chance the baby will have permanent brain damage. Babies born between 28 to 32 weeks have an 80-percent chance of survival and a 90-percent chance of having normal brain development. Beyond 32 weeks, there is more than a 90-percent chance of survival and a 98-percent chance the baby will be born without problems.

> " Preterm labor is definitely scary because they're giving you statistics about what would happen if the baby were to be born. So you're worrying about that and at the same time trying to relax to get the contractions over with."

The main problem with prematurity is the lack of fetal lung development. The lungs develop between 34 and 36 weeks gestation, which is why delivery at an earlier stage is so dangerous. Without mature lungs, the baby does not have the strength to open his airways. With maturity, the lung cells produce surfactant, an oil that coats the small air sacs of the lungs. When the surfactant is present, less effort is needed to inflate the sacs, making breathing possible. A premature baby cannot open air sacs that are void of surfactant, so preemies need to be on a ventilator, which forces air into the lungs. To accelerate the maturation process during pre-term labor, you are given a steroid called betamethasone; if you have already delivered prematurely, your baby is given the steroid. Betamethasone stimulates the lung cells to release surfactant into the airway sacs earlier than normal, allowing your baby to breathe with much less effort.

Immature lungs are not a premature baby's only problem. Babies born before 30 weeks also have an increased risk of bleeding within the brain, which causes seizures and brain damage. Further, the baby's intestinal tract is too immature to absorb food at this stage; the baby must be fed through a vein in the umbilical cord.

TRYING TO PUT ON THE BRAKES

When you understand the gravity of premature birth, you see why more aggressive measures are taken to stop labor the more premature the pregnancy. The initial treatment is to hydrate and sedate. Dehydration is a major cause of pre-term labor, and the combination of hydration and sedation is effective at stopping contractions. You are asked to drink eight cups of water or are given fluids in the hospital through an intravenous line, for hydration. For sedation, you are given morphine or Demerol through the IV or as an injection.

If you continue to have contractions and are 34 to 36 weeks pregnant, an amniocentesis is done to determine if the baby's lungs are mature. If the tests show the lungs are not mature, you are given steroids to hasten maturation. Further, if the lungs are not mature, or you are earlier than 34 weeks, additional medication is used to stop the labor; terbutaline (Brethine) is given as a tablet, or intramuscular injection, or through the IV. Terbutaline binds to receptors in the uterus to prevent contractions. If terbutaline controls the contractions while you are in the hospital, you are sent home and instructed to take the medicine every four to six hours. While at home, you should be on bed rest as much as possible, remain well hydrated by drinking six to eight glasses of water per day, and avoid heavy lifting. Terbutaline causes your heart to race, and you may feel jittery. These side effects decline once you have been

> " I had four weeks of bedrest with the first pregnancy, six weeks for the second, and five weeks with this one. For the first two, I went off the terbutaline and the bedrest at 36 weeks, and they were born at 37 weeks. I'm on bedrest right now with the third one. I'm only 32 weeks. The term they use with me is 'irritable uterus.' "

on the medication for a week. If terbutaline does not work, magnesium sulfate is given through the IV, and it should stop the contractions.

If you still have contractions after receiving these treatments, there is a strong chance you will deliver. In this situation, there is the possibility an infection has developed within the amniotic fluid, and antibiotics will only work once the contents of the uterus are removed. This, unfortunately, could result in the delivery of a very premature baby. In order to determine which bacteria caused the infection, amniocentesis is done, and the amniotic fluid is cultured. Without delivery, both you and your baby could become seriously ill.

WAYS TO AVOID INTRAUTERINE INFECTIONS

🐾 Get regular prenatal care
🐾 Report any problems with urination, such as pain
🐾 Have any abnormal vaginal discharge evaluated

Labor by the Numbers

As we start to review your delivery, let us first review the normal progression through the three stages of labor. The first stage of labor is from the onset of regular contractions until you are completely dilated: Complete dilation is when your cervix is open 10 centimeters. With a first vaginal birth, the average time for the first stage of labor is 10 hours, but it is normal to take up to 24 hours. If this is your second birth or more, the average time for this stage is 8 hours, with about 18 hours being the upper limit of normal.

STAGE ONE

The first stage is broken into three phases: latent, active dilation and deceleration. The latent phase is from the onset of labor until your cervix is 3 to 4 centimeters dilated. During the latent phase, you can remain at home, sitting in a rocking chair or taking a warm bath or shower to help manage the pain. After two hours of contracting every 4 minutes, with each contraction lasting 45 to 60 seconds, you should go to the hospital. Latent labor represents the most variable and frustrating part of labor. You are having very strong contractions, yet there is little progress compared to the amount of pain. Also, this is the time where you do not have the option of epidural anesthesia.

" Labor was definitely easier – and shorter – the second time around. Also, a lot of the fear was gone because I had been through it before."

TIPS FOR MANAGING EARLY LABOR

🐾 *Take a warm shower*
🐾 *Rock in a rocking chair*
🐾 *Have your partner firmly massage your lower back*
🐾 *Pace*
🐾 *Sit still and focus on an object*

The phase of active dilation is from 3 centimeters to 8 centimeters of dilation. You should progress more rapidly through this phase, dilating 1 to 2 centimeters per hour. You may have an epidural at the start of this part of labor. The deceleration phase is from 8 centimeters to complete dilation, and may take up to three hours. If you wait until this point to ask for the epidural, you may not have enough time to receive one, so do not wait until this point to make your wishes known.

STAGE TWO

The second stage of labor – the stage of pushing – is from complete dilation to the delivery of the baby, and the average time is 33 minutes for the birth of your first baby and 9 minutes for future babies. The upper limit of normal on this stage is two hours for the first baby and 45 minutes for subsequent births. However, if you have an epidural and if the fetal heart monitor shows the baby is doing well, you can safely push for three hours. Pushing for more than three hours is associated with an increased risk of shoulder dystocia, where the baby's head has delivered but the shoulders are stuck behind your pubic bone. This situation is managed by pulling your knees up toward your shoulders and applying pressure above your pubic bone until the shoulders are freed. There is a 2-to-5 percent chance the baby will have nerve damage to the arm after shoulder dystocia.

STAGE THREE

The third stage of labor is from the birth of the baby until the delivery of the placenta, or afterbirth. This stage usually takes from five to 30 minutes. While you hold your newborn, you may feel a second sensation of pressure during the delivery of the placenta. This delivery requires little to no effort on your part. In rare cases, the placenta may not separate from the uterus. Your physician must then manually extract it by passing a hand through the vagina and into the uterus. If you have an epidural, this procedure is only mildly uncomfortable. If you do not have an epidural, you may need to be put under general anesthesia to allow removal of the placenta. In fewer than 1 percent of women, the placenta has grown into the muscle of the uterus, preventing separation. In this situation, a hysterectomy is needed to stop the bleeding. In nearly a decade of delivering babies, only once have I had to perform a hysterectomy for this reason, so please do not focus on this possibility too much. In 98 percent of deliveries, the placenta is delivered without notice; in 1 to 2 percent, manual extraction is needed; and hysterectomy is required in less than 1 in 1,000. This information is included to help you understand the stories you may hear in the press about "unnecessary hysterectomies."

What Happens During Vaginal Delivery

If you progress well through labor, the outcome is the delivery of a healthy baby. I am not able to express in words how special this moment is. Regardless of your religious beliefs, it is hard not to stop and give thanks to God for the miracle of birth.

Delivery is a powerful, exciting time; most of the hard work of childbirth is behind you, and you are almost ready to meet your new little miracle. Let's review the details of the delivery process.

PUSH, PUSH, PUSH!

When you are ready to push, you may be positioned on your back with your hands under your knees, pulling your knees up toward your shoulders. Other positions are lying on your side, squatting while holding onto a squatting bar, or in the knee-chest position – on your knees with your chest and head on a pillow, so that you press back while pushing. Regardless of the position, your goal is to generate as much force as possible to push the baby through your birth canal. In order to generate this force, listen to your labor-and delivery-nurse, who will let you know when your efforts are successful or not.

"DO I HAVE TO HAVE AN EPISIOTOMY?"

With time and effort, the baby's head descends to the opening of the vagina. At this point, the delivery table is prepared for the birth. This is a good time to remind your doctor or midwife if your partner wants to cut the umbilical cord, or if you have a particular preference regarding episiotomies. An episiotomy – an incision in the lower part of your vaginal opening – is done to provide more room for the delivery of the baby. If you do not have an episiotomy, this area

> " *The whole time I was pushing, I was thinking, 'I can't wait to get her out to see what she looks like!' So that's what kept me going the whole time. Then when she comes out, you're just overcome by all that emotion. You're happy, and you're crying... The feeling when they put her on your stomach and you feel her warmth – it's just the neatest feeling in the world."*

> " When the nurse found meconium in the fluid, she explained how things would be different at delivery time. I didn't hold my baby until she had been suctioned and checked out, but because I knew what to expect I wasn't too worried."

of the vagina may tear on its own. Your doctor can repair an episiotomy easier than a tear, and usually there is less pain after healing when compared to a tear. However, your skin may be able to stretch without tearing. Also, cutting an episiotomy may allow the skin to tear even deeper. I hope you understand that your doctor must make a clinical judgment at delivery about whether you need and episiotomy. If your skin is not stretching or if your baby is in distress and needs immediate delivery, your physician will do an episiotomy after numbing the area. With either an episiotomy or laceration, you may hear the degree called out to the nurse. The degree refers to the depth of tearing. A first-degree tear is through the vaginal skin only, second-degree (the most common type) is into the supportive tissue below the skin , a third-degree is into the capsule around the rectal muscle, and a fourth-degree is into the rectum. As your baby's head starts to come past the perineum, your physician or midwife holds one hand on the top of the head to prevent excessive tearing of your skin.

HEAD AND SHOULDERS AND THE REST...

Once the head is out, the baby's nose and mouth are suctioned to prevent the baby from aspirating the mucus during his or her first breath. During the suctioning, you are asked not to push for just a moment. When you push again, you must give as much effort as earlier, as you now need to deliver the baby's shoulders. Once the shoulders are out, the rest of the baby is delivered easily.

Now the baby is outside your body, but still attached to the uterus via the umbilical cord. Some doctors and midwives wait for the umbilical cord to stop pulsating, while others immediately cut the cord. The argument for waiting is that it allows more blood to go from you to the baby. However, there is also blood going from the baby to you, so the true gain for the baby is minimal. There is no general consensus on this issue. The cord is clamped with two clamps one inch apart, and your partner can cut the cord between them. Cutting the cord completes the delivery of your baby, and you can now hold this precious gift in your arms for the first time.

Some Special Circumstances

There are three special situations you should be aware of since they may occur during your labor: the presence of meconium in the amniotic fluid, discovery of a nuchal cord, and delivery with the assistance of a vacuum extractor or forceps.

" Her cord was around her neck and she was not breathing well; she was blue, and she had to be resuscitated. She was fine after just a few minutes. But that was scary."

WHEN THE AMNIOTIC FLUID CONTAINS MECONIUM

Meconium-stained fluid is amniotic fluid in which the baby has had a bowel movement. This bowel movement may occur days or weeks before labor, or during labor. Meconium-stained fluid is present more frequently if you go beyond 41 weeks or if the baby is starting to experience stress. Since the baby breathes this fluid while you are in labor, a tube is placed through the vagina and into the uterus. Fluid is passed through this tube to give the baby a bath while still in your uterus. When the baby's head is delivered, a small tube is passed through its nostrils to get any meconium out of its airway before the first breath is taken. You need to resist the desire to push at this time to allow your doctor or midwife a few seconds to suction this fluid out. When the baby is born, the airway is quickly evaluated, and another attempt to suction this fluid is done. During this evaluation, the pediatric team prevents the baby from taking a deep breath. You do not hear your baby cry immediately in this situation, and that is normal. You will be nervous, but please realize this intervention is normal when there is meconium-stained amniotic fluid. Meconium fluid can damage the baby's lungs, and very rarely – less than 1 in 1,000 cases – results in a baby's death after delivery. This is the reason why so much is done to prevent the fluid from getting into your baby's lungs during the first deep breath.

WHEN THE UMBILICAL CORD LOOPS AROUND YOUR BABY'S NECK

"Nuchal cord" describes when the umbilical cord wraps around the baby's neck. There may be one or more loops of cord around the neck. Upon delivery of the head, your doctor or midwife feels for the presence of a nuchal cord. If a loop is noted, you are asked to not push while the cord is pulled over the baby's head. Occasionally the cord is too tight, and it must be clamped and cut to allow immediate delivery of the baby. In this situation, your partner will not have the opportunity to cut the cord, but the baby's health must come first.

WHEN YOU ARE TOO TIRED TO GO ON

There are times when you need help with your delivery. Like every muscle, the uterus has a limited amount of work it is capable of. Just as in running – where you may be able to ask your legs to carry you through a marathon while someone else can hardly run a mile – if your uterus is too fatigued to continue, you may need the help of vacuum or forceps.

The vacuum is actually a suction cup placed on the baby's head, and your physician gently pulls while you push. You do not have to have an episiotomy to use the vacuum. There is a risk that a laceration of your vaginal side wall could occur; if it does, it is repaired just like an episiotomy or other laceration would be. The vacuum might cause a bruise on the baby's scalp, or very rarely – less than 1 in 1,000 cases – a bruise on the brain.

During labor for some women the top of the baby's head forms a cone shape, conforming to the shape of the birth canal. If the baby has developed a cone head from your pushing, the vacuum cup does not fit and this is the time to use forceps to help you deliver the baby. Forceps are instruments shaped like large salad spoons. They are placed around the baby's head just like the doctor's fingers would be if they were long enough. Forceps allow gentle traction to be applied.

The vacuum and forceps should only be used when you have proven your pelvis is large enough to deliver the baby by getting it low enough in your pelvis. Your doctor or midwife will know this by checking your progress. When used appropriately, vacuum and forceps are equally safe. (Before the 1980s, forceps were used when a baby was too high in a woman's pelvis, sometimes resulting in damage to the baby's face and head. Now that forceps are used only when a baby is low in your pelvis, they are very safe.) The progress of your labor is noted by checking the station of your baby's head in your pelvis. The station is the point in your pelvis that the top of the baby's head has reached. It goes from a minus-3 when the baby's head is high up in your pelvis, to 0 when it is midway, to plus-3 when the head can be seen between the labia. You have proven your pelvis is large enough to deliver your baby when you get the baby to a plus-2 station. Therefore, it is safe to use either the vacuum or forceps when you have brought the baby to a plus-2 station.

Other terms you hear include dilation and effacement. Your cervix dilates, or opens, from 0 to 10 centimeters, at which time you are considered "complete" and ready to push out your baby. Effacement refers to the thickness of the cervix as it is drawn up and out of the way, and is expressed in percentages from 0 (very thick cervix) to 100 (paper-thin cervix).

When Cesarean Delivery Makes Sense

A vaginal birth is the birth method of choice if possible. Your physician or midwife will always try to help you have a vaginal delivery, but a cesarean section can be a lifesaver for many children. A cesarean birth involves delivering your child through an incision in your lower abdomen. With modern anesthesia and the availability of blood products, a cesarean section is very safe. A blood transfusion is needed in less than 1 percent of women with vaginal births and in 2 to 3 percent of women with cesarean sections.

On average, 15 to 25 percent of babies are delivered via cesarean section in the United States, and a national effort is underway to lower the incidence of this procedure. (Midwife practices are the exception; their lower c-section rate is due in part to their management of only low-risk pregnancies.) There are practices with c-section rates below 15 percent that congratulate themselves for years, until reviews find high rates of infant damage occurring. The goal of you and your doctor should be to deliver your baby in the safest way possible. Undue pressure from insurance companies and the general public could prevent a doctor from intervening and performing a cesarean section when it should be done.

WHEN THE BABY IS TURNED

There are several indications for a cesarean section. The first indication is if your baby is in a breech (or bottom-first) position. A vaginal birth of a breech baby is possible if this is not your first delivery, if your doctor is trained in the method and if your pelvic bones are large enough based on the results of a CT scan. If you do not meet all of these criteria, you should deliver by cesarean section. The one exception to this rule is when you have twins, and the first baby delivers vaginally and is larger than the second twin, who is breech. In this situation, a vaginal breech delivery is safe.

WHEN THE BABY IS TOO BIG

When your baby is too large to fit through an average pelvis, you should consider a cesarean section. The risk of vaginal birth of a large baby is that the baby's head comes out, but the shoulders can become stuck. This condition is called shoulder dystocia and may cause serious injury to you and the baby. Do not be alarmed, but know that a shoulder dystocia can be serious. You may need a deep episiotomy, and the baby could have nerve damage in the arm, a broken shoulder or possible brain damage and even death. A 9-pound, 9-ounce baby has a 10-percent chance of experiencing shoulder dystocia during delivery (in a diabetic, the risk is 10 percent with a baby who is 8 pounds, 8 ounces). Therefore, if your baby weighs more than this, a cesarean section is better than a trial of labor. Measuring your fundal height (uterine height), taking ultrasound measurements, and evaluating weight gain all help in estimating the weight of the baby. But the estimate of the baby's weight can be off by as much as a pound, which makes the decision to do a cesarean section based on the baby's weight very difficult at times.

FUNDAL HEIGHT

The height of the uterus from the top of the pubic bone to the top of the uterus, in centimeters. This measurement usually correlates roughly with the number of weeks of your pregnancy. For example, most women have a fundal height of about 30 centimeters at 30 weeks.

WHEN LABOR HITS A WALL

A third indication for cesarean birth is arrest of labor, where the cervix does not dilate over two to three hours of active labor. If you do not dilate, your doctor evaluates the strength of your contractions via palpation of your uterus or by passing a small catheter through your vagina and into the uterus. If the contractions are too weak, you will receive oxytocin (Pitocin) to increase their strength. If you still do not dilate, this means that your baby does not fit in your pelvis, and you need a cesarean section. Also, if you have pushed for two to three hours and are unable to bring the baby down low enough in the pelvis to allow the use of the vacuum or forceps, a cesarean section is needed.

" I was overdue and they worried about the baby, so they induced me. But I never dilated – not much, anyway – so I had a cesarean section."

WHEN YOUR BABY NEEDS HELP

When you are in labor, the baby's heart rate is monitored. If the baby is in distress – as indicated by decelerations of the heartbeat – and your doctor does not feel you will deliver within 30 minutes, a cesarean section is indicated. The long-term risks, such as developmental delays, mental retardation or cerebral palsy, are too great to justify avoiding a cesarean section. Most people think birth trauma is the cause for all babies with cerebral palsy. The truth is that birth-related events only account for 20 percent of these problems; the other 80 percent result from some other problem or exposure that occurred during the prior nine months.

WHEN YOU WANT ANOTHER CESAREAN

The last common indication for cesarean section is your personal desire because you have had one in the past. The risk that your scar from a previous cesarean will open during labor is less than 1 percent. If this occurs, there are warning signs, and a cesarean section can then be done. However, you ultimately should have the right to make this decision without undue financial pressure from insurance carriers.

The Good, the Bad and the Ugly: Postpartum Challenges

One of the most important aspects to prepare for in having a baby is the postpartum period. You need to read books and magazines, talk to other women, and get any available help ready. The more prepared you and your partner are, the more you will enjoy this time of bonding with your newborn.

SLEEPING IN THE HOSPITAL: CAN IT BE DONE?

Immediately after delivery, you will be on an energetic high for about two hours; then you feel tremendous fatigue and need to rest. The nursing staff checks your blood pressure and temperature for the first hour, so resting just after birth would be difficult for you anyway. Ideally, you would then get some sleep and wake refreshed to enjoy some very special quiet time with your newborn. Unfortunately, getting rest at the hospital is frequently an exercise in frustration. Between visits from your friends and family, the hospital staff performs such functions as checking your temperature and pressing on your uterus to make sure it is firm and continues to contract down to near its original size. Middle-of-the-night interruptions are not uncommon, either; someone might stop by at 2 a.m. just to make sure you have enough ice (breast-feeding moms especially can become very thirsty).

Getting home is your best bet for getting rest – unless, of course, you have other children at home. In that case, it is your call!

GETTING BACK TO THE BLEEDING

The bleeding pattern you have for the first month depends on whether or not you breast-feed. If you breast-feed, intermittent episodes of bleeding occur just after you feed the baby. Stimulation from suckling makes the brain release the hormone oxytocin, causing the uterus to contract. This contraction expels any blood that has accumulated, but it also stops the slow continuous bleeding from within the uterus for a short time. Therefore, if you breast-feed you will lose less blood over time, even though you see the blood all come out while you feed your baby. The stimulation of suckling also causes painful uterine cramps, which are worse with each child you have.

NEGOTIATING A "CALL SCHEDULE" WITH YOUR PARTNER

No doubt you have heard stories about the "baby blues." The problem is real. Postpartum blues are a mild form of depression that can occur in the first six weeks after birth. Lack of sleep is the number-one cause. Consequently, the best way to reduce this risk is to make sure you get enough sleep. Try to establish certain hours for sleep that are protected for you and your husband. My wife and I both tried to listen for the baby with our firstborn. As a result, both of us were extremely tired and not a great support for each other. With our second child, we set a routine where I listened for the baby during certain hours. If the baby cried then, I knew I was responsible for taking care of her. When you are not "on call" for the baby, you get much better sleep. If you face the common situation in which your husband is going back to work just a few days after the birth of your baby, eat dinner as soon as your husband arrives home from work. After eating, go to bed and sleep until midnight. From midnight on, you are "on call." This schedule assumes you have the opportunity to get a nap during the day. Never allow people to stay with you during this time unless they clearly understand they are there to work. You must not try to entertain guests during this time. Even neighbors with children may wait a month to come visit, because they know how important your sleep is during this first month.

BEATING THE BLUES

If you have a history of depression, you are at increased risk of having postpartum blues. With such a history, it is imperative that you maintain close contact with your counselor to minimize the impact of this time on your depression.

With postpartum blues or depression, you feel sad and cry easily almost all day. Nearly all new mothers have short episodes like this, but you have a problem if you feel this way all the time. Postpartum depression can get so severe that you are unable to care for yourself, much less the baby. It is very important to make every effort to avoid this condition. If you feel you are heading in that direction, contact your physician immediately and explain your feelings. If your obstetrician makes light of the problem, call your family doctor, a psychiatrist or a psychologist, or find another obstetrician.

> " I have never been so tired in my whole life. People in the childbirth classes should warn you how difficult it is when you come home, and how tired you are. I don't think anybody really stressed that – the post-partum part versus the labor part. "

If you come into the office with postpartum blues, we first explore the severity of the problem and review your history for depression. If you have had depression, you are sent to your psychiatrist for counseling and treatment. If you do not have a history of depression and are still functional, we make a plan together. Your partner is important here, because he needs to understand the importance of making adjustments at home to prevent a mild case of the blues from becoming full-blown depression. You need to have no extra demands on you at home. If there is someone visiting who is not helping, he or she must go back home immediately. Also, if there is someone you feel very comfortable with who can come, call him or her and request help. Your partner must make every effort to be home and available to help as much as possible, even if it means taking a family leave from work for two weeks. The blues are usually gone after a few weeks, and you can move on with enjoying your baby. Please know that if you have postpartum blues, it does not mean you do not love your baby. It simply means you have been through too much stress and your body needs time to recover. Mild doses of antidepressants, such as Prozac, are very effective in helping women through this difficult time.

" I had a pretty good recovery. The only thing I didn't anticipate is the difficulty I would have with my first child after my second cesarean section because of my physical ability. I had a child who was still in diapers, and he just needed to be held and changed – things that were physically challenging for me."

CARING FOR INCISIONS

Another postpartum concern is the care of your incision after a cesarean section. You should let your physician know if there is an increase in redness or pain, a discharge that soaks a dressing, or a fever higher than 100.5 degrees Fahrenheit. You should walk every day, but do not try to do strenuous exercise until six weeks postpartum at the earliest. You can walk up stairs, but make sure to hold the handrail. With driving, you can start once you feel you are able to quickly brake. Three weeks is the earliest you should consider driving after a cesarean. You should also shower for the first three weeks, and not take baths.

With an episiotomy or laceration repair, the care of your bottom is important. You can use the Epifoam spray you received at the hospital to help alleviate the discomfort. You can shower to get clean, but then soak your bottom in a tub one-third full of warm water (with two tablespoons of Epsom salts) for ten minutes, twice a day for one week.

GOING BACK FOR A CHECKUP

Your postpartum checkup is done four to six weeks after delivery. During this visit, you have a pelvic exam to make sure your perineum is healing well. During this visit you should get on the best form of contraception available based on your plans for the future. At this visit, women commonly express surprise at how messy the last month has been. You will likely have a bloody discharge of some sort for the entire month, and little time to care for yourself. This is normal. The other surprise is that the pelvic exam done at your postpartum visit is not as uncomfortable as feared. These details to help you prepare for what you may experience.

HAVING SEX AFTER CHILDBIRTH

After the postpartum visit, you are free to resume intercourse. You and your partner must decide the best time to first make love after you have given birth. Speak with your partner about this issue. You may feel so tired and washed out from caring for the baby that you do not have any sexual desire. If that is the case, please make it clear to your partner that you love him dearly, but need some time to regain your sex drive. When you do have intercourse, make sure you communicate about any soreness you have. Pain is most common if you have had an episiotomy or laceration repair. The suture material does not dissolve for two to three months postpartum, so go slow and be gentle. If your partner is on his back, with you in the superior position, you can control the depth, speed and direction of intercourse and minimize the discomfort.

TIPS FOR RESUMING INTERCOURSE

- 🦂 *Communicate with your partner about what feels good or bad*
- 🦂 *Avoid deep penetration or pressure on the episiotomy site*
- 🦂 *Avoid male-superior positions for the same reason*
- 🦂 *Use lubricants*
- 🦂 *Take it slow*
- 🦂 *Keep a sense of humor*

MAKING TIME FOR EACH OTHER

The last issue to discuss is one of the most important, and that is the relationship between you and your partner. There is nothing more important for your newborn than to make sure you and your partner stay happy. Remember this point when you have to decide if you should leave your newborn for a few hours to allow you some personal time as a couple. It does not matter if the time is used to see a movie, take a walk or make love. You must find time to take care of yourself, your relationship with your partner and then your child. In reality, you spend the majority of time in the reverse order, but it is a mistake to neglect yourself or your partner.

Conclusion

The birth of your child is one of the greatest events that will happen to you and your partner. The information in this chapter is intended to help you understand the course you can expect with a vaginal delivery or with a cesarean section. By reducing the stress from the unknown, we hope to increase your ability to focus more on the special bond that starts in the first few minutes after birth. We wish you all the best during this special time.

> " I was emotional about going from being a couple to having a baby in the house – having a little stranger in the house! That was hard because I really missed that couple closeness. In the first few weeks, I felt we'd never be close again, that the baby would always be very demanding and that we would never be a couple again. But the second time, that wasn't an issue anymore."

Resources
Additional Reading

- **Essential Exercises for the Childbearing Year,** *Elizabeth Noble,* Houghton Mifflin, 1988.

- **Conception, Pregnancy and Birth,** *Dr. Miriam Stoppard,* Dorling-Kindersley, 1993.

- **A Good Birth, A Safe Birth: Choosing and Having the Childbirth Experience You Want,** *Diana Korte and Roberta Scaer,* Harvard Common Press, 1992.

- **Mothering the Mother: How a Doula Can Help You Have a Shorter, Easier and Healthier Birth,** *Marshall Klaus, John Kennell and Phyllis Klaus,* Addison-Wesley, 1993.

- **Having Your Baby with a Nurse-Midwife: Everything You Need to Know to Make an Informed Decision,** *Sandra Jacobs and the American College of Nurse-Midwives,* Hyperion, 1993.

- **The Nursing Mother's Companion,** *Kathleen Huggins,* Harvard Common Press, 1995.

- **After the Baby's Birth: A Woman's Way to Wellness: A Complete Guide for Postpartum Women,** *Robin Lim,* Celestial Arts, 1991.

- **Is There Sex after Childbirth?** *Juliet Rix,* Thorsons, 1995.

Organizations

- **La Leche League International, Inc.**
  P.O. Box 4079
  Schaumburg, IL 60168-4079
  (847) 519-7730
  (800) LALECHE
  http://www.lalecheleague.org/

- **Lamaze International**
  1200 19ᵗʰ Street N.W., Suite 300
  Washington, DC 20036-2422
  (800) 368-4404
  E-mail: lamaze@dc.sba.com
  http://www.lamaze-childbirth.com
- **American College of Obstetricians and Gynecologists**
  409 12ᵗʰ Street, S.W.
  P.O. Box 96920
  Washington, DC 20090-6920
  http://www.acog.com/
- **American Academy of Husband-Coached Childbirth**
  Box 5224
  Sherman Oaks, CA 91413-5224
  http://www.bradleybirth.com

Internet Sites

- **http://www.noah.cuny.edu/pregnancy/march_of_dimes/birth/csection.html**
  NOAH (New York Online Access to Health) helps you understand cesarean section – how the procedure is done, what the risks are, what emotional issues surround the procedure, and what you should know about vaginal birth after cesarean.

- **http://www.efn.org/~djz/birth/MT/index.html**
  Midwifery Today, Inc., educations you about midwifery and offers articles on such subjects as breast-feeding and education.

- **http://pregnancy.miningco.com/library/weekly/aa100697.htm**
  This article from the Mining Company compiles many helpful suggestions on how to support a woman during labor.

- **http://www.parentsplace.com/genobject.cgi/readroom/
  pregnant.html**
  *At the ParentsPlace.com Pregnancy and Birth Center, you can "Ask
  the Midwife," read hundreds of birth stories, explore dozens of pregnancy resources and fact sheets, and otherwise immerse yourself in the
  mysteries of childbirth and parenthood.*

- **http://www.parenthoodweb.com/parent_cfmfiles/pregnancy-
  labor.cfm**
  *"Your one-stop shop for everything related to pregnancy and labor"
  features information on vaginal birth after cesarean, natural labor
  techniques, midwives, coaching and comfort during pregnancy.*

CHAPTER SIXTEEN

PAIN MANAGEMENT IN LABOR

Making An Informed Decision

sk any woman preparing for childbirth what her biggest fear is, and you will probably hear variations on the same theme: It's going to hurt! True, only the rare new mother talks about her birth experience without mentioning some discomfort, but few other pains have such a sweet reward – a new life. Like parenthood that follows, labor and delivery are like a journey into the great unknown. Although you cannot be sure in advance how strenuous the journey will be, the good news is that help is available to lighten your load along the way.

The goal of this chapter is to discuss pain management and anesthetic options when you deliver your baby in a hospital under the care of an obstetrician, family physician or midwife with an anesthesiologist. By gathering information from knowledgeable sources, you can reduce the stress often associated with labor. Talking to friends and neighbors is a good way to gain insight, but you also may gain some incorrect information. Reading books such as this one and discussing the subject with qualified health-care personnel are better. Your sense of control, confidence and comfort will grow as you explore your options and become familiar with the safety nets that are in place. As you acquaint yourself with what is available to help you cope with the pain of labor and delivery, it is also important to remain flexible in this ever-changing environment.

Strong opinions abound regarding the management of pain during labor and delivery. Most of the complaints about the pain-relief therapies available are that they make the natural process of childbirth too medical. Your team wants to help make the birth of your child a safe and rewarding experience for you. If that means you want to experience as little pain as possible, so be it. If that means you prefer to use natural methods such as massage, motion and relaxation techniques, that is fine as well. Your physicians or nursing team should not be resistant to any of these possibilities or some combination thereof. The call is yours. Every woman's experience with labor and delivery is different; furthermore, you are not guaranteed the same labor and delivery with your second or third child as you had with your first. And every woman's threshold for pain is her own. What was right for your neighbor, friend, sister or mother may not be right for you, and that person's birth story should not be all you consider when gathering information about pain-relief options for labor and delivery. Nor should your partner's opinion be the only one that decides the matter. The most important opinion is the one you form after discussing the subject with your obstetrician, anesthesiologist, labor-and-delivery nurse and other respected health care personnel and support systems. After all, you are the one giving birth.

" Never say never – about pain medicine for labor or anything else you encounter as a new parent. That's my advice."

You should speak with your physician or midwife during your prenatal visits to develop an idea of your expectations and desires *before* you go into labor. Some women want to minimize the discomfort associated with childbirth, while others want to experience every contraction. Both of these endpoints are perfectly normal, and fortunately, with today's medications and techniques, obtaining the desired result is almost always possible. It is very important that you clearly communicate your desires to the health-care personnel involved with your delivery so they can meet your expectations during this very important event.

Before discussing the medical options for pain control, let us review the non-medical, methods of managing pain in labor.

How to Manage Pain Without Medication

While 90 percent of women in labor take advantage of one or more of the medical methods of pain control, the other 10 percent manage the pain without medication. Even if you plan to have an epidural or IV medication when in active labor, these non-medical pain management options can be useful for you during early labor.

Three criteria must be met if you are to manage labor pain successfully without drugs: you must be motivated, your support person must be educated, and you must know how to distract the brain from the pain.

KNOW YOUR PAIN THRESHOLD

The most important thing is for you to be motivated and educated before labor starts, and very focused and confident through labor. You know your level of commitment to having natural childbirth and your pain tolerance outside of labor. If these levels are high, you are a great candidate for non-medical pain management. If these levels are low, strongly consider having an epidural for active labor. Please do not let someone else make the decision for you to

" I hoped not to have to use any drugs, but I ended up having an epidural. At first, I felt like I had failed. But then I realized I was doing it all natural but with a little help from technology."

deliver without medication, as you then may experience added stress during labor or disappointment in yourself if you later decide to have an epidural. Another option is to try non-medical techniques, accepting that an epidural is a valid option with active labor.

ENLIST SUPPORTIVE HELPERS

For non-medical pain management to be successful, you must also have one or more people committed to giving you active support. Your support person needs to be well educated on the process of labor and how to help you through the pain. He or she has to keep you focused, allow you to vent and constantly attend to your needs. This person makes or breaks the success of this process. A nurse-midwife, a doula, a motivated labor-and-delivery nurse or a well-educated partner can serve this role for you. Most commonly, a team of several of the above would be present.

DISTRACT YOUR BRAIN WITH MASSAGE, MOTION & RELAXATION

The brain receives pain signals from your uterus through nerve fibers that come from the back wall of the uterus and travel through your lower back, up the spine and into the brain. When you experience pain, your brain releases endorphins, a natural form of morphine. These endorphins dull pain naturally. With time, your perception of pain decreases from the release of your natural endorphins.

> " I got a lot of relief during early labor in the shower. When I stood under the warm water during a contraction, the pain seemed to melt away. I only got out when I had used up all the hot water."

In order to dull the pain from uterine contractions as it travels into the spine at your lower back, your partner can actively rub the small of your back during contractions. Other methods include placing a warm compress or sitting in a hot tub with a jet on this same area.

Distracting your brain helps you tolerate the pain of labor. Many hospitals and obstetrics groups offer prepared childbirth classes where you can learn and practice visualization, controlled breathing and other relaxation techniques. Another resource is Lamaze International, an organization that trains childbirth educators (see the Resources list at the end of the chapter for more information). During labor, you can rock in a rocking chair, pace freely in the room or assume any position you desire to decrease the pain (getting on your knees with your head resting on the bed is common). By staying focused and "in control," you keep your body relaxed. This state of relaxation is critical to maintaining good pain control. If you find yourself tensing up during contractions, you note increased pain. Work on relaxation to avoid tension, such as contracting one leg muscle while you take in a deep breath and relaxing it as you exhale.

Do this with any part of your body, and as you relax you find the contractions are more tolerable.

While these methods are useful to everyone for the management of early labor, many women know going into childbirth that they want medical assistance with the pain of active labor. The remainder of this chapter is devoted to educating you about the medical team that cares for you and the options they have available to offer during labor.

Who Is the Anesthesiologist?

Many people are unfamiliar with the identity and the role of the anesthesiologist, for good reasons. Anesthesiologists are hospital-based physicians, and if you have surgery you typically rely on your surgeon to choose the hospital and services instead of choosing an anesthesiologist yourself. Additionally, you are usually rendered unconscious shortly after meeting the anesthesiologist and hearing about the anesthetic plan. You may not be aware of the expertise or vigilance used for administering a safe anesthetic, the anesthesiologist's broad scope of duties and responsibilities, or the amount of training required to practice this specialty.

An anesthesiologist is a physician who has completed medical school and trained an additional four years as a resident in anesthesiology at a teaching hospital. Following residency, he or she enters practice as a board-eligible anesthesiologist. After passing a written and oral exam, he or she is board-certified.

The anesthesiologist acts as a consultant during labor and delivery, assessing your condition and recommending a plan for managing your discomfort in the safest possible manner – which usually involves placing an epidural. If any special circumstances are present, the obstetrician and anesthesiologist discuss the various options with you, and we all agree on a plan tailored to your needs. An anesthesiologist is not called upon for everyone in labor, and you are usually in established labor before one is summoned. A close relationship develops between the members of the delivery team; although the anesthesiologist is not officially consulted until labor is established, he or she generally anticipates the needs of the labor floor by keeping in close contact.

When Labor Has Begun

After your physician or midwife has determined that labor has begun, you undergo an initial assessment on the labor and delivery floor. During this time, your heart rate and blood pressure are measured. A nurse also asks general questions regarding your health. Several items are very important for the anesthesiologist to know, such as allergies to medications or Betadine (iodine) solutions, prior significant medical problems, and a personal or family history of difficulties with anesthesia. Keep your answers complete and concise to help your delivery team provide the best care possible. To prepare yourself to answer these questions, make a list of your medications, allergies, major health problems and prior hospitalizations before labor begins.

WHEN YOU ARE CONSIDERING AN EPIDURAL

If you are considering an epidural, an intravenous catheter, better know as an IV, is also started. An IV catheter provides access to the bloodstream, allowing injection of medications and providing a port for the administration of intravenous fluids.

Before an IV is placed, a tourniquet is wrapped around your arm to cause the vein to "stand up" or dilate. The soft, flexible IV catheter is on a small needle that is introduced into a vein; the catheter is advanced and left in place, while the needle is removed and discarded. Some people fear an IV because they think it involves leaving a needle in their hands. Please note that the rigid needle allows for the placement of the catheter but does not stay in your hand. You need not be afraid to move your hand after the IV is in place. Starting the IV is an important and initial step in pain management and is an important safety net for the anesthesiologist. In the rare event that there is any type of emergency, medicines will be given through the IV to quickly correct the problem.

WHEN YOU DO NOT WANT AN EPIDURAL

Even if you are not planning to have an epidural, most physicians prefer that you at least allow an IV to be inserted and capped off so that you are prepared for any emergency that may occur. Many midwives do not require the IV, and it is this sort of difference that makes many people see the midwife as more natural in her approach to labor. In a way this view is correct, but remember that physicians are trained to care for women in both low- and high-risk pregnancies, and it is the physician's nature to be as prepared as possible. When an emergency occurs, every minute should be focused on the health of you and the baby, not on getting an IV started. Because your physician has seen high-risk deliveries where the life of the baby or mother becomes threatened very quickly, the physician tends to want to be extra careful and prepared. IVs are not inserted in an attempt to take the control of labor away from you, but to satisfy an inherent need most physicians have from many years of experience.

What You Should Know About Intravenous Medication

A simple and common method of pain control during labor involves injecting opioids into the IV catheter. Intravenous pain medications are often the only medications that are needed or desired for the pain of labor. The goal with IV medication is to remove the worst of the pain, to lower the peaks of each contraction. You still feel the contractions, but they are not as intense as before.

HOW THE MEDICINE WORKS

These standard pain medicines circulate through the blood vessels, cross the placenta and distribute through you and your baby. Opioids – frequently referred to as narcotics – change the way your brain interprets the signals coming from the uterus and vagina so that the pain is more tolerable. Over the years, several opioids have been used. The safest and most commonly used are meperidine (Demerol) and butorphanol (Stadol).

WHEN IT IS GIVEN

Intravenous medication is best given during active labor. If you get medication too early, your labor may stop. When you are contracting regularly (at least every five minutes) and your cervix is 3 to 4 centimeters dilated, you are in active labor and these medications should not stop labor. Occasionally, if your pain is severe, we give medicine through the IV early, even though we know it may slow your labor. Once started, the IV medication is given every one to two hours.

THE PROS AND CONS

The advantages of intravenous pain medications are that they are safe, they are simple to administer, they work quickly, and in low to moderate doses, they provide excellent pain relief for mild to moderate pain. A disadvantage is that potentially harmful side effects occur with larger doses. Opioids can slow your breathing, cause excessive sleepiness and decrease blood pressure in you and the baby. If the medication is given just prior to delivery, which can happen if you proceed very rapidly through labor, the baby may not breathe strongly immediately after birth. When this occurs, your physician, midwife or the nursery team ventilates the baby to give him or her oxygen. Your newborn also receives the medication Narcan, which quickly reverses the effects of the narcotic.

" One woman I know said the drugs she got during delivery made her feel as if she had drunk a six-pack of beer in five minutes. That image sticks with me."

Another disadvantage of the IV medication compared to epidurals or "natural," unmedicated childbirth is the way these medications make you feel – drugged-up and not very alert. We have seen women who were controlling their pain well with natural methods, lose the ability to focus once they received IV pain medication. At that point they lose control of the pain as well. After delivery, if you are on narcotics with labor, you are less able to focus and bond with your newborn. For these reasons, IV pain medication is not the form of pain relief most suggested by health-care providers, but this option is available if you are not able to have an epidural. (You may not be able to have an epidural if there is not someone at your hospital trained to place and manage the epidural, or if you have a spinal defect or low platelet count. You should know whether an epidural is an option before labor begins in most cases.)

HOW MUCH DOES IT COST?

One issue to consider when planning for your labor-pain management is the cost involved. Cost may not be a major issue if you have insurance, but if you do not, then the cost is a factor. The cost for having IV medication (Stadol or Demerol) ranges from $20 to $300, depending on how much your hospital charges and how many doses you require. If you have a short labor, there is minimal cost involved with IV medication. If you have an epidural, the cost is from $1,000 to $2,500. That amount includes the hospital charges for supplies, and fees for the anesthesiologist to place the catheter and monitor it throughout labor. These costs can vary greatly from hospital to hospital, and there is nothing wrong with calling local hospitals to find which ones are reasonable before deciding where to go.

What You Should Know About
Epidural Analgesia

HOW IT WORKS

Epidurals work differently than IV pain medications and are the primary tool the anesthesiologist can offer you in labor. Medicine is injected through your lower back, into the epidural space instead of into the IV catheter. The epidural space is an area outside the thick fibrous sac, the dura, that contains the spinal cord and the cerebrospinal fluid in which the cord floats. Because medicine is placed in this enclosed space and not in the IV catheter, it does not cross the placenta and reach your baby to the same degree that IV medications do. The medicine is slowly absorbed into the bloodstream, but the amount of medication in the blood is generally lower than when pain medicines are given directly through the IV.

The medicine used with an epidural is typically a combination of a local anesthetic such as Xylocaine and a narcotic, although, depending on the situation, one or the other can be used alone. The local anesthetic or "numbing medicine" is similar to what dentists use to numb your mouth before filling a cavity. This medicine works by blocking the nerve impulse as it travels up the nerves from the uterus and vagina to the spinal cord. The effect of the epidural is referred to as a "block" because the medicine blocks the movement of the nerve impulse. If the nerve impulse is stopped in the spinal cord and not received by the brain, then it is not experienced as pain. There are several types and concentrations of local anesthetics, and by choosing the appropriate type, the anesthesiologist can control the duration and strength of the block. The opioid works by changing the sensitivity of the spinal cord, thereby dulling the sensations that are experienced.

When an epidural is placed, it not only blocks the pain fibers that supply the vagina and uterus, but it also blocks the nerves that control the size of the large blood vessels in the legs and pelvis, which in turn affects your blood pressure. A stronger or more "dense" block tends to lower the blood pressure more than a weak block. You receive additional fluids through the IV before getting the epidural to counteract this phenomenon. In the rare case when these measures are not totally effective, then additional fluids or medicines are administered by the anesthesiologist, and your blood pressure quickly returns to normal.

The effects of an epidural can be contradictory and need to be balanced during labor. On one hand, the epidural provides pain relief, but increased pain relief is accompanied by increasing weakness that prevents you from effectively pushing the baby out of your vaginal vault. The anesthesiologist can render you completely pain-free at any time during labor, but this is not always the goal or in the best interest of you or the baby. The anesthesiologist and obstetrician work together to minimize pain while maximizing the progression of labor. Fortunately, both goals can be achieved in almost all cases.

WHEN IT IS GIVEN

Many expectant mothers want to know how early an epidural can be placed after the start of labor. The decision is usually made with input from the obstetrician, the anesthesiologist, the nurse providing care, and most importantly, you, the woman in labor. Factors that are considered include the stage of labor, your pre-existing medical conditions, and the preferences and prior experience of the healthcare personnel involved with your case.

In general terms, it is best to place the epidural when the cervix has dilated to at least 4 centimeters, and is no more than 8 centimeters. If a standard epidural is placed before 3 centimeters, it may significantly slow down the progression of labor. If placed after 8 centimeters of dilatation, the epidural may impede your ability to push because of the weakness it produces just after being placed. These are general rules, and each obstetrician has his or her own guidelines as to when to consult the anesthesiologist. For laboring women who are dilated less than 3 centimeters and greater than 8 or 9 centimeters, the alternative techniques discussed below are generally employed.

WHEN AN EPIDURAL IS NOT THE RIGHT CHOICE

There are some situations where it is not in your best interest to have an epidural. If you have a bleeding disorder or a skin infection of the lower back where the needle is placed, if you are experiencing extremely low blood pressure from bleeding or dehydration, or if you do not want an epidural, then you are not a

" When I arrived at the hospital, I was so afraid I would be sent home. My husband says my face just glowed when the doctor told me I was 4 centimeters! I knew I could stay, and I knew that I could have an epidural whenever I asked for one."

candidate for this type of pain relief. Many pregnant women ask if their usual low blood pressure will disallow the use of an epidural. Even if your blood pressure is normally low, it is usually acceptable to use an epidural. The epidural normally lowers your blood pressure by a small percentage, and you and the baby generally tolerate this small change without any problem.

HOW THE EPIDURAL CATHETER IS INSERTED

The placement of an epidural is a source of anxiety and fear for some expectant mothers, and these feelings are magnified by inaccurate or inadequate information. You will worry less if you gain insight into the procedure.

The goal is to place the medicine into the epidural space. For placement of the epidural, you are positioned either sitting or lying on your side, and usually the entire process takes five to 10 minutes and is well-tolerated. Your nurse helps you curve your back in order to widen the area between the vertebrae, or backbones of your lower back. In the sitting position, you are asked to curve your back like "a mad cat" or to slump to help you imagine the correct position. If you are lying on your side, you assume a fetal position by curling around the baby.

Remember that contractions continue during placement. Despite the contractions, concentrate on being as still as possible. It is important to be very still, because this helps the anesthesiologist place the epidural quickly and correctly – *not* because a slip of the needle will result in paralysis or significant nerve damage. The spinal cord ends about two-thirds of the way down your back, whereas the bony part of your spine continues to your hipbones. An epidural is placed *below* the end of the spinal cord, so damage to the spinal cord by the epidural needle is highly unlikely.

Here is what is going on "behind your back" when you are receiving that long-awaited epidural. Your back is swabbed with an antiseptic solution (Betadine) and is draped with a sterile cloth to keep it free of germs. A dime-sized area is "frozen" using a local anesthetic such as lidocaine. This sensation is usually described as a "bee-sting" that lasts for a few seconds. After your skin is numb, the main feeling you have is a sensation of pressure. Then the epidural needle is advanced, and once the epidural space is located, local anesthetic similar to lidocaine is administered through the needle to test the placement of the needle. As the medicine is injected, you may feel some generalized pressure in your lower back that will last a few seconds.

" Sitting still during those contractions was really hard for me, but delivering without an epidural would have been even harder."

Following this "test dose," the nurse wraps an automated blood-pressure cuff around your arm. The cuff remains in place as long as you have the epidural, taking frequent blood-pressure readings that are compared to your normal values. A drop in blood pressure is an important safety issue, so blood-pressure measurements are taken very frequently for the first 15 minutes. The automatic cuff "senses" the pulsation in your arm and determines your blood pressure, freeing health-care personnel to attend to your other needs. Many women comment that the frequent blood-pressure readings are the most uncomfortable part of the entire process, as the cuff squeezes your arm and produces mild discomfort in your hand. To minimize this sensation, hold your arm very still to allow the readings to be made as quickly and infrequently as possible.

Once the soft plastic epidural catheter is advanced through the canal of the epidural needle, the needle is removed and discarded. Occasionally, a woman feels a momentary "funny bone" sensation shoot down one leg or the other as the catheter is advanced through the needle. This sensation is not so uncomfortable as it is surprising if you are not warned in advance. Some women have the impression that the epidural needle remains in the back for the duration of labor, but this is *not* the case. Only the plastic catheter – a soft, flexible tube 1/20 of an inch in diameter – remains. The epidural catheter allows for administration of medicine as either a continuous infusion or as a larger "top-up" dose as needed – determined by the progress of your labor and level of your discomfort. The catheter allows the anesthesiologist to give medicine for the entire length of labor without having to have another catheter placed. The catheter is taped to your back with special glue so the tube will not come out. After the administration of a conventional epidural, you are unable to walk or get out of bed, because your legs might be weak and you could fall.

After delivery, removing the catheter is a very simple process of taking off the tape and gently pulling the catheter out of the epidural space. With the exception of removing the tape (which feels like the removal of a very long adhesive bandage), "pulling" the catheter is essentially painless and is accomplished quickly and easily. The labor-and-delivery nurse removes the catheter just after your delivery.

HOW WELL IT WORKS

The epidural does not provide immediate relief, but you may have significant relief in as soon as five minutes. Within 10 to 15 minutes, you perceive a gradual decrease in the strength and duration of your contractions. Fifteen to 20 minutes after catheter insertion, the contractions feel like "deep pressure" sensations, even though the actual strength of the contractions has not decreased.

In the past, higher concentrations of local anesthetics were used, producing significant lower-leg weakness and numbness. With the introduction of lower concentrations of medicine, you feel slight tingling sensations in your legs but can move your feet and knees without difficulty. The lack of numbness may be surprising if you have not had an epidural in several years. As techniques have advanced, the trend has been to use lower concentrations of local anesthetic – producing less weakness while maintaining adequate pain relief.

To maintain pain relief throughout labor, the epidural catheter is connected to a special pump, and a low concentration of pain medicine and local anesthetic is continuously administered. The local anesthetics include lidocaine, bupivicaine and 2-chloroprocaine, and the pain medicine options include fentanyl, sufentanil, and preservative-free morphine. The pump speed and dose of medicine are adjusted depending on the progression of labor and your comfort level. After you get an epidural, you should rest in preparation for the actual delivery; sleep or spend time with your family while the cervix dilates from 4 to 10 centimeters. If there is a change in your comfort level, the obstetrician or labor-and-delivery nurse calls anesthesia personnel to evaluate the situation. If you are uncomfortable, a "top-up" dose is administered through the catheter. Conversely, if you are too numb or weak, then the pump speed is lowered.

With labor-pain management, it is important to start with a reasonable expectation of the results. The goal with an epidural is to take away the worst of the pain, not to remove all sensations. If labor pain without medication is like climbing Mount Everest, then labor pain with an epidural or IV medication is like walking over rolling hills. If you feel the pain of Everest, please ask your nurse to inform the anesthesiologist.

A doctor trains several years to gain the ability to place an epidural catheter, and all board-eligible and board-certified anesthesiologists are qualified to perform this procedure, as are many obstetricians. Almost all catheters work very well and provide excellent pain relief following this relatively easy and safe procedure. Occasionally, the catheter is difficult to place, moves out of the epidural space or enters a blood vessel, causing the block to be ineffective or gradually wear off after it is established. Rarely, you have pain relief on one side and not the other. You should tell your labor-and-delivery nurse if you feel significantly more pain on one side than the other. This problem is corrected by replacing the catheter, which is usually better tolerated than the initial placement because the insertion site is still numb and you have some degree of pain relief.

" When I had my first child, the epidural was so strong that I couldn't move my legs at all and the only pain I felt was more like a tightness high in my abdomen with each contraction. That was nice, but pushing required some creative visualization on my part. The second time around, I could feel a lot more – including that whole-body urge to push I had heard so much about."

HOW AN EPIDURAL AFFECTS BABY AND YOU

Epidurals have been tested over time and are safe for both baby and mother in labor and delivery. Researchers studying Apgar scores, newborn behavior and blood chemistries have found that these assessments

> " With my first baby, the early stage of labor was extremely long, and I was exhausted. When I finally went to the hospital, the nurse recommended that I get an epidural, get some sleep and have a baby in the morning. That sounded great to me, and that's just what I did."

are not significantly affected by normal epidural analgesia. The major potential effect on the baby comes from changes that can take place with your blood pressure. If your blood pressure drops greatly, your baby gets less blood and oxygen, which can lead to fetal distress. But this scenario is rare, because safety checks and preventative measures are built into the placement of an epidural. Additionally, oxygen, medications and fluids are immediately available to correct this problem quickly.

There are many effects of the epidural on you that have been discussed above. Mild decreases in your blood pressure are normal and are the product of pain relief and changes in the circulation. Low blood pressure also occurs when you lie flat on your back, allowing the weight of the uterus to compress the major blood vessels in the abdomen. To prevent this, you are tilted to one side and supported with a pillow under your hip.

Urination may become difficult following epidural insertion, and a catheter may be used to empty your bladder. Fortunately, the epidural renders insertion of the catheter relatively painless. Other side effects of the epidural include itching and shivering. Itching is a side effect of the narcotic in the epidural, while shivering is thought to be from circulatory and temperature changes associated with the epidural.

HOW AN EPIDURAL AFFECTS LABOR

Many women ask if an epidural will slow or stop labor, making a cesarean section necessary. Answering this question can be very complicated, controversial and difficult. In general terms, the epidural is thought to slow the progression of labor to some degree by slightly decreasing the strength of the uterine contractions, but obviously the benefits outweigh the risks or the procedure would have been abandoned long ago.

Conversely, some studies suggest that an epidural helps speed up labor by decreasing the pain enough to allow you to relax and your cervix to dilate. Many factors come into play, such as the timing of placement, the concentration of local anesthetic, the physician's past experience, and innumerable factors relating to your ability to have a vaginal delivery. These include your height, the size of your pelvic bones, the size of the baby, your weight gain, the presence of diabetes and your prior history of being able to deliver vaginally.

"I had read in some books that advocate unmedicated childbirth that an epidural could affect a baby's ability to nurse. That was not my experience with either of my two children. Both times, the baby latched on and sucked well from the beginning."

WHEN A CESAREAN BECOMES NECESSARY

If delivery by cesarean section is required, the epidural is conveniently used for anesthesia. A stronger concentration of local anesthetic is administered through the catheter, and over several minutes numbness develops from the mid-chest level to the feet. Your legs become numb and very difficult to move. You are able to feel deep pressure sensations, but your ability to feel temperature and sharp pain diminish and then disappear. When you have epidural anesthesia for a cesarean, you are conscious during your baby's delivery and a family member can be in the room to share the experience with you.

WHEN IT IS TOO EARLY OR TOO LATE FOR AN EPIDURAL

If you require pain relief before your cervix has dilated to 3 centimeters, your obstetrician may request a something other than the standard epidural. The **Combined Spinal/Epidural (CSE), or "walking epidural,"** has recently gained popularity. The walking epidural involves the same steps for placing an epidural discussed above, but before local anesthetic or a catheter is placed, a very thin spinal needle is advanced through the epidural needle, and a small amount of narcotic is placed through the spinal needle into the cerebrospinal fluid.

> "I really had the shakes after my baby was born; I couldn't stop shivering for a while. My nurse brought me a blanket from the warmer and wrapped it around my shoulders, and that made me more comfortable."

The spinal needle has a specially designed tip and is so small that it does not produce a spinal headache. This small amount of pain medication has virtually no effect on the baby and will sometimes provide pain relief within two to five minutes. The spinal needle is removed, and the plastic epidural catheter is placed through the needle. Local anesthetic is not yet administered through the catheter. This type of pain management does not slow labor and provides good to excellent pain relief for a variable amount of time. The goal is to provide pain relief until you have dilated to 3 to 4 centimeters, when the usual local anesthetic dose can be administered through the epidural catheter already in place. The advantages of this technique are that you can walk with few restrictions and that the epidural catheter is in place for future use. The disadvantages include variable degrees of pain relief, itching, and the potential for nausea that is associated with this type of pain relief.

If you arrive at the labor-and-delivery floor at 8 to 9 centimeters of dilation, an epidural may not be the best option for pain relief. The anesthesiologist may be able to perform a spinal and place a small amount of local anesthetic, which will very quickly provide good to excellent pain relief for the duration of labor and delivery.

WHEN A SPINAL IS A BETTER CHOICE THAN AN EPIDURAL

If you have an epidural catheter in place during labor and need a cesarean delivery, the epidural is used for anesthesia, as mentioned earlier. If a planned cesarean is necessary, the anesthesiologist may recommend a spinal for your anesthesia.

In the past, a spinal was not the best option because the chance of a spinal headache was high enough to avoid its use. A spinal headache occurs because cerebrospinal fluid leaks from a small puncture made for the spinal. Please remember that with an epidural a spinal headache is very rare, since the needle does not go all the way into the spinal canal where this fluid is, while a spinal needle does. A spinal headache is an intense headache that is much worse when you sit up and is minimal when lying down.

With new developments in spinal needles, these spinal headaches occur only rarely, and performing a cesarean section under spinal anesthesia has become increasingly attractive for several reasons. The spinal is technically easier to perform than an epidural, a fraction of the medicine is used with a spinal, and the incidence of toxic side effects is very rare. Additionally, the spinal is thought to provide a more "dense," or reliable, block.

WHAT CAN GO WRONG WITH AN EPIDURAL

The possibility of a complication exists with all medical procedures, and this fact holds true for pain management during labor and delivery. Fortunately, the probability that you will have a complication is not very great.

Nerve Damage

Perhaps the most prevalent and most erroneous fear is that of being permanently paralyzed by the epidural needle or the medications that are administered through the catheter. As mentioned before, the epidural needle is placed well below the level of the spinal cord, making damage extremely rare. The nerves supplying the legs extend beyond the level of the spinal cord, so it is possible to damage these nerves, but the incidence of nerve damage is very, very low.

There has been much discussion in the anesthesiology literature regarding minor nerve damage following delivery. Minor nerve damage usually refers to small areas of numbness or tingling in various locations on the legs following delivery. When women who have epidurals are compared with those who experience a natural delivery, the incidence of minor nerve damage is about the same. It is thought that this nerve damage may result from the normal stretching of the nerves with hip flexion associated with pushing, or from compression of the nerves as the baby's head descends though the pelvis. Additionally, residual effects of the local anesthetics may temporarily result in minor nerve dysfunction. Fortunately, the vast majority of these problems go away on their own during the first two or three days after delivery. If they persist longer than two or three days, then evaluation by a neurologist may be necessary. Regardless of the severity, it is always a good idea to inform the obstetrician and anesthesiologist so they can evaluate and address the problem promptly.

Placement in a Blood Vessel

If the epidural catheter accidentally enters a blood vessel and local anesthetic is injected into the bloodstream, you can experience dizziness, restlessness, ringing in the ears and seizures. The incidence of this complication has decreased for two reasons. Tests are performed when inserting an epidural catheter to check the placement, and the recent use of weaker concentrations of local anesthetic make this complication less likely than in the past. If it does happen, while waiting for the local to get out of your system, this situation is managed with protection of your airway with intubation if needed (very rare) and support of your blood pressure with IV fluids and medication. This problem usually resolves quickly and without incident.

"I knew something was wrong. I had tingling in my face and I was numb all over, almost unconscious. I was scared for my baby and me."

Inadvertent Spinal

As mentioned earlier, mastering the technique of placing an epidural takes a great deal of time. Occasionally, in about 1 in 300 procedures, the epidural needle is advanced a millimeter too far, and a dural puncture results. In other words, a spinal was performed with an epidural needle, creating a small hole in the dura.

Imagine your spinal column as a water-filled tennis-ball can with several strands of wet noodles hanging from the top. The water is the cerebral spinal fluid; the noodles are the nerve fibers extending from where the spinal cord ended higher in your back, and the plastic of the tennis-ball can is the dura surrounding the spinal column. With an epidural, the catheter is placed just outside this dura. With a spinal, the needle goes through the dura and into the spinal column. If the needle used for an epidural goes through this dura, there is a greater chance of leaking some cerebral spinal fluid. (This fluid is constantly being produced, so that once the small puncture site heals over, the fluid reaccumulates.) If this complication happens, the anesthesiologist has several ways of managing the problem. You are still able to get pain relief, but different concentrations or techniques are used to get the desired results.

A dural puncture can also result in a "spinal headache," which develops over the following 24 hours. This headache, which can be severe at times, is worse when you stand and disappears when you lie down. It is thought to occur because cerebrospinal fluid leaks out of the hole in the dura, leading to mild traction on the structures supporting the brain. A spinal headache can be treated with oral pain medicines, fluids and bed rest. Over one to seven days, the headache goes away as the fluid that leaked is replaced and the hole heals. Administering an epidural blood patch can also treat a spinal headache. The patch is performed by placing another epidural needle and injecting some of your blood through the needle. This procedure is thought to "patch" the hole made by the epidural needle and provides instant relief.

A High Block

If a large amount of local anesthetic gets into the spinal column, a "high block" can occur, resulting in numbness that extends above the level of the chest and is accompanied by low blood pressure and unconsciousness. This complication is not likely with a labor epidural, but when the epidural is used for a cesarean section, the higher concentration of medicine makes this high block a possibility. You are watched very closely by the anesthesia team, which is right there and ready to take care of you and the baby if this complication occurs. The treatment is to support the airway and blood pressure and keep you sedated until the block resolves over two to three hours. In this situation, your partner is asked to step out of the operating room and you are put under general anesthesia, with your airway protected by intubation. With you asleep and your blood pressure stable, the obstetrician proceeds to perform the cesarean section.

Bruising and Soreness

It stands to reason that bruising occurs when the epidural needle is advanced through the skin before reaching the epidural space. Most women experience some soreness at the insertion site for one to three days. You can take oral pain medications if this pain is bothersome. Other causes of lower back pain following delivery include spasm of the muscles that support the spine and strain of the ligaments in the lower back from labor.

Conclusion

The sophistication, effectiveness and safety of pain-relief methods for the laboring woman have improved greatly during the past decade. New techniques allow the anesthesiologist to tailor your pain relief to meet your expectations with a high degree of safety and accuracy. Although knowledge of the potential complications is necessary before undergoing any medical procedure, you should be mindful of how uncommon these complications are. Ninety percent of women in labor use the epidural or spinal as one of their pain-management options. Many women use the non-medical options successfully as their only form of pain control, while most women use these methods to help with the early labor pain, waiting for the epidural for the remainder of labor. The vast majority of women undergo uncomplicated deliveries with excellent pain control and a high degree of satisfaction using today's anesthetic techniques.

The birth of your baby is one of the most special times in your entire life. Plan ahead and enjoy this experience as much as possible.

Resources
Additional Reading

- **Mothering the Mother: How a Doula Can Help You Have a Shorter, Easier and Healthier Birth,** *Marshall Klaus, John Kennell and Phyllis Klaus,* Addison-Wesley, 1993.

- **Epidurals for Childbirth,** *Anne May,* Oxford University Press, 1994.

- **Childbirth: Your Choices for Managing Pain,** *Gillian Van Hasselt,* Taylor Publishing, 1995.

Organizations

- **Lamaze International**
  1200 19th Street N.W., Suite 300
  Washington, DC 20036-2422
  (800) 368-4404
  E-mail: lamaze@dc.sba.com
  http://www.lamaze-childbirth.com

- **The Society for Obstetric Anesthesia and Perinatology**
  1910 Byrd Avenue, Suite 100
  P.O. Box 11086
  Richmond, VA 23230-0090
  (804) 282-5051
  http://www.soap.org/about.htm

Internet Sites

- **http://www.usnews.com/USNEWS/issue/971110/10birt.htm**
  This report from USNews Online's 1997 Health Guide, titled "High-tech and high-touch remedies for easing the pain of childbirth," highlights the walking epidural and hot tub, and provides historical information on pain relief in labor.

- http://www.anesthesia.org/public/guides/lpain01.html
  *"Pain Relief for Childbirth: An Overview of Obstetrical Anaesthesia,"
  produced by Ottawa General Hospital, answers common questions
  about pain relief for childbirth, and includes photographs of an anesthesiologist simulating the "installation" of an epidural.*

- http://gasnet.med.yale.edu/mirror/asa/NEWSLETTERS/1997/
  09_97/MgmtChildPain_0997.html
  *"Management of Childbirth Pain before Anesthesia," an article from
  the newsletter of the American Society of Anesthesiologists, briefly
  highlights the now questionable methods used to help women cope with
  the pain of labor from ancient times through the 1800s.*

- http://www.obgyn.upenn.edu/History/anesanal.html
  *University of Pennsylvania Health System, celebrating "A Century of
  Obstetrics," looks back at developments in obstetrical anesthesia and
  analgesia, from the chloroform mask and "twilight sleep" to the
  epidural.*

- http://www2.ccf.org/ed/pated/kiosk/hinfo/docs/0209.htm
  *"Pain Relief Options During Childbirth," part of HealthNotes from
  the Cleveland Clinic, includes a diagram of where an epidural catheter
  is placed in the spinal column.*

CHAPTER SEVENTEEN

CARING FOR YOUR BABY

Learning the Ropes of Early Parenthood

a newborn infant is wonderful, fragile and in need of constant care and attention. Whether you are an expectant parent, someone who wants to be pregnant, or a bleary-eyed new mom who is looking for her baby's instruction manual, a little information about baby care can go a long way to reduce your worries about this most exciting time.

Before birth, your baby already knows the sound of your voice and soon after, learns your face and touch. You will learn to distinguish your infant's needs by the sound of his cries, and you will be the one who can comfort your baby better than anyone else. The transition to parenthood is an incredible journey!

The purpose of this chapter is to provide you with the knowledge that makes the transition to parenthood smoother and less stressful for you and your family. The first section covers the prenatal visit and things to consider when choosing a physician for your child. The next section covers the newborn period, including care during the hospital stay and beyond. The final section reviews immunizations and follow-up care.

When our son was one month old, my husband asked me how new parents survive without a physician in the family! This chapter is like a private physician at your fingertips. However, if you are not sure about your newborn's actions, make sure you call your baby's doctor.

How to Choose a Physician for Your Infant

You should try to choose your child's physician long before delivery. This choice is such an important one, because you call on this person in times of illness and good health, when you have questions about various aspects of your child's care. Your trust in your child's physician is crucial when you need help and advice.

I strongly encourage you to make several prenatal appointments to interview physicians in your community who provide care for infants and children. Some practices have a charge for this visit, and others do not. Ask in advance in order to avoid confusion. You should start by considering the insurance plan that will cover the baby, and then see if you must use a doctor from your insurance company's list of preferred providers to obtain the maximum coverage. Talk to neighbors and friends about their choice of a physician and their level of satisfaction. Develop a potential list of physicians, and schedule appointments two months prior to your due date so you are not caught unprepared in the event of an early delivery.

" My pediatrician was very highly recommended by a lot of people. He was terrific. He knew when to be nervous about my son's conditions. He made me feel at ease."

In your community, both pediatricians and family practitioners may provide care to newborns. Pediatricians receive three years of training focused on the care of infants and children. Family practitioners receive training in care of adults and children during their three-year residency, and offer the advantage of providing care to your whole family at one visit.

You learn about your infant's potential physician and staff very quickly just by scheduling an appointment. Is the staff courteous and helpful? Do you receive a prompt appointment? Does the staff provide information about the practice prior to your appointment? Remember that the relationship you develop with your child's physician is an important one, and you should feel comfortable talking with the physician. During this prenatal visit, discuss any medical concerns that have arisen during your pregnancy and medications that your doctor may have prescribed. You should also cover any medical problems that might run in your family, your thoughts about breast- or bottle-feeding, and whether or not you plan to have your baby boy circumcised.

You also should learn whether the doctor is certified by the American Academy of Pediatrics or the American Board of Family Practice. You need to know the hospitals in your area at which your physician sees patients, and when to expect to see the doctor at the hospital after your delivery. Other questions should include: office hours, ways to contact a doctor after hours in the event of an emergency, how to obtain advice during regular office hours, and specifics about the office's financial policy and whether or not they will file insurance claims for you.

" I disliked waiting with a newborn. It seemed to take a lot of time before the doctor would come in and check the baby. If you have to wait more than 30 minutes, it gets very difficult because the baby wants to be fed or is crying and you get anxious and sometimes want to leave the office."

The issue of charging for after-hours calls is a sensitive one. Many groups charge for non-emergency calls after hours. The decision about whether the issue is an emergency may be based on whether your baby has to come into the hospital or the office the next day for an evaluation. If you have had an ongoing problem and postpone your call until evening hours, you have a greater chance of being charged for the call. Evening call is for emergencies, so try to call as early in the day as possible if your child seems to be having a problem. This explanation is not meant to communicate a lack of desire to be there for you in a time of need. The opposite is true. Your doctor greatly values your need for having him or her available at all times.

When you conclude your prenatal interviews, you should choose a doctor in whom you feel confident – you feel comfortable talking with this doctor, he or she is on your insurance plan, the location and hours are convenient and the office staff is pleasant. The care of your child is now one of your most important concerns, and you should feel secure your child's physician feels the same.

What Happens to Your Baby During And After Delivery

Immediately after delivery, your newborn's body makes dramatic changes to adapt to life outside the womb. The circulation stops pumping blood through the umbilical cord and starts pumping more blood to the heart and lungs. The lungs were filled with fluid, but at birth expand to fill with air during the baby's first breaths. The infant also has to control his temperature on his own now that he is outside your body.

To ensure your infant is making a smooth transition, a nurse or physician examines your infant immediately after delivery. After you see your newborn, he or she is taken to a special table with a warming light. The baby is dried to help keep him or her from getting cold, and the heart rate and breathing are assessed. We no longer smack a baby's bottom (as you have seen in medical dramas), but we may rub the baby's back and feet to stimulate strong breathing. Your baby is assigned an Apgar score, which rates the baby from 0 to 2 on each of five criteria: heart rate, breathing, color, muscle tone, and grimace (response to stimulation). This score, assigned at one, five and 10 minutes after delivery, gives an indication of the baby's overall well-being. The maximum Apgar score is 10, and there is cause for concern if the score at five minutes is 7 or less.

You have probably been warned that your baby will not look like newborns you see on television. During the journey through the birth canal, the top of your baby's head may have become molded into a cone shape, but it will smooth out on its own. Your baby's hands and feet may be blue, which is also normal. The skin may be covered with a thick, waxy protective coating called vernix, or may be quite wrinkled. The feet are in the position they were when the baby was in the uterus, and will straighten slowly over the first weeks.

It is a wonderful miracle that babies are very alert during the first hours after birth. This very important time allows you to bond with your newborn as you become a new family. If you are able, nurse your baby for the first time in the delivery room. In the next few hours, your baby will become much sleepier – and so will you.

If you have a cesarean delivery with epidural anesthesia, you will be fully awake and alert to see your newborn. You can hold your infant after delivery, and then you will be moved from the operating room to a recovery area. Here you can visit with your newborn and nurse if you plan to breast-feed.

" Seeing my little girl for the first time was an overwhelmingly emotional experience. She was smeared with blood and vernix, but none of that mattered to me. She was perfect just like that."

While in your uterus, the baby can pass a bowel movement, called meconium, into the amniotic fluid. Your doctor knows if your baby has passed meconium because it turns the fluid a greenish color. It is important that the meconium not reach the infant's lungs during the first breaths after delivery. If the baby has passed meconium, your obstetrician uses a special tube to remove any fluid in the baby's mouth and nose before delivery is completed. Then, your infant's physician immediately examines the baby's throat with a special light and removes any meconium that might be in the baby's airway. While this is being done, the baby is not able to cry. Do not be alarmed if you do not hear the baby cry just after delivery. The physician expects this and is taking care of your baby. After a few minutes, you will have the baby in your arms.

After delivery, your baby's eyes are treated with an antibiotic eye ointment to prevent infection. In order to prevent a bleeding disorder, your infant receives an injection of Vitamin K. The nurses monitor your baby carefully to make sure he or she stays warm without the assistance of a warming light. Then the nurse gives your baby a bath.

While in the delivery room, the nursery nurse places a cord clamp one inch from your baby's abdomen to shorten the cord. Once in the nursery, the nurses check the baby's temperature with a rectal thermometer. They document the baby's heart rate and respiration (breathing rate), and examine the baby from head to toe. The cord is painted with triple dye, an antibiotic solution. After 24 hours the cord clamp is cut off, and the stump is treated with alcohol three times a day. Once you go home, treat the stump with alcohol with each diaper change. The baby should have a sponge bath and not a tub bath until the cord comes off. The stump should fall off within about 15 days.

If your baby boy has been circumcised, the way the procedure was done determines how you care for the penis as it heals. Two devices are commonly used in circumcision – the plastic "bell" and the Gomco clamp. The bell includes a plastic ring that is placed over the head of the penis, and the extra skin is cut off over this ring. No special care is required with this method. The ring should fall off on its own within 15 days. During the Gomco procedure, a metal device is placed over the head of the penis, and the foreskin is pinched between two pieces of metal and cut off. When your baby has the Gomco circumcision, he will come back from the nursery with Vaseline gauze around the head of the penis. After 24 hours, you must loosen the gauze from the penis by placing a damp cloth in the diaper for five minutes, and then gently remove the gauze. At home, place a small amount of Vaseline on the tip of the penis with each diaper change for the first five days. Before you go home from the hospital, your physician and nursery nurse will review their instructions with you about care of the umbilical stump and circumcision.

How to Fill Your Baby's Hungry Little Stomach

After delivery, your hospital stay is devoted to your safe recovery and helping your baby adapt to this new world. Whether you are breast- or bottle-feeding, the hospitals nursery staff can provide a lot of information during this time. No question is silly, and they are happy to help with anything you need while learning to feed your baby.

WHEN YOU ARE BREAST-FEEDING

A decision to breast-feed provides your baby with many benefits. Perhaps the most important of all is the wonderful bond between the nursing mother and baby. The physical closeness of you and your baby, and the miracle of growth provided only by mother's milk, leave you with special, treasured memories of your infant's early days. In addition, cells and proteins in the breast milk give your infant valuable protection against diseases. Breast-feeding also provides protection against common viral illnesses that cause infant diarrhea and ear infections. Even if you plan to return to work, your child's physician can help you develop a nursing schedule that is right for you. Each day that you breast-feed, you are giving your child an important gift.

Babies are born with the innate knowledge of how to nurse, but you and the baby must learn over the first few days how to work together. Nurses and lactation consultants can help you position the baby at the breast. One of the most common and comfortable positions is the "football hold." With this position, you sit up in bed or in a chair and support your elbow on a pillow. Rest the baby's head in the palm of your hand, with the body under your arm and feet behind you. Your baby probably will seem sleepy during the first day, and show increased interest in nursing over the next days. During the first two days, your baby receives a fluid called colostrum from your breasts. This thin, watery fluid contains proteins and cells that protect your baby from disease. During the third and fourth days after delivery, your body produces milk for the baby. The milk changes from watery gray to white in color. As your milk

" I took the convenience of breast-feeding for granted until I visited a friend who bottle-fed her baby. Every morning, she had to mix all those bottles of formula and refrigerate them, then re-heat them one by one. Then there were bottles and nipples to scrub and sterilize. And during the night, she had to get up and heat a bottle. Breast milk is always ready and always the perfect temperature."

> *" The first couple of weeks of breastfeeding were hard. My nipples were very sore. Other than that, it was really very easy. I breast-fed for seven months."*

comes in, your breasts can become very full and engorged. If you are uncomfortable from engorgement or you have trouble getting your infant to latch onto the breast, please call your lactation consultant or pediatrician for advice. You can also try wearing a supportive bra, feeding the baby very frequently (every 2 hours) and massaging your breast while the baby is feeding.

One of the greatest sources of anxiety for a breast-feeding mother is wondering whether her baby is getting enough milk. A newborn should nurse eight to ten times daily. I suggest that you feed your baby on demand and keep a record of feedings, wet diapers and bowel movements over the first few days. You can look for signs that your baby is hungry before he begins to cry – when he smacks his lips or "roots" (tries to find a nipple to suck on your shoulder or whatever his mouth touches). When this occurs, you can offer the breast. The baby should nurse at least five to ten minutes on each side, and the interval between feedings is timed from the beginning of one feeding to the beginning of the next. Don't be alarmed if it seems that you are feeding the baby "all the time" – every two hours or so. (When we say you are feeding your baby "every two hours," you are spending about 20 minutes of that time feeding.) These frequent feedings help refill your baby's small stomach, satisfy the urge to suck, and build your milk supply.

The baby's first bowel movements are thick, sticky and black, and these are called meconium stools. As your milk comes in, the stools change to greenish-brown, and then to a loose mustard yellow. The stools occur once to several times with each feeding. Infants should make at least three bowel movements and three wet diapers daily as a sign that they are getting enough milk. You should call your child's physician for advice if you find the baby has not had a bowel movement for 18 to 24 hours.

One of the best ways to know your infant is getting enough milk is to follow the baby's weight. All newborns can lose 10 percent of their birth weight during the first few days after birth, and should regain their birth weight by the end of the first or second week. Your child's physician will advise you when to bring the baby into the office for the first examination. If you have any questions about your baby's milk intake, feel free to call your physician to schedule a visit to weigh the baby and review your feeding progress.

> *"Breast-feeding went well, except my daughter wanted to eat all the time. During the day, she would eat about every hour and a half. It would drive me crazy. But the good news was she slept well at night."*

WHEN YOU ARE BOTTLE-FEEDING

If you are bottle-feeding, ask your child's physician in advance about a choice of formula. Common formulas are derived from cow's milk or soy protein. Both types of formula are equally nutritious for your baby, but your baby may tolerate one formula better than another. Signs that your baby is having trouble with a formula include excessive spitting or fussiness after feedings. Initially, your baby may take one ounce or less at each feeding. Most bottle-fed babies eat every three or four hours, and should be taking 18 to 20 ounces per day within a few days. Like breast-fed babies, bottle-fed babies should be fed on demand. Unlike breast-fed babies, however, those fed from a bottle will not need to eat every two hours around the clock (unless your child's physician advises for medical reasons such as prematurity or jaundice). Formula is harder to digest than breast milk, so your bottle-fed baby feels satisfied longer. Please burp your baby after every ounce.

Please discuss any formula changes with your child's physician prior to making a switch. Your physician can advise you whether any symptoms your baby is experiencing are from a formula problem or part of normal infant behavior.

What Happens Before Your Baby Leaves the Hospital

Your child's physician visits your infant daily while in the hospital and is available to talk to you. If this is your first baby, you do not know what to expect, so ask questions. Answers to your questions help you feel less anxious when you are discharged to go home.

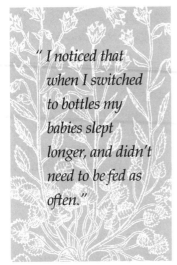

" I noticed that when I switched to bottles my babies slept longer, and didn't need to be fed as often."

THE CIRCUMCISION DECISION

If you have a boy, you should decide about circumcision prior to your discharge. Circumcision is the removal of the foreskin that covers the end of the penis. This procedure is not medically necessary, and is done for cosmetic and religious reasons. The circumcision is performed by your child's physician or your obstetrician. Most often, the circumcision is performed before you go home from the hospital. The skin heals in a few days, and your physician may instruct you to use petroleum jelly or antibiotic ointment until the healing is complete, depending on the method used to do the circumcision, as discussed earlier in this chapter.

SCREENING FOR DISEASES

Your state laboratory screens newborns for a variety of medical problems, such as thyroid disease and an inability to break down fats or proteins (phenylketonuria or PKU). The test involves applying a small amount of blood from your baby's heel to a filter paper. The results are sent to your baby's caregiver within three weeks. Any abnormal results are reported immediately to your child's physician by telephone or certified mail. Please rest assured that no news is good news! Your physician can confirm your child's normal newborn screening results within a few weeks.

HEPATITIS B VACCINATION

All parents dread their child's first immunizations. The first recommended vaccine, for hepatitis B, is administered prior to discharge. Hepatitis B is a serious and often chronic infection of the liver. Newborns can be exposed to hepatitis B through the birth canal of an infected mother or by close personal contact with an infected person, and lifelong infection can lead to liver failure. The vaccine does not contain any live virus; it is composed of proteins made in a laboratory. Three doses are necessary to provide immunity; the first is given at birth and the others at ages one month and six months. You can expect only slight soreness at the vaccine site, but no other side effects.

Vaccine recommendations keep changing – for the better. Immunizations continue to improve in terms of safety. There are new vaccines available, such as the one for chicken pox. Your physician should be able to keep you up to date as new information becomes available.

INSTALLATION OF YOUR BABY'S CAR SEAT

You must have an appropriate car safety seat for your infant. The seat should be easy to use and fit your car's seat-belt system. Please read the manufacturer's information to ensure you have installed the seat correctly. The safest position for an infant is in the rear of the car (in the center seat, if possible). Mirrors are available that allow you to see your infant in the back seat. The child should be in the rear-facing position until 20 pounds. If your child weighs 20 pounds before one year of age, the child should remain in the rear-facing position in an infant/toddler seat. A rear-facing child safety seat should never be placed in the front seat of a car equipped with a passenger-side air bag. The infant should recline at a 45-degree angle so the head does not flop forward. The hospital staff is happy to inspect your car seat prior to discharge to make sure it is safely installed.

" Even with the car seat installed correctly, the baby seemed to lean forward too much for my comfort. I think I kept my hand on her forehead all the way home."

Caring for Your Baby: Learning the Ropes of Early Parenthood

What to Know During Those First Weeks at Home

It is amazing to think about how much confidence you gain in caring for your newborn during the weeks after discharge. Bonding during this period establishes a lifelong relationship with your child. Your baby quickly learns your gentle touch, and is already familiar with the sound of your voice. The newborn can see clearly for six to eight inches, and prefers to look at the human face more than anything else. Face-to-face conversations with your newborn are quite soothing. It is a wonderful feeling of satisfaction when your newborn calms easily with your voice or touch.

Please remember that your child's physician and staff are available to you by telephone to answer any urgent questions you may have. If you are worried about your baby, obtain medical advice. You will always know your baby better than anyone else, and you need to pay attention to that sense that tells you something is wrong. Often, your physician can put your mind at ease, but only if you call!

KEEPING VISITORS UNDER CONTROL

Frequently, the number of family members and friends visiting immediately after discharge can be overwhelming to a fatigued new mother. Try to limit the number of visitors during the first week, and respect the need for both mother and baby to rest. All people handling the baby should wash their hands first, and any ill persons should stay away from the baby.

" The first days were hard. I especially remember the first day coming home. The baby was hungry, he had to be changed and I had to go to the bathroom, too. I felt overwhelmed."

HELPING BABY LEARN THAT NIGHTS ARE FOR SLEEPING

During this time, your baby may sleep as much as 20 hours per day, waking only to eat. Most new babies prefer to sleep all day and spend their waking hours at night. Fortunately, with a little help, babies can learn to sleep at night. Sleep is a learned behavior, and by reducing stimulation during nighttime feedings, you can help the baby learn to sleep at night. Keep the lights low and conversation to a minimum during the night. Try to put the baby down after the feeding, even if he or she is still awake. As long as the baby is not crying, it is fine to let him or her fall asleep alone, and it encourages later sleep patterns. However, it is important to soothe a crying baby, and don't let anyone tell you that you will "spoil" him!

The recommended sleep position for newborns is on their backs. This position reduces the occurrence of Sudden Infant Death Syndrome (SIDS). Your baby should sleep on a firm mattress and never on a soft pillow. Use a firm support cushion to keep your baby in position if needed. Sleeping on the back has not been shown to cause choking if the baby spits up; however, you should discuss this issue with your caregiver if your child's vomiting is excessive. If your physician advises you to position your baby on the side, it is important to switch sides each night to avoid flattening the face.

"My baby startled easily, and it wasn't always easy to keep her swaddled. But the hardest part about positioning her on her back was putting up with what my mom had to say about that. 'What if she spits up?' 'She'd feel more secure if she could snuggle up on her tummy.' I told her about the SIDS research and held my ground."

Watching Your Baby Grow

During the first two months, your baby gains approximately one ounce per day. Periods of alertness increase steadily, and your baby begins holding up his or her head. He or she should focus on your face and watch your movements. By the end of the second month, he or she is smiling responsively, cooing, noticing his or her hands, and beginning to reach out for objects.

Visiting the Doctor

> "I asked a lot of questions when my babies were sick, and I was always interested in the growth chart to make sure they were growing well."

Well-child check-ups are the best way to preserve health and prevent illness. Your child's physician provides valuable information at each visit. During these visits, the doctor reviews your child's development and discusses what your child should be doing in the coming months. The doctor plots your child's growth on a chart and asks you about feedings, sleep and bowel patterns. At these visits, any question you want to ask is fair game. You may want to keep a pad and pen by the changing table to note questions as they arise.

Please find out whether your insurance policy covers well-child exams. Unfortunately, many policies cover only a limited number of check-ups annually, and you are not reimbursed for every visit during the first year.

Immunizations are an important part of your child's care. The dreaded shots protect your child from serious illness. As I suggested before, the recommendations change quite often, so please discuss all immunizations with your child's physician. Written information concerning the risks and benefits of each vaccine is available. You also receive a permanent immunization card that you should keep as a record of your child's immunizations.

Conclusion

Congratulations upon creating a new life. You are also born again because your life will never be the same – it is richer for your labor of love with your child. Parenting is one of the most intense experiences that you will ever have. I hope this information helps ease your anxiety. Remember that your child's physician and staff are a valuable asset when you have questions and concerns.

I wish you much happiness along the way with your child.

Resources
Additional Reading

- **Bestfeeding: Getting Breastfeeding Right for You,** *Mary Renfrew, Chloe Fisher and Suzanne Arms,* Celestial Arts, 1990.

- **The Nursing Mother's Companion,** *Kathleen Huggins,* Harvard Common Press, 1995.

- **The Expectant Father: Facts, Tips and Advice for Dads-to-Be,** *Armin A. Brott and Jennifer Ash,* Abbeville Press, 1995.

- **Bringing Baby Home: An Owner's Manual for First-Time Parents,** *Laura Zahn,* Down to Earth Publications, 1993.

Organizations

- **March of Dimes Birth Defects Foundation**
  National Office
  1275 Mamaroneck Avenue
  White Plains, NY 10605
  (888) MODIMES (663-4637)
  E-mail: publiceducation@modimes.org
  http://www.modimes.org

Internet Sites

- **http://www.dfcreations.com/nh.html**
  This commercial site offers 10 helpful hints for naming your baby.

- **http://www.modimes.org/pub/newborn.htm**
  This March of Dimes information sheet explains newborn screening tests.

- **http://healthguide.com/newborn/default.htm**
  HealthGuide Online's "Newborn Care" section covers all the basics and then some — feeding, bathing, dressing, changing and more issues that occupy new parents.

- **http://pregnancy.tqn.com/msub14.htm**
  "Newborn Resources" from the Mining Company include a fun, clickable image map of a newborn's body, advice on car-seat selection, and a searchable database called "kidsDoctor."

CHAPTER EIGHTEEN

PREGNANCY AFTER 35

Considering the Risks & Rewards

regnancy after age 35 is as wonderful and special as pregnancy at any other age. In certain ways it can be even more special than at younger ages, because you and your partner may have been waiting for a long time to start a family. There are many reasons you may have waited to have a child – getting a career established, waiting to get married (or be married to the right person), or just not being sure that you wanted to have a child until now. If you are single and want to have a baby without a partner (or have a sterile partner or a female partner), we encourage and support your desire to have a child. Children need love and support, and your ability to give these two things is the most important factor to consider when deciding if you should be a parent. You also may be pregnant after age 35 because this is your second, third, fourth or fifth baby. Whatever the reason, please feel confident that you can have a wonderful pregnancy and a healthy child.

What You Need to Know

There are some special concerns many women have when starting a family at a more mature age. These concerns include a fear of not being able to conceive, as the risk of infertility is increased for women over age 35. You may also be concerned about the increased chance of having a miscarriage. Then there are the worries about having a baby with a chromosome problem, having twins, or delivering your baby prematurely. These are all appropriate thoughts, but it is important to have a clear understanding of these and other issues related to pregnancy after age 35.

The goal of this chapter is to give you important knowledge

about having a baby at a mature age, while at the same time relating great optimism that you can have a wonderful pregnancy and a normal outcome. You should be excited about having a baby if this is the right time in your life. Our desire is to help you understand why a pregnancy at this time of your life is special and requires additional considerations when compared with a pregnancy in a woman younger than 35.

> "I wouldn't have been happy raising a child in my 20s because I had other projects. For me, it was the right choice to wait until I was in my early 30s to start, and then have the second one now. For me, I'm just more settled in my life and more mature, and a more well-rounded person. I think that's good for the children. I'm now ready to stay around and be satisfied to hang around with my kids."

Let us go ahead and tell you that the medical term applied to a pregnancy in a woman over 35 is **advanced maternal age (AMA)**. We feel this is a poor choice of words, considering we are in our 30s and do not consider this age "advanced." However, special counseling is appropriate after age 35. I hope this chapter helps you understand this counseling. Please discuss what you read with your caregiver before making any final decision regarding your plans to conceive.

Our discussion of pregnancy after age 35 focuses on the risks involved. However, there are also some benefits when you start a family later in life. These include greater maturity to help handle the demands of children. Also, you may be in a stronger relationship than when you were very young. Your financial situation may be better, reducing the monetary stress of having to provide for a new member of the family. Please do not get the feeling that all is doom and gloom, but be informed as you approach a decision of this importance.

How Your Age Affects Your Fertility

Beyond age 25, your ability to become pregnant declines. As you age, the eggs within the ovaries are aging as well. Just as you can no longer do the tumbling you could at age 7, your older eggs are no longer able to conceive a baby as easily. There is no effect on your chance to get pregnant based on your husband's age. A man's is testes continuously produce new sperm throughout life. You, on the other hand, have the greatest number of eggs within your ovaries when you are a fetus within your mother's uterus. Starting at birth, the number of eggs available for reproduction constantly declines. We do not clearly understand why there is a greater rate of infertility, miscarriage and chromosome problems with advancing maternal age.

Infertility is the inability to conceive after one year of unprotected intercourse. The chance you are infertile if you are under age 30 is around 1 in 20. Between the ages of 30 and 35, the chance you are infertile increases to 1 in 10. By 35 to 40, the risk is 1 in 5. Beyond age 40, the risk is 1 in 2 or 1 in 3. Very young women who are trying to decide when to get pregnant are probably not reading this chapter. However, this information is useful to very young women. During the busy years of establishing ourselves personally and professionally, it is easy to postpone starting a family. There is a very real risk you take if you delay too long. We encourage you to consider increasing incidence of infertility with advancing age when you are trying to plan your family. One truism is that there is never an ideal time to have a child. Please consider sharing these statistics with the younger members of your family, even if they are clearly many years away from wanting to start their own families.

If you are in your 30s and are starting or expanding your family, please do not be discouraged. Simply use this information to help you establish realistic expectations about how fast you will become pregnant. Conception normally takes place within one year. If your periods are not regular, or if you are older than 30 and have tried to get pregnant for six months, we encourage you to discuss this with your physician and not wait for a full year.

While infertility is more common after age 35, there are procedures available to help you conceive if you have a problem. These are discussed in the next chapter, "Infertility."

How Miscarriage Becomes More Likely

Once you are pregnant, the fear of having a miscarriage becomes very real. You may find that you develop an unbelievably strong bond as soon as you know you have a baby growing within your womb. (There is nothing wrong with you if you don't feel the strong bond immediately. That is no reflection on your suitability for motherhood.) Even when the embryo inside you is only an inch long, your visions and dreams are about that little baby boy or girl who will grow into a companion for you throughout your life. The degree of love that develops at this early stage of pregnancy is remarkable and powerful. This quick and strong bond is also what makes the thought of having a miscarriage unbearable for many women.

However unpleasant the topic, the issue of miscarriage must be addressed in this chapter, because the older you are, the greater your risk. During your 20s and early 30s, your risk of having a miscarriage is 1 in 10. From 35 to 40, the risk is 1 in 5. If you are over 40, the risk increases to 1 in 3 or 4. Therefore, the chance your pregnancy will end in a miscarriage is 10 percent before age 35, 20 percent at 35 to 40, and 30 to 40 percent after age 40.

FATHERS AND MISCARRIAGE

The man's age does have a small effect on your risk of having a miscarriage; the risk increases slightly if your baby's father is over age 40.

And while we are on the topic of fathers: we have observed that fathers and mothers seem to bond differently with their unborn children. We have described the intense bond you have as soon as you are pregnant. This same degree of bonding does not tend to occur with the fathers until farther into the pregnancy or once your baby is born. Of course, this is not true for all men; some husbands grieve more over miscarriage than their wives. I share this observation to help you understand why your partner may not be feeling as much apprehension about having a miscarriage as you are during this early phase of pregnancy.

Whenever your baby's heartbeat is found, your risk of having a miscarriage declines to less than 5 percent. Ultrasound shows the heartbeat at eight weeks, and the Doppler picks it up by 15 weeks. (The Doppler is the small instrument that we place on your lower abdomen to allow us to hear the sound of your baby's rapid heartbeat.)

This information about miscarriage is not intended to add to your fear of pregnancy, but to increase your knowledge of the issues involved. This information is very important for someone in her 20s or early 30s to know when making a decision to postpone starting a family. If you are already over 35, we wish we could present this topic without adding to your fears. However, these facts are part of pregnancy at this age, and we believe most women are already aware of them. we hope this information puts real numbers to the risks, and thereby lowers your apprehension. Without the facts, our imaginations can paint a much worse scenario than is appropriate. Please speak to your caregiver to get the details as they relate to you.

When Chromosomal Abnormalities Become More Common

Another concern for all women over age 35 is the risk of having a baby with a chromosomal problem. A normal child has 46 chromosomes – 23 from the mother and 23 from the father. Your egg that is released with ovulation carries 23 chromosomes. Each of your partner's sperm carries 23 as well. When one sperm enters the egg, the egg's outer cover changes and becomes impenetrable to additional sperm. This combination of chromosomes makes each of us unique and special. If the chromosomes do not join perfectly, there is a chromosomal abnormality.

Sperm carry one copy of chromosomes 1 to 22 and either an X or Y chromosome. The egg carries its own copy of chromosomes 1 to 22, and then an X. If a sperm with an X joins the egg, the baby will be a girl (46XX); if a sperm with a Y joins the egg, the baby will be a boy (46XY). Therefore, since all eggs carry the X chromosome, it is the sperm that determines the sex of the baby. If the egg or sperm carries more than one copy of any of the 23 chromosomes, the baby will have three copies of that particular chromosome instead of the usual two. The addition results in abnormalities. These abnormalities may cause minor problems, or they may be life-threatening. With severe defects, fetal development stops at an early stage, and the pregnancy ends in a miscarriage.

" I was very nervous waiting for the results of the CVS, because I was thinking, 'What am I going to do if it's bad news?' I have worked with children who are handicapped for almost 20 years now, and a handicap wouldn't be a big problem for me unless it was the kind of birth defect where you knew the baby would die very quickly. But my husband has never had any experience with handicapped children. I am definitely more prepared than my husband, but in marriage, it's not just me; I have to think of both of us. I think the one big reason we had the test done is because if there was bad news, then we would have had time to find out more about the problem – how bad it was; you know, and all the kinds of things we would have had to deal with. "

The most common chromosomal defect is Down's syndrome (Trisomy 21), where there is an extra chromosome number 21. The extra copy comes from the mother's egg in two-thirds of the cases and the fathers' sperm in one-third of the cases. The baby is born with the normal two copies of all the other chromosomes except number 21; there are three copies of chromosome 21. Children with Down's syndrome usually have a protruding tongue; small, low-set ears; a prominent forehead; a flat, wide nose bridge; heart defects; and some degree of mental retardation. Their average IQ is 50. Many of these individuals function very well in society.

While Down's syndrome is the most common chromosomal defect, it is not the most severe. Most infants with Trisomy 13 and Trisomy 18 die within a few months. A baby with an extra chromosome 13 (Trisomy 13) has mental retardation, a cleft lip and palate, holes between the chambers of the heart, small eyes, extra fingers, clenched fists, and toes that arch up. More than 50 percent of these babies die within one month of life. With Trisomy 18, a baby has mental retardation, a prominent forehead, small jaw, low-set ears, a short chest bone and clenched fists. Babies with Trisomy 18 die with a few months of birth from the heart abnormalities common to this chromosomal defect.

Your risk of having a baby with a chromosomal defect increases exponentially with your age. The risk is small at age 20, near 1 in 600. At age 30, the risk is 1 in 400; at 40, it is 1 in 60. You see how the risk increases rapidly after age 30. This fact is important to consider when choosing the best time in your life to have children. While you should never have children when you are not prepared, you also should not put off starting your family without understanding this issue. If you do not clearly understand this fact, please speak with your doctor.

" I don't want to be very old when I see my kids growing up. So 35 was my own limit. And the risk of increase of Down's syndrome – that was pretty scary to me. But I've had tests – I've had a CVS – just to check that everything was OK, and it was."

How Genetic Testing is Performed

There are two tests available to determine the chromosomal makeup of your child. These tests are CVS and amniocentesis.

CVS

CVS, or chorionic villus sampling, is performed between weeks 9 and 12 of pregnancy. The chorion refers to the placenta, and villus refers to the small protrusion of the placenta that attaches to your uterus. This test involves passing an instrument through the cervix and collecting a sample from this placental tissue. The results are back within 10 days in most cases. Passing a needle through your lower abdomen is another way to do the CVS. The risk of losing the pregnancy because of the test is 1 to 2 percent.

AMNIOCENTESIS

An amniocentesis is performed between weeks 15 and 20. You are placed on an examination table where you first have an ultrasound. This ultrasound is done to make sure your baby is fine and to locate the placenta. The placenta is avoided if possible, but if not, it is safe to pass the catheter through this tissue. Once an area of fluid is located on ultrasound, your abdomen is cleaned with a sterile solution such as Betadine. The ultrasound head is covered with a sterile drape and placed on the area where the amniocentesis is to be done. A very thin needle is passed through the skin and into the sac of fluid. The needle is visible on the ultrasound the entire time, making sure the baby is not hurt. The needle collects a sample of amniotic fluid, which contains the baby's skin cells. Chromosome tests are performed on those skin cells.

Before the needle is passed through your skin, the doctor may numb your skin with lidocaine. Many doctors do not numb the skin because the numbing is sometimes more uncomfortable than passing the amniocentesis needle. This should give you an idea of how little discomfort you can expect with an amniocentesis. The amount of time needed for the amniocentesis is 30 minutes, with only one minute for the actual procedure with the needle and the rest for the ultrasound and preparation. The risk of losing the baby due to an amniocentesis is ½ percent.

" I had the CVS because I am close to 40 years old, and the doctor shared with me that beyond 40, there's the highest chance of birth defects. We wanted to have some knowledge; in case there was a problem, we could get prepared and deal with it. They told me what they were going to do ahead of time, and it was like having a Pap done in a way. They had a monitor so I could watch what was going on, and that really helped me. I have had Pap smears that were more painful than this. Actually, it was not painful. I was just very nervous and needed to relax. The catheter is so small... I mean, it's very, very tiny; I didn't even feel it when they put it in. I was nervous about the baby; I didn't want to lose the baby."

HOW TO USE THESE TESTS

The reason age 35 is chosen for defining advanced maternal age is that the risk of having a baby with a chromosomal problem at age 35 (1 in 200) is close to the risk associated with an amniocentesis or CVS. With both of these tests, there is the risk of rupturing the amniotic sac, resulting in the loss of amniotic fluid. Also, bacteria could be introduced, resulting in an infection within the uterus, causing the delivery of the baby (miscarriage). In order to minimize your chance of having a miscarriage after an amniocentesis or CVS, avoid strenuous activity for one week after the procedure. The symptoms of an impending miscarriage are spotting or bleeding like a period, and cramping in your lower abdomen. If you notice either of these problems, please call your doctor.

The advantage of having a CVS is that the results are known much earlier in the pregnancy. If there is a chromosomal defect and you decide to terminate the pregnancy, an abortion is much easier physically and emotionally at this earlier stage. The advantage of an amniocentesis is the lower risk of a miscarriage after the procedure. Therefore, if you have experienced infertility, have an amniocentesis, whereas if you do not have such a history, have the CVS.

> " I had an amnio with my second baby, so I know what it was like to wait for test results. I had anxiety like I've never had in my whole life. And a week after the amnio, I had such anxiety that I had to see a doctor. I had no energy and I would be crying all the time – and that was the anxiety I was keeping in."

IS GENETIC TESTING THE RIGHT CHOICE FOR YOU?

Genetic testing with either amniocentesis or CVS is not for every woman over age 35. You may feel the risk of miscarriage, even though small, is too great to accept. You also should consider what you would do with the information before you have the test. If a termination, or abortion, is not an option for you, you may not want to go through the testing. The only advantage in that situation is to help you and your family prepare for the birth of a baby with special needs. In terms of preparation, you can read information about your baby's problem, speak to other parents who have already gone through what you are about to experience, allow your religious leaders to know so you will have support, and inform your other children and family members.

If you are younger than 35, there is a screening test to determine if you should consider chromosomal testing. This test, called the triple screen, is a blood test done at 15 weeks of pregnancy. The triple screen

measures the level of three hormones: HCG (human chorionic gonadotropin), AFP (alpha-fetoprotein) and estrogen. Through a calcula-
tion of these levels, you are given a risk of having a baby with a chromosomal defect. If that risk is the same as a woman at age 35, consider
having an amniocentesis.

If you are over 35, you may be asking if you should take the triple
screen and wait to see if you are at risk of having a baby with a chromosomal defect. Many physicians not support this plan, as the triple
screen is not that good at making sure the chromosomes are normal.
Your age alone tells us you are at increased risk. Women younger than
35 should use the triple screen to see who needs an amniocentesis. A
woman older than 35 should not use the triple screen to reassure herself that there is no concern over chromosome problems.

Obviously the issue of having a baby with a chromosome defect
is serious. You need to be educated about this topic when deciding the
best time to start your family. Also, when pregnant, you have to decide if having CVS or amniocentesis is best for you. The topic of abortion is too personal and complicated to cover in this book, but you
need to know the options that you will be presented during your pregnancy if you are over 35.

What Else We Know About Pregnancy After 35

The ability of your uterus to provide a strong blood supply to
the baby at the end of your pregnancy may be impaired if you are
over age 35. In order to make sure this is not occurring, your baby is
tested each week after 34 weeks. This test, a non-stress test (NST),
involves listening to the baby's heartbeat while you note any movements. The baby is fine if there are accelerations in the heart rate,
especially if they are associated with the baby's movements. There
is cause for concern about the baby if there are decelerations or dips
in the heart rate. If this occurs, your baby is tested with a biophysical
profile (discussed below), or the baby is delivered through induction of labor or cesarean section.

If you are older than 40, the risk of these problems at the end of pregnancy is slightly higher, and the test started at 34 weeks is a biophysical profile. A biophysical profile includes a NST as well as an ultrasound evaluation of the baby's breathing movements, level of amniotic fluid, main body and limb movements. The biophysical profile is scored from 0 to 10, with 2 points possible for each of the above factors. If the baby scores an 8 or 10, everything is fine. If the score is 6, the test is repeated within 48 hours, or your labor is induced if you are near your due date. If the score is 4 or less, serious consideration is given to delivering your baby regardless of where you are in the pregnancy.

The incidence of preterm birth and twins increases only minimally with AMA, and therefore they should not change the management of your pregnancy. Also, they should not influence your decision on when to start your family.

Conclusion

This chapter is a serious discussion of the issues you need to be aware of if you are pregnant after age 35. This information is very important for the couple trying to decide when to start a family. However, we do not want to make pregnancy at this age sound like a miserable experience. In fact, many women over age 35 are able to enjoy pregnancy more than their younger counterparts because of their greater maturity. Pregnancy is a wonderful blessing that should be cherished, regardless of your age.

As obstetricians we marvel at the miracle of fetal development and birth. It is an honor to share this experience with so many couples. However, we must make sure you are fully informed of the issues related to having a baby at this stage of life. Please do not read this as a warning to not get pregnant if you are over 35, but rather be prepared to address the issues we have discussed. This information is also useful to young women who may be deferring starting their family. Talk to your doctor about what you have read. Enjoy the pregnancy experience!

Resources

Additional Reading

- **Birth over 35,** *Sheila Kitzinger,* Penguin USA, 1995.
- **Your Pregnancy after 30,** *Glade B. Curtis,* Fisher Books, 1996.
- **Surviving Pregnancy Loss: A Complete Sourcebook for Women and their Families,** *Rochelle Friedman and Bonnie Gradstein,* Citadel Press, 1996.

Organizations

- **March of Dimes Birth Defects Foundation**
  National Office
  1275 Mamaroneck Avenue
  White Plains, NY 10605
  (888) MODIMES (663-4637)
  E-mail: publiceducation@modimes.org
  http://www.modimes.org

Internet Sites

- http://www.noah.cuny.edu/pregnancy/march_of_dimes/
  pre_preg.plan/after30.html
  Review how your age affects such things as infertility, miscarriage, genetic problems and delivery with this information from the New York Online Access to Health (NOAH) project.

- http://www.noah.cuny.edu/pregnancy/march_of_dimes/genet-ics/gcbooklt.html
  This NOAH site provides a full description of how chromosomal problems occur and which tests best determine if your baby is genetically normal.

- http://www.midlifemommies.com/
  Do you think you are the only woman in her 40s who is pregnant? Think again. Midlife Mommies offers health, business and parenting advice for mature moms.

CHAPTER NINETEEN

INFERTILITY

Overcoming the Obstacles To Conception

Having a child is not for everyone, but for most of us, it is one of the most important things that ever happens in life. We look forward to having a newborn to love and cuddle, a toddler to watch as a little personality evolves, a child to help us remember our own youth, an adolescent to guide through the challenges of becoming an adult, and finally an adult to share our golden years with as a family. The desire to be a "family" makes us want to have children. We know we never truly die as long as we have offspring to carry on our family genes. For these reasons and many more, it is very painful to want a child but be unable to conceive. The stress can affect how you feel about yourself and your partner. Many wonderful marriages have ended over this issue.

This chapter can help you and your partner understand why infertility occurs and how it can be treated. Please keep the lines of communication open so that you two can face this difficulty as a couple. If you feel that infertility is adversely affecting your relationship, either take a break from trying to get pregnant or seek guidance from a psychologist. As with the other chapters in this book, use the information here to help reduce your fears and concerns.

Infertility affects about 10 percent of the population, and the incidence may be increasing as women elect to defer

" I have times when I feel like the whole world is falling apart. And every month I'm hoping, 'Well, maybe I pulled it off this month.' I told my husband, 'You don't understand.' It's like losing a game, and then the consolation prize you get – a period – is so bad! It's like you lose twice."

childbearing because of career demands or personal choice. There are other factors suspected as well, such as environmental toxins, which are believed to decrease sperm counts. Approximately 60 percent of the recognized factors contributing to infertility originate in the female, and 40 percent originate in the male; usually a contribution of some degree from both partners causes a couple to be infertile. Fortunately, many advances in this field of medicine allow couples more options than ever when faced with infertility.

" When my sister-in-law got pregnant, she had been trying about as long as we had. Her pregnancy was very difficult for me. I would also find excuses not to go to church or something because everybody would be pregnant. There were constantly baby showers going on..."

Infertility, as medically defined, is the inability to conceive after one year of unprotected intercourse. Many couples do not realize that achieving pregnancy may take many months under normal circumstances. While we often assume that pregnancy will soon follow discontinuing birth control, this is not always the case. Unfortunately, this misunderstanding may provoke undue anxiety, which can become counterproductive to your efforts to conceive by interfering with sexual function or by disrupting your normal cycles.

The purpose of this chapter is to discuss the normal sequence of events surrounding the initiation of a pregnancy. We review the role hormones play in your reproductive cycle, the anatomy that allows an egg and sperm to meet, ways to increase your chances of getting pregnant, the known factors of infertility, and their evaluation and treatment.

How Hormones Control A Normal Menstrual Cycle

To understand pregnancy, and therefore problems with getting pregnant, you must first understand the normal menstrual cycle. Under normal circumstances, your cycle is under tight and somewhat complex hormonal control. Female hormones are found in different amounts at varying times of the menstrual cycle. The brain sends the hormones FSH (follicle stimulating hormone) and LH (luteinizing hormone) to the ovary to make it work. The ovary produces an egg and releases it at the proper time (ovulation). The ovary also sends estrogen and progesterone to the uterus to make the lining ready to receive the baby. If there is no pregnancy, the lining is shed during menstruation. Once the ovary has released the egg (ovulation), it begins to produce progesterone from the area that used to hold the egg. This area is the corpus luteum.

If a pregnancy occurs, the hormone of pregnancy, human chorionic gonadotropin (hCG), keeps the corpus luteum active. Therefore, the production of progesterone from the corpus luteum continues. With elevated levels of progesterone during pregnancy, the uterus expands and supports the developing baby. Progesterone is also responsible for the bloated, achy feelings many women experience during the last half of their cycle after ovulation. Progesterone plays a major role in premenstrual syndrome.

LH and FSH are present in very small amounts during most of the menstrual cycle. These hormones control the development of a new egg each month in the ovary. There is a surge of LH from the brain just prior to ovulation. It is this surge of LH that the commercially available ovulation kits detect, and display as a color change on the test strips. You ovulate the same day or the day after the color change with these urine ovulation-prediction kits.

Many women are concerned they may not be ovulating correctly. If you have a regular monthly menstrual cycle, this is strong support that you must be ovulating well. A normal cycle requires that you ovulate, form a corpus luteum, produce progesterone and do not get pregnant. The length of a normal cycle varies from every 26 to 32 days. If your cycle is shorter than 26 days, your ovary may

" I had a range of emotions, from the excitement and anticipation of possibly getting pregnant to the absolute lows of the day I started my period and realized that we had to start all over again. Infertility is the epitome of emotional hell."

not produce enough progesterone; if the cycle is more than 32 days, you may not release the egg (ovulate) appropriately. Therefore, you can see how having a normal cycle tells you a lot about your hormones. If the cycles are normal, your hormones are probably normal.

How Sperm Meets Egg: The Anatomy of Conception

In order to understand infertility, you also must understand how your body allows an egg and sperm to meet. At the top of the vagina there is the opening of the uterus called the cervix. The uterus is pear-shaped, with two fallopian tubes extending off the sides. Just beyond the tubes on each side is an ovary.

Inside an ovary during each normal cycle, a follicle containing the egg to be ovulated begins to grow under the influence of FSH. As the follicle develops, it produces more estrogen. When the follicle is mature, the estrogen produced by the follicle causes a rise in the LH level. This rise in LH causes ovulation, where the ovary releases the egg. Finger-like projections at the end of the fallopian tube collect the egg, which then travels down the fallopian tube, where it meets sperm in its mid-section. It is here in the middle of the fallopian tube that sperm and egg join. Thus fertilization occurs. At fertilization, the sperm and egg become a conceptus. The conceptus ultimately develops into a baby.

The conceptus continues down the tube to enter the uterus, where it implants on the wall of the uterus and grows. If any obstruction in the tube prevents the conceptus from entering the uterus, it will begin to grow within the tube itself. This is how an ectopic pregnancy occurs.

Sperm are produced in a man's testicles. (Problems involved with the production of sperm are detailed in the section of this chapter on male infertility). With ejaculation, millions of sperm are deposited in the top of the vagina. The sperm then swim through the cervix into the uterus. Once in the uterus, sperm swim into the fallopian tubes to try to meet an egg.

In a cycle in which fertilization does not occur, the egg disintegrates and is flushed from the body with the menstrual flow.

A NARROW WINDOW

Mucus in the cervix changes consistency at different times of the menstrual cycle. In a way, the cervical mucus is like a protective gate that is only open for a short time to allow sperm into the uterus. During most of your menstrual cycle, there is not an egg waiting in the fallopian tube. During this time, the mucus in the cervix is very thick. This thick mucus acts as a protective barrier to decrease the risk of bacteria getting up into the uterus and causing an infection. However, just after ovulation, when an egg is in the fallopian tube, the cervical mucus becomes very watery and thin, allowing sperm to swim through and get to the egg. A couple of days after ovulation, the cervical mucus changes back to being very thick.

How to Optimize Your Chances of Getting Pregnant

HAVE INTERCOURSE OFTEN ENOUGH

As is apparent from the discussion of the menstrual cycle, timing is essential for pregnancy to occur. Sperm are able to fertilize an egg for about 72 hours, and the egg is available for fertilization for only 24 hours after ovulation. Therefore, if you are trying to conceive, most physicians recommend intercourse every other day, beginning several days before the anticipated ovulation. Ovulation occurs 14 days before menstrual flow begins. If your cycle is usually 28 days, ovulation occurs in the middle of the cycle. In a 30-day cycle, ovulation occurs on day 16 (30 minus 14 equals 16). Remember that day one of a menstrual cycle is the first day of flow.

With intercourse every other day near ovulation, sperm should be available whenever an egg is released. Another option is to have intercourse the day of ovulation as well as the day before and after ovulation. Since millions of sperm are released with each ejaculation, but only a few hundred actually reach the egg, a borderline or low sperm count can be detrimental to achieving pregnancy. The use of lubricants during intercourse is discouraged when you are trying to conceive, as some are toxic to the sperm. After intercourse, rest on your back to maximize the contact between the pool of sperm and the cervix.

KNOW WHEN YOU OVULATE

By Feel

In order to determine the best time for intercourse, you might use one of several methods of detecting ovulation. Some women can feel when they ovulate. There is frequently some degree of pain on one side or the other of your lower abdomen. This is called *Mittelschmerz*.

By Temperature

Another way to determine ovulation is to take your temperature each morning as soon as you wake, before getting out of bed. This reading is called the basal body temperature. An increase in temperature occurs one day after ovulation. The problem with this routine is that it tells you a day late that you should have had intercourse the prior day. There should be a dip in your temperature just before ovulation, but this dip is rarely of such a degree that you can confidently predict ovulation. Some physicians have you chart your basal body temperature to make sure you are ovulating. As we have already discussed, if you have a regular menstrual cycle, you should be ovulating. Therefore, charting the basal body temperature provides little helpful information, and is a chore to perform each day. The increased frustration created with recording the basal body temperature is not justifiable for many couples. However, you may feel more in control of the process by taking these readings, and there is no harm involved.

By Cervical Mucus

A very natural way to know when you are ovulating is to check the cervical mucus and vaginal discharge. Around ovulation, the cervical mucus becomes very thin and watery, and you can stretch it between two fingers. During the rest of the month, the mucus is very thick and will not stretch. You quickly learn to notice the difference. When the mucus is very watery, this is the best time to have intercourse if you want to get pregnant.

By Predictor Kit

One of the most common methods for knowing when ovulation is going to occur is to use a urine ovulation kit, also known as a urine predictor kit. You test your urine each morning to detect a rise in LH. A rise in LH occurs the day before ovulation. When this test changes color, indicating a rise in LH, you should plan to have intercourse that day and the next day. These test kits are expensive. Once you document ovulation is occurring at the correct time in your cycle (14 days before your menstrual cycle), you can stop using them.

> " The stress of infertility kills my sex life. He has to stay on stand-by all the time for whenever I get the will!"

TRY TO KEEP THE STRESS LEVEL DOWN

Having discussed all the methods for timing intercourse, one important issue remains. It is important to keep sex fun and natural. Do not make intercourse a science project strapped with stress and tension. Numerous couples have given up on getting pregnant after years of infertility procedures. Once they relax about this issue, many have become pregnant within months. We feel tension can have a major negative impact on a couple's ability to become pregnant. That is not to say that a woman with obstructed fallopian tubes is going to get pregnant if she and her partner just relax. However, there are many couples with unexplained infertility who need to keep this advice in mind.

CAN YOU CHOOSE YOUR BABY'S GENDER?

Many people are interested in the issue of gender selection with timing of intercourse. Sperm determine the sex of a baby; the egg has no influence on your having a boy or a girl. One theory is that intercourse before ovulation is more likely to produce a female, while intercourse occurring after ovulation is more likely to produce a male. This theory is based on the fact that sperm that will produce male babies, because of less weight in the chromosomal material they carry, can swim faster. Therefore, if the sperm are deposited before ovulation, the sperm for a male baby will have already swum up to, and possibly out of, the tubes before the egg arrives. The sperm for a female baby will be the only ones remaining available to fertilize the egg. However, many physicians doubt this theory, and this method is not reliable. There is a procedure that can separate the sperm, allowing a sample containing almost all of one sex or the other to be placed up around the egg. However, this method is costly and also not guaranteed.

What Causes Infertility, and How You Are Evaluated

As previously noted, the causes for infertility are found in the male 40 percent of the time and in the female 60 percent. There also are occasions where the cause of infertility cannot be determined. Problems that lead to infertility in men all involve damage to the production of sperm, or to the transport of sperm. A woman's problems come from the cervix, uterus, fallopian tubes or ovaries. We will discuss the problems that occur in each of these areas, and describe the simple tests used in the evaluation of infertility. The approach most physicians advocate in the evaluation of infertility is to begin with the most simple tests and progress to the more complex. Often, testing is completed within several months, and usually a diagnosis or explanation can be found. If you have had one year of unprotected intercourse and are not pregnant, you and your partner should see your gynecologist or family physician.

When the Male Contributes to Infertility

The production of sperm occurs in the male's testicles. The process requires several months from initial development to the act of ejaculation. Once sperm have been made, they are stored and mature in glands that sit on the testicles called the epididymis. During ejaculation, sperm rapidly move from the epididymis out through the penis. Damage can occur at any point in this system, with infertility as a result.

PROBLEMS IN THE TESTICLE

Damage to the production of sperm in the testicle can result from mumps infection, injuries to the testicle, exposure to toxic chemicals, hernia operations, and prolonged exposure to heat in the workplace or from a sauna or whirlpool. Also, a mass of dilated blood vessels around the testicles, called a **varicocele**, raise the temperature within the testicle, resulting in damage to sperm production.

A MISPLACED URETHRAL OPENING

With ejaculation, sperm are normally placed at the top of the vagina, near the cervix. In some men, the opening of the urethra is not at the tip of the penis. Instead, it opens lower down on the backside of the penis, closer to the base. This condition is called **hypospadias**. If a man has a normal urine stream from the top of his penis, he does not have this problem. If the stream is abnormal, he should see a urologist for further evaluation.

RETROGRADE EJACULATION

As part of ejaculation, sperm from the testicle join the urethra near the base of the penis. At the base of the penis is the prostate gland, which adds seminal fluid to the sperm to produce the ejaculate. The urethra normally carries urine from the bladder, through the penis to the outside. In a few men, the ejaculate travels in the wrong direction, and goes into the bladder. This is retrograde ejaculation. You cannot become pregnant if your partner's sperm end up in his bladder after intercourse. Retrograde ejaculation occurs in men with diabetes mellitus, prior spinal damage or surgery on the prostate.

DECREASED SPERM COUNT

Smoking and drinking alcohol are two habits that lower a man's sperm count. Also, a simple viral illness can lower the number of sperm available. It takes three months to replenish a low volume of sperm. Therefore, if your partner has had a viral illness or recently stopped smoking and drinking, his sperm count will be lower than normal for a few months.

WHAT SEMEN ANALYSIS LOOKS FOR

In order to test the male system, a semen analysis is done. Your gynecologist arranges to have your partner tested at a special lab. After two days of avoiding ejaculation, your partner produces a sperm sample. Without using lubricants, he ejaculates into a sterile cup. Some labs insist that the sperm be produced in their facility. Others allow a man to produce the sample at home and then bring it immediately to the lab. To be considered normal, there should be at least 20 million sperm in the ejaculate. Also, the sperm are evaluated for their ability to swim in a forward direction. If there are any problems, your partner is sent to a urologist for a complete physical. If the sperm count is normal, that basically completes the evaluation of the male. If your partner has poor sperm production or no sperm, you can have artificial insemination with donor sperm. This procedure is discussed in detail under the section about your cervix in this chapter. Another option is to have one of your husband's sperm injected directly into your egg. Once the egg is fertilized, it is placed back into your uterus.

When Ovulatory Problems Are the Source of Infertility

After you have a complete history and physical, your initial testing is begun. The purpose of testing is to show that the ovary is releasing the egg, the fallopian tube is open, and the uterus and cervix are normal. The order of testing is not critical, and several tests may be done during the same menstrual cycle. Let us first look at problems with ovulation and how they are treated.

We have already reviewed how to tell if you are ovulating correctly. Indicators include a normal monthly cycle, a mid-cycle change in cervical mucus, and a mid-cycle LH surge (measured by urine predictor kits). Once ovulation has occurred, the ovary produces the hormone progesterone. If the level of progesterone on cycle day 21 is normal, this also confirms a normal ovulation. Another way to make sure enough progesterone is being produced is for your doctor to do a biopsy of your uterus just prior to a menstrual cycle. By looking at the lining of your uterus under the microscope, a pathologist can tell if you are producing enough progesterone. When you do not ovulate normally, then we need to find out why. The most common reasons women do not ovulate are stress, thyroid problems, prolactin problems, and polycystic ovarian syndrome. Below is an explanation of each of these and how they are treated.

It is important to note that for many women there is no clear reason why they do not ovulate. Ovulation occurs in only one ovary each month. With each monthly cycle there is an equal chance ovulation will occur in the right or left ovary.

STRESS AS THE CAUSE OF NOT OVULATING

A normal monthly menstrual cycle, and therefore normal monthly ovulation, are under the control of the brain. The brain sends two hormones to the ovaries to cause ovulation to take place each month. These hormones are FSH and LH. If you are under a great deal of stress, your brain is unable to release FSH and LH in the correct amounts.

Women today may be under more stress then ever before. Many carry full loads at work, continue to be the primary caregiver at home, and still maintain active relationships with their friends, family and partner. Many women push themselves to the point of self-destruction to keep up with their schedules. Under normal circumstances, this stress leads to fatigue and mild depression, alerting you to back off on the demands. However, if you are trying to get pregnant, the result may be infertility. The stress blocks the brain's ability to stimulate a normal ovulation from the ovary.

If you are feeling stretched to the breaking point, the treatment for this problem is to first recognize the effect stress is having on your body. It may be best to see a psychologist to help develop a less stressful routine. A psychologist may be able to help you realize your personal limits. Once you set limits with work, friends and family, you can begin to find time to take care of yourself. You must always find some time to care for yourself in order to continue your other responsibilities. This is simple to state, but very difficult to accomplish. That is why you should seriously consider having a psychologist help guide you through this process. Stress is one of the least appreciated reasons couples have a difficult time getting pregnant.

THYROID PROBLEMS AS A CAUSE OF NOT OVULATING

The thyroid gland is located in the front of your neck. This gland produces a hormone that regulates your body's rate of metabolism. If there is a problem with the production of this hormone, the brain is not able to stimulate the ovary to ovulate. Infertility is the result.

As part of a routine evaluation for infertility, a blood test is done to make sure your thyroid gland is working correctly. If a problem is noted, you are placed on medication to return your thyroid hormone level to normal. When you take this medication, your brain can stimulate the ovary to ovulate.

PROLACTIN PROBLEMS AS A CAUSE OF NOT OVULATING

Prolactin is a hormone produced in the pituitary gland, which is located at the base of your brain. The body uses prolactin to stimulate milk production with breast-feeding. With either an overactive pituitary gland or a tumor in the pituitary gland, inappropriately elevated levels of prolactin may be released. The overproduction of prolactin blocks the brain's ability to control ovulation of an egg from the ovary. Women with this problem may also have visual problems, headaches and leakage of breast milk.

The level of prolactin in your blood is checked as part of the routine work-up if you are experiencing infertility. If the level is elevated, additional tests are needed. Once the problem is defined, the usual treatment is medication to bring the level of prolactin back to normal. With a normal prolactin level, the brain stimulates the ovaries to ovulate again.

PCO AS A CAUSE OF NOT OVULATING

Sometimes the hormonal stimulation from the brain is normal, the ovaries make an egg each month, yet the egg is not released from the ovary – ovulation does not occur. This condition is called PCO, or polycystic ovaries. With time, all the unreleased eggs create small cysts within the ovary, thus the name. This syndrome is commonly seen in obese women who are experiencing abnormal menstrual cycles and infertility. A thin woman with PCO has a higher chance of having unrecognized diabetes.

PCO is diagnosed with an ultrasound of the ovaries. Before you are diagnosed with PCO, you first should be tested for a thyroid problem or prolactin problem, and these results should be normal. PCO is also known by the names chronic anovulation and Stein-Leventhal Syndrome. The treatment of PCO is with medication that forces the ovary to release the egg each month. This medication, Clomid, is discussed in the section below.

HOW OVULATION PROBLEMS ARE TREATED

If you have problems with ovulation, the cause of the problem guides your treatment. If the problem is related to the thyroid gland or prolactin level, you receive medication to correct the problem. You then should start ovulating again without any other treatment needed. However, if no cause for the problem is found, or if you have polycystic ovaries, you need medicine to stimulate the ovaries to ovulate. The most common medication used to stimulate ovulation is Clomid. This medication is given either on days five through nine or days four through eight of the menstrual cycle.

The dose of Clomid is initially low, but if ovulation does not occur, a higher dose is used each month. Therefore, it may take several months to find your correct dose.

Clomid, like all other medications used to stimulate ovulation, increases the chance to 10 percent that you will have twins or triplets, due to the release of multiple eggs. These drugs can also cause painful cysts to develop on the ovaries. Recent studies suggest that prolonged use of these medications is associated with an increased risk of developing ovarian cancer. This link is being studied very carefully, and the results are showing no significant increase risk of ovarian cancer. For now, we still need to realize this is a potential risk. A more definitive answer should be available in three to five years.

When the Fallopian Tubes and Uterus Impair Fertility

Having assessed ovulation, many physicians who are evaluating infertility next make sure your fallopian tubes and uterus are normal. The fallopian tubes carry the egg from the ovary to the uterus. In the tubes, sperm and egg meet, resulting in fertilization. Fertilization is the beginning of a new baby. Therefore, a baby is first made in the fallopian tube, and carried to the uterus where it grows for nine months. If there is blockage in the tubes, the egg and sperm never meet, resulting in infertility. If there is partial damage to the tube, the egg and sperm may join, but the baby may not be able to get to the uterus. Then you have an ectopic pregnancy – one that lodges and grows in the fallopian tube. The baby has no chance of survival, and the situation is very dangerous for you.

HOW THE FALLOPIAN TUBES ARE TESTED

In order to test your fallopian tubes, a hysterosalpingogram, or HSG, is performed. In this procedure, your cervix is cleaned, a tiny tube with a balloon is inserted into the cervix, and a special dye is used to fill the uterine cavity and fallopian tubes. If your tubes are normal, dye is seen spilling out of the ends on X-ray. (Because X-rays are used, an HSG is scheduled in the first part of the menstrual cycle, before ovulation takes place, to avoid exposing a newly forming baby to radiation.) During HSG, your physician is looking for abnormalities in the shape of the uterus, which can cause both infertility and repeated miscarriage. If the fallopian tubes are blocked at their ends, an outpatient surgical procedure is done with the laser to reopen them. Should there be scar tissue in the uterus, this is removed through the cervix by a technique called hysteroscopy.

HOW THE UTERINE LINING IS ASSESSED

Besides the structure of the uterus, the readiness of the lining of the uterus to accept a fertilized egg is very important. The hormones that control reproduction affect not only the release of the egg, but also the receptiveness of the uterine lining. The hormones stimulate the blood vessels in the lining of the uterus to make it ready to accept a developing baby. If the hormone levels are not correct, a fertilized egg will not implant in the wall of the uterus. The result is miscarriage.

The condition of the uterus is evaluated by an endometrial biopsy. A small sample of the uterine lining is obtained just before a period is expected. In this procedure, a very small, usually flexible tube is passed through the cervix, and suction is applied to the tube. A few cells of the uterine lining are aspirated and analyzed. The chance of disturbing an early pregnancy is quite small, and any discomfort in the procedure is mild and passes quickly. Numbing medicine is sometimes given during this procedure. If the test shows that the lining of the uterus is not prepared for acceptance of the fertilized egg, treatment options include ovulation medication or progesterone suppositories.

" I had the test where they check to see if your fallopian tubes are clear. And we found that one wasn't. The ink went to the end of one, then it wasn't coming out. After that, they did a laparoscopy. One ovary had scar tissue around it. They did the surgery and I got pregnant right away. I never even had a period."

When the Cervix Hinders Fertilization

The cervix plays an important role in the reproductive process by supplying the cervical mucus, in which the sperm swim to reach the uterus and fallopian tubes. If problems occur with this mucus, your ability to become pregnant may be hampered.

Infertility: Overcoming the Obstacles to Conception

The cells that produce cervical mucus may be destroyed if you have had surgery on your cervix, such as a cone biopsy. A cone biopsy involves the excision of a part of the cervix to remove pre-cancerous cells.

The mucus may have antibodies within it that destroy your partner's sperm as they try to enter the uterus. This second condition is routinely tested for in the initial evaluation of an infertile couple. The test is called a **post-coital test**. For this test, you and your partner have intercourse without using lubricants, and then you come into the office within two to eight hours. A sample of your cervical mucus is then evaluated under the microscope. A normal result shows many active, motile sperm still alive within the mucus. An abnormal result shows no sperm or only dead sperm. If no sperm are found, your partner is tested to make sure he is producing sperm. If he has a normal sperm test, and only dead sperm are found in the cervical mucus after a post-coital test, then the mucus probably has antibodies that are killing the sperm.

If your cervical mucus is found to be a cause of infertility, it is bypassed through artificial insemination. Your partner's sperm are prepared at a special lab and placed into a plastic catheter. (A donor sperm sample also can be used.) You are positioned the same as for a Pap smear. The catheter is passed through your cervix, and the sperm are placed within the uterus. From there, sperm are able to get into the fallopian tube to meet the egg coming from the ovary. After insemination, you rest on your back for 10 minutes. Artificial insemination is done at the time of ovulation. You can best time this procedure by use of the ovulation-prediction kits. With a color change in these kits, you should come in for the insemination that day or the next day.

𝒰𝓃𝑒𝓍𝓅𝓁𝒶𝒾𝓃𝑒𝒹 𝒥𝓃𝒻𝑒𝓇𝓉𝒾𝓁𝒾𝓉𝓎: 𝒲𝒽𝒶𝓉 𝒩𝑒𝓍𝓉?

If blood tests, semen analysis, HSG and the post-coital test are all normal, you and your partner are said to have unexplained infertility. At this point, consideration is given to **laparoscopy**. In this outpatient surgical procedure, a lighted tube is inserted in a tiny hole made below your belly button so the surgeon can see inside your abdomen and pelvis. If endometriosis is present, it is removed with the laser. Endometriosis is a condition in which tissue similar to the lining of the uterine wall is located outside the uterus. Women with endometriosis frequently have very painful periods and pain with intercourse. However, some women have advanced endometriosis and have no complaints other than infertility. Endometriosis causes scarring, distortion of the normal shape of the fallopian tubes, and interference with the normal transport of the egg for fertilization. The laser is a very useful tool for removing the spots of endometriosis that can be seen. This type of surgery requires two to three days off work to recover, and leaves a very small scar.

Sometimes all of the tests, including laparoscopy, are normal. There are several options to consider at this time. If you are younger than 30, and you and your partner have been trying for only one year, you may want to take no further action if the tests show your systems are normal. After another six months, if you still are not pregnant, you can move on to the next options.

If you are 30 to 35, you may want to try six months of treatment with an ovulation-inducing drug (Clomid), then artificial insemination. If after four to six months a pregnancy has not occurred, you and your partner are best served by consulting with a reproductive endocrinologist. These physicians are able to do IVF (in-vitro fertilization), where the sperm and egg are joined within a special solution outside your body. The fertilized egg is later placed within your uterus.

If you are older than 35 and have unexplained infertility, you should go directly to the care of a reproductive endocrinologist for evaluation and consideration of IVF. Although expensive, IVF has allowed many couples to conceive who would otherwise have been unable. A more recent achievement is the ability of doctors to directly inject sperm into the egg, thus replicating fertilization. This new procedure is called ICSI (intracytoplasmic sperm injection) and is used when there is a problem with your partner's sperm or you have unexplained infertility.

There also are some very special options you should consider. If

" I think the hardest thing for me is, I'm just at that age and we've been married enough years that people ask me, 'When are you going to start a family?' And I don't have any answer for them."

> " During those three years, I had just the total – fear of never having a child to love who was a creation of me and my husband, never coming home to that ribbon on the mailbox that announces to the world that I am a Mom."

you have had your uterus removed, surrogate parenting is now an option. Your partner's sperm and your egg are combined outside your body, and the newly formed baby is placed into the uterus of another woman. The baby is formed from you and your partner, but carried by another woman. In most states, the baby legally belongs to you because you donated the sperm and egg. Before participating in a program with a surrogate mother, you should make sure your state's laws make it clear who has the rights to the baby. This subject is very complex, and every physician offering this has a comprehensive program you must go through before you can consider using a surrogate mother.

The alternative of adoption may make sense if you are unable to conceive or do not wish to go through all of the previously mentioned tests. Many couples have found the satisfaction of having children through this method. You may tend to focus your desire to become a parent on having your egg and your partner's sperm combine to produce a baby. In reality, a lot of what defines a couple as parents has more to do with how you devote yourself to caring for your children as they grow.

Conclusion

The emotional and financial burdens of infertility are serious. You experience feelings of inadequacy that are difficult to discuss, even in the best of relationships. Infertility is more than a medical condition, there are sensitive emotional aspects as well. Therefore you should find a physician with an excellent reputation in all of these areas. Evaluate the physician not only on how successful he or she is at helping patients become pregnant, but also on his or her level of compassion. Go to infertility meetings in your region and ask other couples for names of physicians they like.

Even if you feel you want to do "whatever it takes" to have a baby, the infertility testing process can take its toll on you. Semen analysis is embarrassing for many men. Your evaluation with a post-coital test, hysterosalpingogram, day-21 progesterone, endometrial biopsy and laparoscopy is strenuous. Both you and your partner may need to take a mental break, and you should support each other is this becomes necessary. Please do not let infertility damage or destroy a healthy and happy relationship. If you are having difficulty getting pregnant, take heart in knowing that the options for helping infertile couples have never been better. This chapter serves only as a broad outline of the techniques used to help the infertile couple. Please discuss your individual situation with your physician, and best of luck!

Resources
Additional Reading

- **The Couple's Guide to Fertility: With the Newest Scientific Techniques to Help You Have a Baby,** *Gary S. Berger, M.D., Marc Goldstein, M.D., and Mark Fuerst,* Doubleday, 1995.

- **How to Be a Successful Fertility Patient: Your Guide to Getting the Best Possible Medical Help to Have a Baby,** *Peggy Robin,* Quill, 1993.

- **Getting Pregnant: What Couples Need to Know Right Now,** *Niels H. Lauerson, M.D., Ph.D., and Colette Bouchez,* Fawcett Columbine, 1992.

- **Preventing Miscarriage: The Good News,** *Jonathan Scher, M.D., and Carol Dix,* HarperPerennial, 1991.

- **The Infertility Book: A Comprehensive Medical and Emotional Guide,** *Carla Harkness,* Celestial Arts, 1992.

Organizations

- **RESOLVE, Inc.**
  1310 Broadway, Somerville, MA 02144-1731
  Business office: (617) 623-1156
  HelpLine: (617) 623-0744
  http://www.resolve.org

- **InterNational Council on Infertility Information (INCIID)**
  P.O. Box 6836, Arlington, VA 22206
  (520) 544-9548 or (703) 379-9178
  Fax: (703) 379-1593
  E-mail: INCIIDinfo@inciid.org
  http://www.inciid.org

- **American Society for Reproductive Medicine**
  1209 Montgomery Highway
  Birmingham, AL 35216-2809
  (205) 978-5000
  Fax: (205) 978-5005
  E-mail: asrm@asrm.com
  http://www.asrm.com

- **National Adoption Center**
  1500 Walnut Street, Suite 701, Philadelphia, PA 19102
  (215) 735-9988
  E-mail: nac@adopt.org
  http://nac.adopt.org/nac/nac.html

Internet Sites

- **http://ferti.net/na/index.htm**
  The Ferti.Net Worldwide Fertility Network offers general infertility information, including male testing and diagnosis, as well as links to many helpful sites.

- **http://www.rxlist.com/cgi/generic/clomiph.htm**
  Rx List, the Internet Drug Index, gives an excellent overview of the action and side effects of the ovulation-stimulating drug Clomid.

- **http://www.adoption.com**
  Adoption.com's many features include adoption news, support, products and services.

INDEX

Order Form

To Order Additional Copies Of
"Women's Health: Your Guide to a Healthier and Happier Life,"
Simply choose one of the convenient ways to order listed below.

FAX ORDER LINE: **704/948-7119**
CALL TOLL FREE: **888/919-6636**
                         Have your AMEX, Discover, VISA or MasterCard ready.
ON-LINE ORDERS: *www.womensbooks.com*
POSTAL ORDERS: **Better Health Publishing**
                         1235 East Barden Road
                         Charlotte, NC 28226
                         704/365-3867

Name _____

Address _____

City _____ State _____ Zip _____

Telephone _____

Quantity _____

Sales Tax _____

Shipping _____

Total _____

Sales Tax:
Please add 6% for books shipped within North Carolina.

Shipping:
$4.00 for the first book and $2.00 for each additional book

Payment:
_____ Cheque
_____ Credit Card   VISA   MasterCard   AMEX   Discover
Card Number: _____
Name on Card: _____ Exp. Date: _____

Please allow 4 to 6 weeks for delivery.

I understand that I may return the book(s), that I have ordered by mail, for a full refund–for any reason, as long as the book(s) are returned in good condition.

CALL TOLL FREE TO ORDER NOW!

Order Form

To Order Additional Copies Of
"Women's Health: Your Guide to a Healthier and Happier Life,"
Simply choose one of the convenient ways to order listed below.

FAX ORDER LINE:	**704/948-7119**
CALL TOLL FREE:	**888/919-6636**
	Have your AMEX, Discover, VISA or MasterCard ready.
ON-LINE ORDERS:	*www.womensbooks.com*
POSTAL ORDERS:	**Better Health Publishing**
	1235 East Barden Road
	Charlotte, NC 28226
	704/365-3867

Name _____

Address _____

City _____ State _____ Zip _____

Telephone _____

Quantity _____

Sales Tax _____

Shipping _____

Total _____

Sales Tax:
Please add 6% for books shipped within North Carolina.

Shipping:
$4.00 for the first book and $2.00 for each additional book

Payment:
_____ Cheque
_____ Credit Card   VISA   MasterCard   AMEX   Discover
Card Number: _____
Name on Card: _____ Exp. Date: _____

Please allow 4 to 6 weeks for delivery.

I understand that I may return the book(s), that I have ordered by mail, for a full refund–for any reason, as long as the book(s) are returned in good condition.

CALL TOLL FREE TO ORDER NOW!